MEDICAL PSYCHIATRY

Series Editor Emeritus

William A. Frosch, M.D.
Weill Medical College of Cornell University, New York, New York, U.S.A.

Advisory Board

ASPERGER'S DISORDER

Edited by

Jeffrey L. Rausch
The Medical College of Georgia
Augusta, Georgia, USA

Maria E. Johnson
Gracewood State School and Hospital
Gracewood, Georgia, USA

Manuel F. Casanova
University of Louisville
Louisville, Kentucky, USA

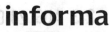

informa
healthcare

New York London

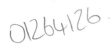

Informa Healthcare USA, Inc.
52 Vanderbilt Avenue
New York, NY 10017

International Standard Book Number-10: 0-8493-8360-9 (Hardcover)
International Standard Book Number-13: 978-0-8493-8360-1 (Hardcover)

Library of Congress Cataloging-in-Publication Data

Asperger's disorder / edited by Jeffrey L. Rausch, Maria E. Johnson, Manuel F. Casanova.
    p. ; cm. — (Medical psychiatry ; 40)
   Includes bibliographical references and index.
   ISBN-13: 978-0-8493-8360-1 (hardcover : alk. paper)
   ISBN-10: 0-8493-8360-9 (hardcover : alk. paper) 1. Asperger's syndrome.
I. Rausch, Jeffrey L. II. Johnson, Maria E. III. Casanova, Manuel F. IV. Series.
   [DNLM: 1. Asperger Syndrome. 2. Case Reports. W1 ME421SM v.40 2008 /
WS 350.6 A8387 2008]
   RC553.A88A4884 2008
   616.85′8832—dc22

                            2008022551

For Corporate Sales and Reprint Permissions call 212-520-2700 or write to: Sales Department, 52 Vanderbilt Avenue, 7th floor, New York, NY 10017.

**Visit the Informa Web site at
www.informa.com**

**and the Informa Healthcare Web site at
www.informahealthcare.com**

2 3 AUG 2010

To John, Gloria, and June; To Manuel Casanova and Elisa Soto de Casanova

Foreword

For me, the opportunity to practice in academic medicine has been one of the finest rewards of a medical career. It has given me the privilege to teach, to interact with great minds, and to meet so many fine people. As Ralph Waldo Emerson stated, "a chief event of life is the day in which we have encountered a mind that startled us."

Hans Asperger described his childhood cases as "little professors," so maybe it's fitting to describe the professorial phenotype, at least the academic medicine version, because in academic medicine you'll meet all kinds: the pedantic stuffed shirts, rigid, poker-faced, retentive of divulging any unnecessary information, the hypercritical, the critically minded, and sometimes even the rather uncritical (usually constrained to the youngsters, one would hope). There are the social climbers, the snobs, the one-upmanship types, the regular guys ("guys" includes the gals here), the salt of the earth types, transparent, genuine, unassuming, the phonies, the posers, the cavalier, the fearful, the timid, the worriers, the self-effacing, the highly dedicated, those dedicated to their patients, their careers, those dedicated to the advancement of their fields, the adventurers who take thrill in the discovery of new knowledge, the mensches on the high road you can always count on, as well as the meshuggeners, the just plain crazies, the paranoid, and the grandiose, as well as the family types, the perennial student types, the spiritual, the devout, the atheistic, the agnostic, the over-whelmed, the underwhelmed, the introverted, the extroverted, the geniuses (a few), the brilliant, the bright, the outstanding, the remarkable, the not-so-remarkable, and the gifted. Some are driven by neurosis, and some are driven by love; all are driven by hope.

Most of us constitute some combination of the above, but don't get the idea that I've got everyone pegged; it's in the perception of the beholder, and both phenotype and perception can be fluid over time. I can think of more than one time over the years that a nemesis became a best friend.

This book then is much about the labeling of social and perceptual phenotypes and their fluidity potential over time.

It's been among some of the best of this lot that we've had the pleasure to work in the writing of this book. I first met Dr. Manuel Casanova in 1991, a fine and dedicated and straightforward gentleman, just after we'd been recruited to the Medical College of Georgia (MCG), Manny from the National Institute of Mental Health and I from University of California at San Diego. Manny had already earned an international reputation when I'd first met him.

In 1998, we both, under separate circumstances, also first met Dr. Maria E. Johnson, at that time, a freshman medical student looking to do research. Most freshman medical students at MCG are doing all they can to survive passing their classes, so I was skeptical at first about whether she would be able to do both things, but Maria asked me to consider her. She said she needed freshman research work to prevent boredom, and besides, she had entered medical school "to write books about the brain." Both statements astonished me. A struggle to survive in medical school may be unpleasant in various respects, but boredom usually isn't one of them. Moreover, I had never heard of anyone going to medical school to "write books" (even though they later may). All of it was enigmatic to me, especially coming from someone gratified and dedicated in her work with patients, an outstanding clinician. She worked both in Dr. Casanova's laboratory and in mine at different junctures, the result of which was several published papers.

Dr. Elizabeth Sirota played an important role in our group's increasing interest in Asperger's disorder. Dr. Sirota had practiced psychiatry in Russia for many years before immigrating to the United States, where she had to reenter training to get her United States certification eligibility. Dr. Uta Frith has only recently translated Dr. Asperger's work into English; however, since reading German was common in Russian medical schools, Elizabeth knew a lot about Asperger's disorder.

Elizabeth was working with an adult Asperger's group when I was assigned as her training supervisor. Her adult Asperger's patients sounded much like patients with schizotypal personality or residual schizophrenia, and we began an intellectual argument about diagnosis. That debate led to a systematic comparison of the diagnostic criteria, the results of which are now published in this book.

We concluded that most, or all, of the DSM-IV symptoms of Asperger's disorder are much like those described as the "negative symptoms" of schizophrenia. Elizabeth was interested in my doing research into an effective pharmacologic treatment for her patients. There was little information on the subject at the time. One of the more authoritative articles at the time stated that "no pharmacologic treatment was effective," although the fact of the matter was that there simply weren't any data.

Having observed the likeness to negative schizophrenic symptoms, we realized that it seemed straightforward to postulate that a treatment with efficacy for such symptoms in schizophrenia should be tried in Asperger's. We started such a project, Elizabeth matriculated and went to New York, while Maria returned to MCG for a research fellowship and helped complete and publish the work. Dr. Donna Londino had since joined the project and was instrumental in her clinical and research skills in helping us make it happen.

A few months after the *Journal of Clinical Psychiatry* published our work, Susan B. Lee, from Informa, somehow found me at the American Psychiatric Association meeting and told me that her publisher was interested in publishing a medical textbook on Asperger's disorder. She had researched the books available on the subject and identified that there was no medical textbook available on Asperger's disorder.

Through the course of our studies, I was convinced of the great need for an informed understanding of the condition. I was equally struck by how much lack of understanding there was out there. Dr. Casanova had been doing original and well-regarded work on Asperger's and autistic spectrum disorders. Dr. Johnson had amassed an expertise on the subject as well; she was still keen to write her first book and worked hard to make the book happen.

Having honed our interests and received our commission, we set out to find the best experts we could as contributors to our work. Again, we found them gratifyingly among the best of the lot, giving us some quite good and provocative reading.

The *cauldron academe* forges consolidation and distillation of knowledge into a matrix, as a precursor into its denser crystallization, understanding. Knowledge and understanding are gems respectively precious and rare. Emerson told us, "Every man supposes himself not to be fully understood; and if there is any truth in him... I see not how it could be otherwise." "To be great is to be misunderstood," he said. Although this above sort of academic alchemy is subject to competing impurities in modern medicine, with time, in science, the metaphorical gold evolves apparent. In this pursuit, the book is one such increment of this iterative process.

Jeffrey L. Rausch, M.D.

Preface

We're not broken in need of fixing. We're different in need of acceptance.

A post by morning_after on WrongPlanet.net, an Asperger's website

Although we were commissioned to write on Asperger's disorder, several of our contributors weighed in favor of titling our book *Asperger's Syndrome* instead. Prof. Baron-Cohen argued that "syndrome" (a group of symptoms) is a "more neutral terminology," suggesting that the term "syndrome" is one more respectful of those with the condition than is the term "disorder" (a disturbance of function or structure).

The question about the book's title was within the context of a field's nosology like the Tower of Babel. Diverse, often strongly held views on nomenclature were, and are, pervasive. Our contributors, as it turned out, were a representative sample. Preferred nomenclature includes the DSM-IV term "Asperger's disorder" and the ICD-10 term "Asperger's syndrome"; "Asperger syndrome" is just as popular. Moreover, others prefer to discuss the topic of high-functioning autism, or autistic spectrum disorder.

With the original contributions of Lorna Wing, Asperger syndrome is now very well recognized and defined as an identity that came into existence only after Hans Asperger described his case series. One ardent lay advocate speaker lecturer prompted consideration as to whether the initial definition created a condition despite the historical precedence of people with similar symptomatology (see, for example, *Autism in History* by Houston and Frith).

This connection between history and phenomenology exemplifies how definitions are framed by a vocabulary and set of thinking that emphasize observation and sensory experience. The advancement of DSM-III from DSM-II was primarily to empirically define clusters of behavioral symptoms devoid of causal inference. The "neuroses" disappeared from the DSM as it progressed to empirical observation and classification of observed behavioral symptoms. Classifications based on theoretical causality that could be directly observed were considered an impediment to scientific empiricism at the time.

Pavlov and his successor Skinner founded behavioral science through strict empiricism. Data in test of a scientific or clinical hypothesis were to be observed without inference, without mixing the hypothetical inference with the data used to test it. However, one should remember that empiricism descriptive of populations need not presume such determinism for a given individual. After all, there is a large amount of behavioral variability within the naturalistic setting, and many complex traits typically occur within a spectrum linking extremes of severity and normality.

The need for clarification and distinction of these terms that could be served by our book became immediately apparent, yet still left us with two questions. What should we title a book about Asperger's disorder if the term itself is perceived to be disrespectful or pejorative within a contingent of the Asperger's community? Second, once deciding on terminology, what should we do about standardizing it in our text, among contributors who present interesting and cogent arguments to the alternatives, and thus enrich the discussion and give dimension to contemporary debate?

A study of the arguments against using the term "disorder" reveals objection to application of the term to those without disturbance of function, albeit those with a cluster of Aspergian symptoms, but without impairment in social or occupational functioning. Folks in this category could understandably object to their unique, unimpaired differences being considered psychopathology. DSM-IV would not qualify such individuals for Asperger's disorder pathology either.

Freud originally defined for us the hallmark of psychopathology: an impairment in the ability to love and (or) work (P. 26), now termed "impairment in social or occupational functioning." As medical professionals, our attention is not sought except for concern of pathology, and our publisher's commission was to write a medical text. This book is written to inform professionals and the public on current understanding and care of a condition for which people seek treatment and understanding.

Thus the title was resolved. But secondly, how could the text maintain standardized nomenclature? Some contributors presented interesting and cogent arguments to the alternatives thus enriching the discussion and giving dimension to contemporary debate.

Consequently, we chose to leave the nosological terminology what each author contributed. As a result, there is information as several variants of the Asperger's phenotype contained within.

It is said in medical schools that patients are often the best teachers, and it was evident in our association with the Asperger's community that there is a strong sense that diagnostic criteria alone do not convey what Asperger's is. We are fortunate to have, in addition to our clinical science chapters, both a patient and a teacher tell of their Asperger's experience, providing us with a more pictorial image of the condition, appealing to other aspects of our sense of it.

The possibility that human naïveté or ignorance could inhibit the unfolding of development calls for close examination of this issue of diagnostic clarity and stigmatization. Empirical investigation increases strength and resiliency of the individual and society and may assist societal accommodations for those with Asperger's. The book, at least for those of us writing it, might have been titled *Asperger's Discovery*. We hope the reader will find it an Asperger's discovery as well.

Jeffrey L. Rausch
Maria E. Johnson
Manuel F. Casanova

Contents

Contributors

Saurabh Aggarwal   Vascular Biology Center, Medical College of Georgia, Augusta, Georgia, U.S.A.

Fayeza S. Ahmed   Department of Psychology, University of Georgia, Athens, Georgia, U.S.A.

Carrie Allison   Autism Research Centre, Department of Psychiatry, University of Cambridge, Cambridge, U.K.

Hans Asperger   University Children's Hospital, and University of Vienna, Vienna, Austria,

Simon Baron-Cohen   Autism Research Centre, Department of Psychiatry, University of Cambridge, Cambridge, U.K.

John Smith Boswell   Medical College of Georgia, Augusta, Georgia, U.S.A.

Manuel F. Casanova   Department of Psychiatry, University of Louisville, Louisville, Kentucky, U.S.A.

Michael Fitzgerald   Department of Psychiatry, Trinity College, Dublin, Ireland

Seth D. Friedman   Department of Radiology, University of Washington, Seattle, Washington, U.S.A.

Christopher Gillberg   Department of Child and Adolescent Psychiatry, Institute of Neuroscience and Physiology, Göteborg University, Göteborg, Sweden

David S. Janowsky Department of Psychiatry, University of North Carolina, Chapel Hill, North Carolina, U.S.A.

Maria E. Johnson BrainScience Augusta and Developmental Disability Psychiatric Consultation-Liaison, Gracewood Hospital, Augusta, Georgia, U.S.A.

Allan M. Josephson Division of Child and Adolescent Psychiatry, Department of Psychiatry and Behavioral Sciences, University of Louisville, Louisville, Kentucky, U.S.A.

Natalia M. Kleinhans Department of Radiology and Autism Center, University of Washington, Seattle, Washington, U.S.A.

Donna L. Londino Department of Psychiatry and Health Behavior, Medical College of Georgia, Augusta, Georgia, U.S.A.

Grace Mathai Department of Pediatrics, University of Louisville, Louisville, Kentucky, U.S.A.

Diana Mattingly Department of Psychiatry and Health Behavior, Medical College of Georgia, Augusta, Georgia, U.S.A.

L. Stephen Miller Clinical Psychology Program; Bio-Imaging Research Center; and Neuropsychology and Memory Assessment Laboratory, Department of Psychology, University of Georgia, Athens, Georgia, U.S.A.

Jeff Munson Autism Center, University of Washington, Seattle, Washington, U.S.A.

Jeanne Rausch Columbia County Public School System, Evans, Georgia, U.S.A.

Jeffrey L. Rausch BrainScience Augusta and Department of Psychiatry and Health Behavior, Medical College of Georgia, Augusta, Georgia, U.S.A.

Lisa A. Ruble Department of Educational and Counseling Psychology, University of Kentucky, Lexington, Kentucky, U.S.A.

Cary Sanders Medical College of Georgia School of Medicine, Augusta, Georgia, U.S.A.

Peter Tanguay   Division of Child and Adolescent Psychiatry, Department of Psychiatry and Behavioral Sciences, University of Louisville, Louisville, Kentucky, U.S.A.

Sara J. Webb   Autism Center; Department of Psychiatry and Behavioral Sciences; and Center on Human Development and Disability, University of Washington, Seattle, Washington, U.S.A.

Jennie Westbrook   Department of Psychiatry and Health Behavior, Medical College of Georgia, Augusta, Georgia, U.S.A.

Autism: Asperger's Syndrome—History and First Descriptions

Michael Fitzgerald

Department of Psychiatry, Trinity College, Dublin, Ireland

INTRODUCTION

Hans Asperger (1) was the first pioneer of autism research, and not Leo Kanner (2). I have no doubt that Leo Kanner was aware of Hans Asperger's 1938 paper because he mentions that "since 1938, there have come to our attention a number of children.... " Sadly he did not mention Hans Asperger's name. This is plagiarism, Asperger and Kanner spoke the same language and came from the same city, Vienna. During World War II, Leo Kanner had much contact with medical refugees from his native country.

Nonattribution or in this case plagiarism is always sad and is usually exposed even if it takes 60 years, as in this case (3).

There is no doubt that Hans Asperger was unaware that Leo Kanner had taken over his ideas, and indeed in his paper in 1944 (4), as translated by Uta Frith (5) and published in this book specifically, he states that autism "has not yet been described." World War II made it impossible for Asperger to be aware of Kanner's paper.

Hans Asperger (4) in his paper *Autistic Psychopathy in Childhood* translated by Uta Frith (5), which I am using in this discussion, describes Fritz V. This is the most brilliant description of autism I have ever read. There is no better paper that anyone coming to autism for the first time could read. For me, autism and Asperger's syndrome (6) are part of autism spectrum disorders. Personally,

I use Asperger's syndrome when the IQ is above 70, and autism criteria are met also for those below IQ 70. In *Diagnostic and Statistical Manual of Mental Disorders-Fourth Edition-Text Revision* (DSM-IV-TR) (7), there is an unsatisfactory hierarchical rule, which does not allow Asperger's syndrome diagnosis to be made if autism (another specific pervasive developmental disorder) criteria have already been met. It is possible that DSM-V will change the criteria for Asperger's syndrome and allow mild cognitive delay and language difficulties, e.g., semantic pragmatic problems, which occur very commonly (8).

In relation to Fritz V., it is likely that his brother had a mild form of autism (autistic psychopathy) or what we would call today pervasive developmental disorder not otherwise specified (7). Fritz V. himself would meet the criteria for autism (7) rather than Asperger's syndrome (7). His language difficulties were noticed very early, with his talking "like an adult" and talking before he walked.

In 1971, van Krevelen (9) emphasized this walking before talking in his description of early infantile autism, while he suggests that in autistic psychopathy the child walks late and speaks earlier. This would be consistent with Hans Asperger's description of Fritz V.

Oppositional defiant disorder (7) is a very common comorbidity, with autism and Asperger's syndrome. There is no doubt that Fritz V. had many of the features, while conduct disorder (7) would be a more accurate diagnosis. He never did "what he was told," did "the opposite of what he was told," and was "intentionally spiteful."

In terms of conduct disorder (7) Fritz V. met the criteria. He bashed and attacked other children. It seems fairly clear that he got sadistic pleasure from this. This behavior is something that has been much misunderstood by many writers on autism (10,11). He was also threatening and intimidating to others and indeed lashed out "with a hammer."

Fritz V. showed evidence of autistic language and autistic narrative (8). He showed evidence of expressive language problems. He spoke "very slowly," with much reduced content. It was hard to get answers to questions from him, and there was much reduced content to his speech. He was paying more attention to his own thinking than to the questioner. He enjoyed using repetitive language, as did Ludwig Wittgenstein who had Asperger's syndrome (12). Fritz V. showed the typical tone of voice of persons with Asperger's syndrome.

Fritz V. had sensory integration problems. To reduce human sensory input he would look out the corner of his eyes. He also had unusual traits—pica—eating "lead or paper." He also liked to lick the table. Physical demonstrations of affection upset him. He also enjoyed chewing wood and making noise using wood.

He showed the typical social interactional difficulties of persons with autism and Asperger's syndrome. He showed a gross lack of empathy, and lack of an ability to "read" or understand in detail other minds. He tended to "objectify" people. People were there to be used for his purposes. While he was an "outsider" much focussed on introspection and his thoughts, he picked up more from the environment than was realized. He did enjoy his sadistic behavior toward people. He was tactless and socially very immature. As a child, he had severe deficits in playing skills. He was not interested in other children, which goes with autism rather than Asperger's syndrome, according to Luke Tsai (13). He had great difficulty understanding anger and kindness.

He could not manage the standard emotional interactions of the classroom, and teachers had to use the strategy in the classroom of turning off "affect" and making it a structured mechanical kind of classroom.

He did at times show inappropriate affection, further evidence of his poor social skills and social know-how. It was clearly critical for the Austrian teacher to take his social and emotional deficits into account and to find ways around them in teaching him. Not all teachers have what Asperger calls "inner strength and confidence" to teach these children. A few "autistic traits" in teachers themselves can help them to identify with these children. Hans Asperger suggests giving a teaching instruction "not as personal requests but as objective impersonal law." It is clear that Hans Asperger wanted teachers to be thoroughly familiar with autism.

Fritz V. showed evidence of Dyspraxia, which is supposed to be more common in Asperger's syndrome than autism (8). Nevertheless it has never been possible to make clear differentiation between autism and Asperger's syndrome. Fritz V. showed evidence of stereotyped motor mannerisms, which were pleasurable but also came on as a result of stress. There is overlap between autism/Asperger's syndrome and attention deficit hyperactivity disorder (ADHD) (14).

Fritz V. showed evidence of poor attention (except to what interested him), restlessness, often did not respond when spoken to directly, often did not follow through on teachers instructions, and was easily distracted. He could hyperfocus on what interested him and progressed well academically in the long term when he was dealing with subjects that interested him.

While novelty seeking is mostly associated with ADHD, there is also an autistic type of novelty seeking described (15). This seeking of originality is part of this autistic novelty seeking. It is associated with narrow interests, which Fritz V. had.

In terms of family history there is much evidence of autism and Asperger's syndrome.

A sister of the maternal grandfather was a great scholar, eccentric, reclusive, and would appear to have Asperger's syndrome. Certainly some of the multiple genes associated with autism and Asperger's syndrome came down the female line. Mother also appeared to have Asperger's syndrome and was a strange person and a "loner." She had an awkward walk and had poor hygiene, something which is common in persons with Asperger's syndrome. Indeed some of these multiple genes associated with Asperger's syndrome also would seem to come from Fritz V.'s father who was "withdrawn," "reticent," was "pedantic," "distant," and reluctant to speak about himself. It is not unusual for the maternal and the paternal line to be relevant.

In terms of cognitive educational assessment the usual problems in conducting this accurately were seen. In my experience, psychological tests in persons with autism often seriously underestimate IQ levels. The profile of Fritz V. was uneven. He showed "an extraordinary calculating ability." Persons with Fritz V.'s profile are often very good at mathematics (16).

Fritz V. was also autodictatic, which is typically the way persons with Asperger's syndrome learn (17).

Hans Asperger discusses the possibility of childhood schizophrenia as a differential diagnosis and correctly rules against it. Unfortunately in adult psychiatry today many persons with Asperger's syndrome are misdiagnosed as having schizophrenia with the great negative consequences associated with this misdiagnosis (18).

AUTISTIC INTELLIGENCE

Hans Asperger showed profound insights into creativity and autistic intelligence, which have never been superseded. This is hardly surprising, as Hans Asperger, a very creative person, had his own syndrome (3,19).

Hans Asperger stated that "autistic children are able to produce original ideas." Hans Asperger also recognized how creativity and disability are linked, as in Sophocles writing on Philoctes (20), where the great man was wounded and had a limp. I believe autism and creativity (8) are two sides of the same coin. Hans Asperger appreciated this in the 1930s when he first recognized autism.

Hans Asperger noted that persons with autistic intelligence were "linguistically original." Indeed Ludwig Wittgenstein, the greatest philosopher of the 20th century (12,21), had Asperger's syndrome and specialized in language. Hans Asperger also noticed this "abstruse" language and this was certainly true of Ludwig Wittgenstein. Hans Asperger also notes their "rare maturity of taste in art." This was certainly true in the case of the visual artists with Asperger's syndrome, e.g., Lowry, Warhol, van Gogh (22).

Hans Asperger might be thought of contradicting himself when he described persons with autism as being "a judge of character." Nevertheless there is some support for this in relation to Stanley Kubrick, who also had Asperger's syndrome (23). They can be massive observers.

In terms of what Hans Asperger describes as "clarity of vision," Einstein (13,14), "Stonewall" Jackson (24), Alan Turning (25), Michael Ventris (26) would be examples.

Unfortunately because of poor services even talented persons with Asperger's syndrome have trouble progressing (27).

REFERENCES

1. Asperger H. Das psychisch abnormale kind. Wiener Klinische Wochenschrift 1938; 51:1314–1317.
2. Kanner L. Autistic disturbances of affective contact. Nervous Child 1943; 2: 217–253.

3. Lyons V, Fitzgerald M. Asperger (1906–1980) and Kanner (1894–1981) the two pioneers of autism. J Autism Dev Disord 2007; 37:2022–2023.
4. Asperger H. Die "Autistischen Psychopathen" im Kindesalter. Archiv für Psychiatrie und Nervenkrankheiten 1944; 117:76–136.
5. Frith U, ed. Autism and Asperger's Syndrome. Cambridge, UK: Cambridge University Press, 1991.
6. Wing L. Asperger's syndrome—a clinical account. Psychol Med 1981; 11:115–129.
7. American Psychiatric Association. DSM-IV-TR. Washington, DC: APA, 2000.
8. Fitzgerald M. Autism and Creativity: Is there a link between autism in men and exceptional ability? New York: Brunner Routledge, 2004.
9. Van Krevelen AD. Early Infantile Autism and Autistic Psychopathy. Journal of Autism and Child Schizophrenia 1971; 1(1):84–85.
10. Fitzgerald M. Callous-unemotional traits and Asperger's syndrome? J Am Acad Child Adolesc Psychiatry 2003; 42(9):1011.
11. Fitzgerald M. Callous and unemotional traits in autistic psychopathy. Br J Psychiatry 2007; 191:265.
12. Fitzgerald M. Did Ludwig Wittgenstein have Asperger's syndrome? Eur Child Adolesc Psychiatry 2000; 9:61–65.
13. Tsai L. From Autism to Asperger's disorder. Presented at: the American Academy of Child and Adolescent Psychiatry Conference, Hawaii, October 2001; 5–6.
14. Fitzgerald M, Bellgrove M, Gill M. Handbook of Attention Deficit Hyperactivity Disorder. John Wiley & Sons, 2007.
15. Fitzgerald M. The Genesis of Artistic Creativity. London: Jessica Kingsley, 2005.
16. Fitzgerald M, James I. The Mind of the Mathematician. Baltimore, MD: Johns Hopkins University Press, 2007.
17. Fitzgerald M. Did Isaac Newton have Asperger's disorder? European Child Adolesc Psychiatry 1999; 8:244.
18. Fitzgerald M. Antecedents to Asperger's syndrome. Autism 1988; 2(4):427–429.
19. Lyons V, Fitzgerald M. Did Hans Asperger have Asperger's syndrome? J Autism Dev Disord 2007; 37:2020–2021.
20. Lee M. Wagner: The Terrible Man and His Truthful Art. Toronto: University of Toronto Press, 1999.
21. Fitzgerald M. Einstein: Brain and behaviour. J Autism Dev Disord 2000; 620–621.
22. Harpur J, Lawlor M, Fitzgerald M. Succeeding in College with Asperger's Syndrome. London: Jessica Kingsley, 2004.
23. Lyons V, Fitzgerald M. Asperger's Syndrome Gift or Curse? New York: Nova Biomedical Books, 2005.
24. Arshad M, Fitzgerald M. Did 'Stonewall' Jackson have Asperger's syndrome? Irish Psychiatrist 2003; 3(6):223–224.
25. O'Connell H, Fitzgerald M. Did Alan Turing have Asperger's syndrome? Ir J Psychol Med 2003; 20(1):28–31.
26. Arshad M, Fitzgerald M. Michael Ventris: a case of high functioning autism? Irish Psychiatrist 2004; 5(1):28–30.
27. Harpur J, Lawlor M, Fitzgerald M. Succeeding with Interventions for Asperger's syndrome and Adolescents. London: Jessica Kingsley, 2006.
28. McCarthy P, Fitzgerald M, Smith M. Prevalence of childhood autism in Ireland. Ir Med J 1984; 77(5):129–130.

2

The Case of Fritz V.*

Hans Asperger[†]

University Children's Hospital, and University of Vienna, Vienna, Austria

Translated and annotated by Uta Frith Institute of Cognitive Neuroscience and Department of Psychology, University College London, London, U.K.

This is the first case described by Hans Asperger. It is reported that he followed Fritz V. into adulthood and that Fritz V. became a professor of astronomy, solving an error in Newton's work.

The following selection of Die 'Autisitic Psychopahten' im Kendesalter is reprinted from the text Autism and Asperger Syndrome (copyright 1991) with permission from Cambridge University Press.

FRITZ V.

We start with a highly unusual boy who shows a very severe impairment in social integration. This boy was born in June 1933 and came for observation to the Heilpädagogische Abteilung (Remedial Department) of the University Paediatric Clinic in Vienna in the autumn of 1939.[1] He was referred by his school as he was considered to be 'uneducable' by the end of his first day there.

Fritz was the first child of his parents. He had a brother two years younger who was also somewhat difficult but not nearly as deviant as Fritz. Birth was normal. Motor milestones were rather delayed. He learnt to walk at fourteen months, and for a

---

[†]Dr. Asperger died October 21, 1980.

[1]This famous clinic was founded in 1918 by Erwin Lazar and pioneered a combination of special education and paediatrics.

long time was extremely clumsy and unable to do things for himself. He learnt the practical routines of daily life very late and with great difficulty.[2] This will be looked at in more detail later. In contrast, he learnt to talk very early and spoke his first words at ten months, well before he could walk. He quickly learnt to express himself in sentences and soon talked 'like an adult'.[3] Nothing was reported about unusual childhood illnesses and there was no indication of any brain disease.

From the earliest age Fritz never did what he was told. He did just what he wanted to, or the opposite of what he was told. He was always restless and fidgety, and tended to grab everything within reach. Prohibitions did not deter him. Since he had a pronounced destructive urge, anything that got into his hands was soon torn or broken.[4]

He was never able to become integrated into a group of playing children. He never got on with other children and, in fact, was not interested in them. They only 'wound him up'. He quickly became aggressive and lashed out with anything he could get hold of (once with a hammer), regardless of the danger to others. For this he was thrown out of kindergarten after only a few days. Similarly, because of his totally uninhibited behaviour, his schooling failed on the first day. He had attacked other children, walked nonchalantly about in class and tried to demolish the coat-racks.

He had no real love for anybody but occasionally had fits of affection. Then he would embrace various people, seemingly quite unmotivated. The effect, however, was not at all pleasant. This behaviour never felt like the expression of genuine affection, instead, it appeared to be as abrupt as a fit. One could not help thinking that Fritz might never be able to love anyone and would never do something solely to please somebody else. He did not care if people were sad or upset about him. He appeared almost to enjoy people being angry with him while they tried to teach him, as if this were a pleasurable sensation which he tried to provoke by negativism and disobedience.[5]

Fritz did not know the meaning of respect and was utterly indifferent to the authority of adults. He lacked distance and talked without shyness even to

---

[2] Practical routines include self-help skills such as washing, dressing and, generally, keeping clothes and body clean, and probably also some typical social skills, such as eating properly at table, and sitting still and paying attention at school. Toilet training is never mentioned while it looms large as a problem in Kanner's cases.

[3] Donald, Kanner's first case, also appears to have had rather early and unusual development of speech. By the age of two, he was said to be able to name large numbers of pictures and to recite poetry and prose. Asperger's descriptive phrase 'talking like an adult' suggests oddness over and above precocity.

[4] While conduct problems are highly prominent symptoms in Asperger's cases, they are not in Kanner's sample although the problems mentioned there do include aggressive and destructive behaviour. This difference can perhaps be explained by the more child-centred attitudes prevalent in the United States at the time, while in Europe the instilling of respect and discipline had remained a major aspect of education.

[5] The social impairment described here closely resembles the picture of the 'odd' rather than the 'aloof' or 'passive' type, using Wing and Gould's (1979) terminology.

strangers. Although he acquired language very early, it was impossible to teach him the polite form of address ('Sie'). He called everybody 'Du'. Another strange phenomenon in this boy was the occurrence of certain stereotypic movements and habits.[6]

Family History

The mother stemmed from the family of one of the greatest Austrian poets. Her side of the family were mostly intellectuals and all were, according to her, in the mad-genius mould. Several wrote poetry 'quite beautifully'. A sister of the maternal grandfather, 'a brilliant pedagogue', lived as an eccentric recluse. The maternal grandfather and several of his relatives had been expelled from state schools and had to attend private school. Fritz strongly resembled this grandfather. He too was said to have been an exceptionally difficult child and now rather resembled the caricature of a scholar, preoccupied with his own thoughts and out of touch with the real world.

The mother herself was very similar to the boy. This similarity was particularly striking given that she was a woman, since, in general, one would expect a higher degree of intuitive social adaptation in women, more emotion than intellect. In the way she moved and spoke, indeed in her whole demeanour, she seemed strange and rather a loner. Very characteristic, for instance, was the situation when mother and son walked to the hospital school together, but each by themselves. The mother slouched along, hands held behind her back and apparently oblivious to the world. Beside her the boy was rushing to and fro, doing mischief. They gave the appearance of having absolutely nothing to do with each other.[7] One could not help thinking that the mother found it difficult to cope not only with her child but with the practical matters of life. She was certainly not up to running the household. Even living, as she did, in the upper echelons of society, she always looked unkempt, unwashed almost, and was always badly dressed.[8] She was also, clearly, not coping with the physical care of her son. It has to be said, however, that this was a particularly difficult problem. The mother knew her son through and through and understood his difficulties very well. She tried to find similar traits in herself and in her relations and talked

---

[6] Examples later on show that Fritz's stereotypic (repetitive) movements and habits include jumping, hitting and echoing speech. The critical feature of such activity is its fragmentary nature. Often it seems to be generated without external provocation.

[7] It is interesting to compare Kanner and Eisenberg's (1955) description of the autistic boy George and his mother: 'As they come up the stairs, the child trails forlornly behind the mother, who does not bother to look back'. Here the authors seem to sympathise with the child while being somewhat censorious of the mother. Asperger instead points out the similarity of mother and son In the way they ignore each other.

[8] Kanner and Eisenberg's (1955) account of George's mother again strikingly similar: 'His mother, a college graduate, looked bedraggled at the time oj the first visit. She felt futile about herself, was overwhelmed, by her family responsibilities and gave the impression of drabness and ineffectualness.'

about this eloquently. She emphasised again and again that she was at the end of her tether, and this was indeed obvious as soon as one saw them both together.

It was clear that this state of affairs was due not only to the boy's own internally caused problems, but also to the mother's own problems in relating to the outside world, showing as she did a limited intuitive social understanding. Take the following typical trait: whenever things became too much for her at home she would simply walk out on her family and travel to her beloved mountains. She would stay there for a week or more at a time, leaving the rest of the family to struggle for themselves.

The boy's father came from an ordinary farming family, with no reported peculiarities. He had made a successful career for himself, eventually becoming a high-ranking civil servant. He married late and was fifty-five years old when his first child was born. The father was a withdrawn and reticent man who did not give much away about himself. He clearly hated to talk about himself and his interests. He was extremely correct and pedantic and kept a more than usual distance.

Appearance and Expressive Characteristics

The boy was of a rather delicate build and very tall, 11 cm above the average height for his age. He was thin, fine-boned and his musculature was weakly developed. His skin was of yellowish-grey pallor. The veins were clearly visible on the temples and upper parts of the body. His posture was slouched, his shoulders slumped, with the shoulder blades protruding. Otherwise his appearance was unremarkable. The face showed fine and aristocratic features, prematurely differentiated in a six-year-old. Any baby features had long since gone.

His eye gaze was strikingly odd.[9] It was generally directed into the void, but was occasionally interrupted by a momentary malignant glimmer. When somebody was talking to him he did not enter into the sort of eye contact which would normally be fundamental to conversation. He darted short 'peripheral' looks and glanced at both people and objects only fleetingly. It was 'as if he wasn't there'. The same impression could be gained of his voice, which was high and thin and sounded far away. The normal speech melody, the natural flow of speech, was missing. Most of the time, he spoke very slowly, dragging out certain words for an exceptionally long time. He also showed increased modulation so that his speech was often sing-song.

The content of his speech too was completely different from what one would expect of a normal child: only rarely was what he said in answer to a

---

[9] Kanner (1943) does not dwell much on peculiarity of gaze in his first case descriptions, but a clear reference to the same phenomenon that Asperger describes appears in the case of Virginia: 'She responded when called by getting up and coming nearer, without even looking up to the person who called her. She just stood listlessly, looking into space.'

question. One usually had to ask a question many times before it registered. When he did answer, once in a while, the answer was as short as possible. Often, however, it was sheer luck if he reacted at all! Either he simply did not answer, or he turned away while beating a rhythm or indulging in some other stereotypic behaviour. Occasionally, he repeated the question or a single word from the question that had apparently made an impression on him; sometimes he sang, 'I don't like to say that . . .'.

Behaviour on the Ward

Posture, eye gaze, voice and speech made it obvious at first glance that the boy's relations to the outside world were extremely limited. This was instantly apparent also in his behaviour with other children. From the moment he set foot on the ward he stood out from the rest of the group, and this did not change. He remained an outsider and never took much notice of the world around him. It was impossible to get him to join in group play, but neither could he play properly by himself. He just did not know what to do with the toys he was given. For instance, he put building blocks in his mouth and chewed them, or he threw them under the beds. The noise this created seemed to give him pleasure.[10]

While appropriate reactions to people, things and situations were largely absent, he gave full rein to his own internally generated impulses. These were unrelated to outside stimuli. Most conspicuous in this respect were his stereotypic movements: he would suddenly start to beat rhythmically on his thighs, bang loudly on the table, hit the wall, hit another person or jump around the room. He would do this without taking any notice of the amazement of those around him. For the most part, these impulses occurred out of the blue, but sometimes they were provoked, for instance, when certain demands were made which acted as undesirable intrusions into his encapsulated personality. Even when one was able to get him to respond for a short time, it was not long before he became unhappy, and there would eventually be an outburst of shouts or odd stereotypic movements. On other occasions, it was sheer restlessness which seemed to drive him to engage in stereotypic behaviour. Whenever the ward was in a noisy, happy or restless mood, for instance, when there was a competitive game going on, then one could be sure that he would soon break out of the group and start jumping or hitting.

In addition to these problems there were also various nasty and unacceptable habits. He 'ate' the most impossible things, for example, whole pencils, wood and lead, or paper, in considerable quantities. Not surprisingly, he frequently had stomach problems. He was in the habit of licking the table and then playing around with his spit. He also committed the mischievous acts which are

---

[10] In comparison, Donald (Kanner's-first case, described in 1943) 'had a disinclination to play with children and do things children his age usually take an interest in'. Further, 'he kept throwing things on the floor, seeming to delight in the sounds they made.'

characteristic of this type of child.[11] The same boy who sat there listlessly with an absent look on his face would suddenly jump up with his eyes lit up, and before one could do anything, he would have done something mischievous. Perhaps he would knock everything off the table or bash another child. Of course he would always choose the smaller, more helpless ones to hit, who became very afraid of him. Perhaps he would turn on the lights or the water, or suddenly run away from his mother or another accompanying adult, to be caught only with difficulty. Then again, he may have thrown himself into a puddle so that he would be spattered with mud from head to foot. These impulsive acts occurred without any warning and were therefore extremely difficult to manage or control. In each of these situations it was always the worst, most embarrassing, most dangerous thing that happened. The boy seemed to have a special sense for this, and yet he appeared to take hardly any notice of the world around him! No wonder the malicious behaviour of these children so often appears altogether 'calculated'.[12]

As one would expect, the conduct disorders were particularly gross when demands were made on him, for instance, when one tried to give him something to do or to teach him something. This was regardless of whether he was in a group with other children or on his own. It required great skill to make him join some physical exercise or work even for a short while. Apart from his intransigence to any requests, he was not good at PE because he was motorically very clumsy. He was never physically relaxed. He never 'swung' in any rhythm. He had no mastery over his body. It was not surprising, therefore, that he constantly tried to run away from the PE group or from the work-table. It was particularly in these situations that he would start jumping, hitting, climbing on the beds or begin some stereotyped sing-song.

Similar difficulties were encountered when one worked with him on his own. An example was his behaviour during intelligence tests. It turned out that it was impossible to get a good idea of his true intellectual abilities using standard intelligence tests. The results were highly contradictory. His failure to respond to particular test questions seemed to be a matter of chance and a result of his profound contact disturbance. Testing was extremely difficult to carry out. He constantly jumped up or smacked the experimenter on the hand. He would repeatedly drop himself from chair to floor and then enjoy being firmly placed back in his chair again. Often, instead of answering a question, he said 'Nothing at all, nobody at all', grinning horridly, Occasionally he stereotypically repeated the question or a meaningless word or perhaps a word he made up. Questions and

---

[11] Kanner (1943) does not talk of mischievous behaviour. However, Donald showed behaviour that Asperger would almost certainly have labelled spiteful: 'He still went on chewing on paper, putting food on his hair, throwing books into the toilet, putting a key down the water drain, climbing onto the table and bureau, having temper tantrums.'

[12] One of the most controversial of Asperger's ideas is his contention that the autistic children he describes display intentionally spiteful or malicious behaviour. This idea has to be seen together with his other observations of the children's general indifference to other people's feelings. Examples that Asperger gives suggest that the child had only a physical effect in mind, not a psychological one, as, for instance, when Fritz provoked his teacher because he enjoyed seeing her display anger.

requests had to be repeated constantly. It was a matter of luck to catch him at exactly the moment he was ready to respond, when he would occasionally perform considerably in advance of his age. Some examples are given below.

CONSTRUCTION TEST (a figure made out of sticks, and consisting of two squares and four triangles, is exposed for a few seconds and has to be copied from memory). Even though he had only half-glanced at this figure, he correctly constructed it within a few seconds, or rather, he threw the little sticks so that it was perfectly possible to recognise the correct figure, but he could not be persuaded to arrange them properly.

RHYTHM IMITATION (various rhythms are beaten out to be copied). In spite of many attempts he could not be persuaded to do this task.

MEMORY FORDIGITS He very readily repeated six digits. One was left with a strong impression that he could go further, except that he just did not feel like it. According to the Binet test, the repetition of six digits is expected at the age of ten, while the boy was only six years old.

MEMORY FOR SENTENCES This test too could not be properly evaluated. He deliberately repeated wrongly many of the sentences. However, it was clear that he could achieve at least age-appropriate performance.

SIMILARITIES Some questions were not answered at all, others got a nonsensical answer. For instance, for the item tree and bush, he just said, 'There is a difference'. For fly and butterfly, he said, 'Because he has a different name', 'Because the butterfly is snowed, snowed with snow'; asked about the colour, he said, 'Because he is red and blue, and the fly is brown and black'. For the item wood and glass, he answered, 'Because the glass is more glassy and the wood is more woody'. For cow and calf, he replied, 'lammerlammerlammer . . .'. To the question 'Which is the bigger one?' he said, 'The cow I would like to have the pen now'.

Enough examples from the intelligence test. We did not obtain an accurate picture of the boy's intellectual abilities. This, of course, was hardly to be expected. First, he rarely reacted to stimuli appropriately but followed his own internally generated impulses. Secondly, he could not engage in the lively reciprocity of normal social interaction. In order to judge his abilities it was therefore necessary to look at his spontaneous productions.

As the parents had already pointed out, he often surprised us with remarks that betrayed an excellent apprehension of a situation and an accurate judgement of people. This was the more amazing as he apparently never took any notice of his environment. Above all, from very early on he had shown an interest in numbers and calculations. He had learnt to count to over 100 and was able to calculate within that number-space with great fluency. This was without anybody ever having tried to teach him — apart from answering occasional questions he asked. His extraordinary calculating ability had been reported by the parents and was verified by us. Incidentally, we found, in general, that the parents had an excellent understanding of their child's intellectual abilities. Such knowledge as the boy possessed was not accessible by questioning at will. Rather, it showed itself accidentally, especially during his time on the ward, where he was given individual tuition. Even before any systematic teaching had begun, he had mastered calculations with numbers over ten. Of course, quite a number of bright children are able to do this before starting school at six. However, his ability to use fractions was unusual, and was revealed quite incidentally during his first year of instruction. The mother reported that at the very beginning of schooling he set himself the problem — what is bigger $1/16$ or $1/18$ — and then solved it with ease. When somebody asked for fun, just to test the limits of his ability, 'What is $2/3$ of 120?', he instantly gave the right answer, '80'. Similarly, he surprised everybody with his grasp of the concept of negative numbers, which he had apparently gained wholly by himself; it came out with his remark that 3 minus 5 equals '2 under zero'. At the end of the first school year, he was also fluent in solving problems of the type, 'If 2 workers do a job in a certain amount of time, how much time do 6 workers need?'

We see here something that we have come across in almost all autistic individuals, a special interest which enables them to achieve quite extraordinary levels of performance in a certain area. This, then, throws some light on the question of their intelligence. However, even now the answer remains problematic since the findings can be contradictory and different testers can come to different intelligence estimates. Clearly, it is possible to consider such individuals both as child prodigies and as imbeciles with ample justification.[13]

Now, a word about the boy's relations to people. At first glance, it seemed as if these did not exist or existed only in a negative sense, in mischief and aggression. This, however, was not quite true. Again, accidentally, on rare occasions, he showed that he knew intuitively, and indeed unfailingly, which person really meant well by him, and would even reciprocate at times. For instance, he would declare that he loved his teacher on the ward, and now and then he hugged a nurse in a rare wave of affection.

Implications of Remedial Education

It is obvious that in the present case there were particularly difficult educational problems. Let us consider first the essential prerequisites which make a normal child learn and integrate into school life, in terms not just of the subject matter taught, but also of the appropriate social behaviour. Learning the appropriate behaviour does not depend primarily on intellectual understanding. Well before the child can understand the spoken words of his teacher, even in early infancy, he learns to comply. He complies with and responds to the glance of the mother,

---

[13] Asperger and Kanner were both impressed by the isolated special abilities found in almost all their cases. Fritz shows superior rote memory and calculating ability; Donald likewise has excellent rote memory and could count to 100 at the age of five.

the tone of her voice, the look of her face, and to her gestures rather than the words themselves. In short, he learns to respond to the infinitely rich display of human expressive phenomena. While the young child cannot understand this consciously, he none the less behaves accordingly. The child stands in uninterrupted reciprocity with his care-giver, constantly building up his own responses and modifying them according to the positive of negative outcome of his encounters. Clearly, an undisturbed relationship with his environment is an essential requirement. In Fritz's case, however, it is precisely this wonderful regulating mechanism which is severely disturbed. It is a sign of this disturbance that Fritz's expressions themselves are abnormal. How odd is his use of eye contact! Normally, a great deal of the outside world is received by the eye and communicated by the eye to others. How odd is his voice, how odd his manner of speaking and his way of moving! It is no surprise, therefore, that this boy also lacks understanding of other people's expressions and cannot react to them appropriately.[14]

Let us consider this issue again from a different point of view. It is not the content of words that makes a child comply with requests, by processing them intellectually. It is, above all, the affect of the care-giver which speaks through the words. Therefore, when making requests, it does not really matter what the care-giver says or how well-founded the request is. The point is not to demonstrate the necessity of compliance and consequence of non-compliance — only bad teachers do this. What matters is the way in which the request is made, that is, how powerful the affects are which underlie the words. These affects can be understood even by the infant, the foreigner or the animal, none of whom is able to comprehend the literal meaning.

In our particular case, as indeed, in all such cases, the affective side was disturbed to a large extent, as should have become apparent from the description so far. The boy's emotions were indeed hard to comprehend. It was almost impossible to know what would make him laugh or jump up and down with happiness, and what would make him angry and aggressive. It was impossible to know what feelings were the basis of his stereotypic activities or what it was that could suddenly make him affectionate. So much of what he did was abrupt and seemed to have no basis in the situation itself. Since the affectivity of the boy was so deviant and it was hard to understand his feelings, it is not surprising that his reactions to the feelings of his care-givers were also inappropriate.[15]

---

[14] Recent findings of an impairment in the understanding of emotion in voice and face confirm Asperger's impression. See Hobson (1989) for a review of research and theoretical interpretation. Asperger believed autistic children to have a disturbed relation to the environment in general, and not merely to the social environment. It follows that their lack of emotional understanding is a consequence of the same underlying problem (that is, contact disturbance) which also results in their helplessness in practical matters of everyday life. Kanner (1943), instead, contrasts the 'excellent relation to objects with the non-existent relation to people', a highly influential view which has become the basis of many theories of autism.

[15] From Asperger's descriptions throughout it is clear that he believed autistic children to be capable of having strong feelings, and to be disturbed only in their ability to manifest such feelings appropriately.

In fact, it is typical of children such as Fritz V. that they do not comply with requests or orders that are affectively charged with anger, kindness, persuasion or flattery. Instead, they respond with negativistic, naughty and aggressive behaviour. While demonstrations of love, affection and flattery are pleasing to normal children and often induce in them the desired behaviour, such approaches only succeeded in irritating Fritz, as well as all other similar children. While anger and threats usually succeed in bending obstinacy in normal children and often make them compliant after all, the opposite is true of autistic children. For them, the affect of the care-giver may provide a sensation which they relish and thus seek to provoke. 'I am so horrible because you are cross so nicely', said one such boy to his teacher.

It is difficult to know what the appropriate pedagogic approach should be. As with all genuine teaching, it should not be based primarily on logical deduction but rather on pedagogic intuition. Nevertheless, it is possible to state a few principles which are based on our experience with such children.

The first is that all educational transactions have to be done with the affect 'turned off'. The teacher must never become angry nor should he aim to become loved. It will never do to appear quiet and calm on the outside while one is boiling inside. Yet this is only too likely, given the negativism and seemingly calculated naughtiness of autistic children! The teacher must at all costs be calm and collected and must remain in control. He should give his instructions in a cool and objective manner, without being intrusive. A lesson with such a child may look easy and appear to run along in a calm, self-evident manner. It may even seem that the child is simply allowed to get away with everything, any teaching being merely incidental. Nothing could be further from the truth. In reality, the guidance of these children requires a high degree of effort and concentration. The teacher needs a particular inner strength and confidence which is not at all easy to maintain!

There is a great danger of getting involved in endless arguments with these children, be it in order to prove that they are wrong or to bring them towards some insight. This is especially true for the parents, who frequently find themselves trapped in endless discussions. On the other hand, it often works simply to cut short negativistic talk: for example, Fritz is tired of doing sums and sings, 'I don't want to do sums any more, I don't want to do sums any more', the teacher replies, 'No, you don't need to do sums', and continuing in the same calm tone of voice, 'How much is. . .?' Primitive as they are, such methods are, in our experience, often successful.

There is an important point to be made here. Paradoxical as it may seem, the children are negativistic and highly suggestible at the same time. Indeed, there is a kind of automatic or reflex obedience. This behaviour is known to occur in schizophrenics. It could well be that these two disorders of the will are closely related! With our children we have repeatedly found that if one makes requests in an automaton-like and stereotyped way, for instance, speaking softly in the same sing-song that they use themselves, one senses that they have to obey, seemingly unable to resist the command. Another pedagogic trick is to announce any educational measures not as personal requests, but as objective impersonal law. But more of this later.

I have already mentioned that behind the cool and objective interaction with Fritz and all similar children there needs to be genuine care and kindness if one wants to achieve anything at all. These children often show a surprising sensitivity to the personality of the teacher. However difficult they are even under optimal conditions, they can be guided and taught, but only by those who give them true understanding and genuine affection, people who show kindness towards them and, yes, humour. The teacher's underlying emotional attitude influences, involuntarily and unconsciously, the mood and behaviour of the child. Of course, the management and guidance of such children essentially requires a proper knowledge of their peculiarities as well as genuine pedagogic talent and experience. Mere teaching efficiency is not enough.

It was clear from the start that Fritz, with his considerable problems, could not be taught in a class. For one thing, any degree of restlessness around him would have irritated him and made concentration impossible. For another, he himself would have disrupted the class and destroyed work done by the others. Consider only his negativism and his uninhibited, impulsive behaviour. This is why we gave him a personal tutor on the ward, with the consent of the educational authority. Even then, teaching was not easy, as should be clear from the above remarks. Even mathematics lessons were problematic when, given his special talent in this area, one might have expected an easier time. Of course, if a problem turned up which happened to interest him at that moment (see previous examples), then he 'tuned in' and surprised us all by his quick and excellent grasp. However, ordinary mathematics — sums — made for much tedious effort. As we will see with the other cases even with the brightest children of this type, the automatisation of learning, that is, the setting up of routine thought processes, proceeds only with the utmost difficulty. Writing was an especially difficult subject, as we expected, because his motor clumsiness, in addition to his general problems, hampered him a good deal. In his tense fist the pencil could not run smoothly. A whole page would suddenly become covered with big swirls, the exercise book would be drilled full of holes, if not torn up. In the end it was possible to teach him to write only by making him trace letters and words which were written in red pencil. This was to guide him to make the right movements. However, his handwriting has so far been atrocious. Orthography too was difficult to automatise. He used to write the whole sentence in one go, without separating the words. He was able to spell correctly when forced to be careful. However, he made the silliest mistakes when left to his own devices. Learning to read, in particular sounding out words, proceeded with moderate difficulties. It was almost impossible to teach him the simple skills needed in everyday life. While observing such a lesson, one could not help feeling that he was not listening at all, only making mischief. It was, therefore, the more surprising, as became apparent occasionally, for example through reports from the mother, that he had managed to learn quite a lot. It was typical of Fritz, as of all similar children, that he seemed to see a lot using only 'peripheral vision', or to take in things 'from the edge of attention'. Yet these children are able to analyse and retain what they catch in such glimpses. Their active and passive attention is very disturbed; they have difficulty in retrieving their knowledge, which is revealed often only by chance. Nevertheless, their thoughts can be unusually rich. They are good at logical thinking, and the ability to abstract is particularly good. It does often seem that even in perfectly normal people an increased distance to the outside world is a prerequisite for excellence in abstract thinking.

Despite the difficulties we had in teaching this boy we managed to get him to pass successfully a state school examination at the end of the school year. The exceptional examination situation was powerful enough to make him more or less behave himself, and he showed good concentration. Naturally, he astounded the examiners in mathematics. Now Fritz attends the third form of a primary school as an external pupil, without having lost a school year so far. Whether and when he will be able to visit a secondary school we do not know.

Differential Diagnosis

Considering the highly abnormal behaviour of Fritz, one has to ask whether there is in fact some more severe disturbance and not merely a personality disorder. There are two possibilities: childhood schizophrenia and a post-encephalitic state.

There is much that is reminiscent of schizophrenia in Fritz: the extremely limited contact, the automaton-like behaviour, the stereotypies. Against this diagnosis, however, speaks the fact that there is no sign of progressive deterioration, no characteristic acute onset of alarming florid symptoms (severe anxiety and hallucinations), nor are there any delusions. Although Fritz shows a very deviant personality, his personality remains the same and can largely be seen as deriving from father and mother, and their families. In fact, his personality shows steady development, and on the whole this is resulting in improved adaptation to the environment. Lastly, the complex overall clinical impression, which cannot be pinned down further, is completely different from that of a schizophrenic. There, one has the uncanny feeling of a destruction of personality which remains incomprehensible and incalculable, even if it is perhaps possible to some extent to stave off disintegration through pedagogic means. Here, however, there are numerous genuine relationships, a degree of reciprocal understanding and a genuine chance for remedial education.

One has also to consider the possibility of a post-encephalitic personality disorder. As we shall see below, there are a number of similarities between autistic children and brain-damaged children who either had a birth injury or encephalitis. Suffice it to say here that there was no reason for thinking this applied in the case of Fritz. There were certainly none of the symptoms that are always present in post-encephalitic cases (though these are sometimes easily overlooked). There was not the slightest evidence of neurological or vegetative symptoms such as strabismus, facial rigidity, subtle spastic paresis, increased salivation or other endocrine signs.

3

Diagnosis of Asperger's Disorder

Jeffrey L. Rausch

BrainScience Augusta and Department of Psychiatry and Health Behavior, Medical College of Georgia, Augusta, Georgia, U.S.A.

Maria E. Johnson

BrainScience Augusta and Developmental Disability Psychiatric Consultation-Liaison, Gracewood Hospital, Augusta, Georgia, U.S.A.

INTRODUCTION

Understanding the diagnosis of Asperger's disorder is important. Without proper diagnosis, Asperger's individuals can be misunderstood, misinterpreted, and deprived of informed support, care, and understanding of their condition.

Individuals with Asperger's disorder may have a great deal of potential with respect to long-term developmental outcomes. As a group, they may have both special needs and special abilities. It has been argued, for example, that Michelangelo met the criteria for Asperger's disorder (1). Some data suggest, for another example (discussed below), that abstract reasoning ability, i.e., "fluid intelligence," may be superior in Asperger's disorder, compared with normal individuals (2).

Although some individuals with Asperger's may achieve social and financial independence, perhaps even high degrees of achievement, many experience isolation, anxiety, and depression, unmitigated without knowledgeable support (3–5). As a group, they are often understudied and underserved in current therapeutic programs (6).

Early diagnosis and referral to treatment are key to outcome, yet the literature suggests that many medical providers may lack the training to recognize, diagnose, treat, or make appropriate treatment referral for the condition where indicated. Adding to the difficulties in diagnosis are controversies about the existence, the criteria for diagnosis, and a relative lack of discussion and emphasis outside of child psychiatry.

Providers unacquainted with the clinical diagnosis and context for identification may find it difficult to evaluate the unusual symptoms of the disorder. It is common for individuals with Asperger's to be misdiagnosed as having schizophrenia or other disorders (7). Developmental pediatricians to date, relative to psychiatrists/primary care physicians, neurologists, and psychologists, may make diagnoses earlier and be more likely to provide important information to those individuals and families affected by the disorder (8).

Lacking adequate information at times from health care providers, affected individuals, parents, caregivers, and teachers often report having to turn to the media (i.e., television, Internet, books, etc.), or peers, to acquire the necessary information to best support those affected (8). In view of the availability of treatments and the deleterious effect of the untreated condition in the sensitive years of personality development, and, recognizing the considerable "burden of disease" (9), early recognition and diagnosis of Asperger's are of utmost importance (10).

In this chapter, we will first consider the *distinctions* relevant to a specific diagnosis of Asperger's disorder in contrast to other similar disorders, with attention to current complexities and controversies of consideration in diagnosis. In the second half of this work, we consider how *similarities* of symptom clusters, "endophenotypes," between Asperger's disorder and other disorders that may share certain categories of symptoms in common—autism, certain symptoms of schizophrenia, and the schizotypies (11), e.g., schizotypal personality or schizoid personality—may advance our understanding of the diagnosis and thereby treatment of Asperger's disorder.

Discussed in the latter half of this work is evidence for a group of diagnoses within a "negative symptom spectrum." The negative symptom spectrum diagnoses arguably share similarity in receptive and expressive deficits in emotion processing coupled with stereotypies in cognition and behavior. We discuss consideration of such cross-diagnostic endophenotypes that may not only share certain categorical neuropsychological symptomatologies but also share potential common biological diatheses and responses to treatment.

DIAGNOSTIC CHALLENGES

Aside from the task of differential diagnosis discussed below, there are additional challenges to making a correct diagnosis of Asperger's disorder. These include delays in the recognition of the presence of the condition, evaluation of the potential presence of common comorbidities, and evaluation of the role of psychosocial factors as stressors or protective factors. A substantial aspect of the diagnostic challenge lies within interpretation of current diagnostic criteria and debate about their application.

Delays in the Age at Recognition

The typical impairment of social communication may be difficult to identify in early childhood and can be camouflaged in adulthood by compensatory learning (12). Neurocognitive impairments in Asperger's are more strongly associated with psychiatric symptoms at school rather than home (13). Although Asperger's disorder is an illness that begins in childhood, the diagnosis is often not made until later stages.

The presence of common symptoms between Asperger's and other psychiatric disorders as well as the possible existence of comorbidity may lead to an incorrect or late diagnosis (14). The diagnosis of autism has been found to be made at earlier ages than Asperger's disorder (8,15). For example, the average age of diagnosis in one study was three years for children with autistic disorder, and seven years for Asperger's disorder (16).

Recognition of Comorbidity and Associated Features

Not only are early recognition and treatment important but also important is the recognition of its comorbidities. Clinicians should be sensitive to the auxiliary conditions such as motor dysfunction, sensory, and sleep disturbances during the early stages of life (17). A variety of comorbid conditions may deserve evaluation at different stages, while at the same time carrying the potential to confound initial diagnosis. Professor Gillberg's excellent review in chapter 4 discusses comorbidity; associated features, in addition to complementary discussion about diagnosis.

Recognition of Psychosocial Stressors

Although the core social deficits of Asperger's and other autistic spectrum disorders (ASDs) may often seem resistant to involvement from the outer world, psychosocial stressors often facilitate the appearance of the comorbid anxiety, depression, dissociative or delusional thinking, and suicidal (18) or antisocial behavior (19). Perhaps consistent with better emotion perception, Asperger's individuals may tend toward greater anxiety indicators than high-functioning autistic subjects (20). In addition to evaluating the prognostic impact of protective psychosocial factors, it is important to recognize and aggressively intervene in psychosocial predisposing factors, as discussed by Ruble and colleagues in chapter 14.

Diagnostic Criteria for Asperger's Disorder

One of the impediments to common diagnosis of Asperger's disorder is the relatively recent establishment of formal diagnostic criteria for Asperger's disorder. The American Psychiatric Association's diagnostic criteria for Asperger's disorder were first published in 1994, in the DSM-IV (Diagnostic and Statistical Manual, fourth edition), with a text revision, DSM-IV-TR, published in 2000, which expanded the descriptive text for Asperger's disorder. Below, "DSM-IV" is used to refer to diagnostic criteria, whereas "DSM-IV-TR" is used to refer to descriptive text included in it. DSM-IV criteria for Asperger's disorder are reviewed in Table 1.

Controversy over which features best distinguish Asperger's compared with that of autism constitutes another challenge to diagnosis. An implicit concern about current diagnostic limitations is whether the Asperger's syndrome originally described is captured by present diagnostic criteria.

One group asserts that the four cases that Hans Asperger originally presented in his seminal paper met DSM-IV criteria for autism, rather than Asperger's

Table 1   DSM-IV Diagnostic Criteria for Asperger's Disorder

A. Qualitative impairment in social interaction, as manifested by at least two of the following:
  1. marked impairment in the use of multiple nonverbal behaviors such as eye-to-eye gaze, facial expression, body postures, and gestures to regulate social interaction;
  2. failure to develop peer relationships appropriate to developmental level;
  3. a lack of spontaneous seeking to share enjoyment, interests, or achievements with other people (e.g., by a lack of showing, bringing, or pointing out objects of interest to other people); and
  4. lack of social or emotional reciprocity.
B. Restricted repetitive and stereotyped patterns of behavior, interests, and activities, as manifested by at least one of the following:
  1. encompassing preoccupation with one or more stereotyped and restricted patterns of interest that is abnormal either in intensity or focus;
  2. apparently inflexible adherence to specific, nonfunctional routines or rituals;
  3. stereotyped and repetitive motor mannerisms (e.g., hand or finger flapping or twisting, or complex whole-body movements); and
  4. persistent preoccupation with parts of objects.
C. The disturbance causes clinically significant impairment in social, occupational, or other important areas of functioning.
D. There is no clinically significant general delay in language (e.g., single words used by age 2 yr, communicative phrases used by age 3 yr).
E. There is no clinically significant delay in cognitive development or in the development of age-appropriate self-help skills, adaptive behavior (other than social interaction), and curiosity about the environment in childhood.
F. Criteria are not met for another specific pervasive developmental disorder or schizophrenia.

Source: From Ref. 44.

disorder (21). However, a subsequent study of 74 clinical case records of children with "autistic psychopathy" diagnosed by Asperger and his team at the Viennese Children's Clinic and Asperger's private practice revealed that 68% of the sample did meet ICD-10 (International Statistical Classification of Diseases) criteria for Asperger's syndrome, although they construed that 25% fulfilled diagnostic criteria for autism (22).

Asperger's disorder is defined in DSM-IV as a pervasive developmental disorder characterized by severe and sustained impairments in social interaction and the development of restricted, repetitive patterns of behavior, interests, and activities. Asperger drew attention to the fact that such individuals show some of the core features of autism, yet in the presence of high verbal intelligence. In distinction to autism, language acquisition, cognitive development, learning skills, and even most adaptive behaviors are largely preserved in Asperger's disorder.

Two sets of diagnostic criteria for Asperger's disorder, one by Szatmari et al. (23) and another by Gillberg and Gillberg (24) preceded the publication of DSM-IV-TR consensus criteria. These 1989 criteria essentially agree both with the original observations of Hans Asperger and other important early researchers (25–29) as well as with that of DSM-IV-TR. However, some of the features are given different emphasis in prior descriptions, leaving potential for question whether DSM may necessarily best capture each aspect of the finer points of diagnostic distinction.

Insights into evolution of observations on the nature of Asperger's disorder may be gleaned from comparison of the respective criteria. Table 2 compares the main features of Asperger's disorder as summarized by Szatmari et al., Gillberg and Gillberg, and DSM-IV-TR.

DSM-IV-TR added the lack of a clinically significant delay in cognitive development, the lack of spontaneous seeking to share enjoyment, and a persistent preoccupation with parts of objects to the prior diagnostic criteria of Szatmari et al. and Gillberg and Gillberg. A reliance on rote memory and motor clumsiness was noted by Gillberg and Gillberg. Although not included in DSM-IV criteria, these features appear in the DSM-IV-TR descriptive language.

Szatmari et al. emphasized oddities of expressive language, such as abnormal inflection, verbosity or taciturnity, lack of cohesion, idiosyncratic diction, and repetition. Gillberg and Gillberg noted abnormalities of both expressive language and language comprehension and that persons with Asperger's disorder often have expressive speech skills that exceed their abilities to interpret spoken language.

The DSM-IV-TR criteria note the absence of a "clinically significant general delay in language," although several studies note abnormalities of speech in Asperger's disorder (30) not as markers of developmental delay in communication but as often presenting as relatively constant and enduring features of the disorder. The DSM-IV-TR text observes that conversation, for example, may be marked by a preoccupation with certain topics and verbosity.

ICD-10 criteria characterize "Asperger's syndrome" as "a disorder of uncertain nosological validity," differing from autism primarily in that there is no general delay or retardation in language or in cognitive development.

Table 2 Comparison of Features of Asperger's Disorder According to Szatmari et al., Gillberg and Gillberg, and DSM-IV-TR

Feature	Szatmari et al, 1989	Gillberg and Gillberg, 1989	DSM-IV-TR
Social interaction	Impaired • Solitary, no close friends • Limited facial expression, unable to read facial expressions • Unable to give message with eyes; does not look at others • One-sided responses to peers • Does not use hands to express self • Clumsy social approach • Avoids others; no interest in making friends; approaches only for need • Difficulty sensing feelings of others; detached • Comes too close to others	Severe impairment • Odd and socially or emotionally inappropriate behavior • Little or inappropriate facial expression; coldness; emotional bluntness or immaturity • Extreme egocentricity • Unintentional play acting • Stiffness • Limited, clumsy gestures • Inability to play reciprocally • Lack of appreciation of social cues	Qualitative impairment • Impaired nonverbal behavior in social interaction • Impaired eye contact, facial expression, body posture, gestures • Failure to develop peer relationships appropriate to developmental level • Lack of spontaneous seeking to share enjoyment, interests, achievements with others • Lack of emotional reciprocity
Behavior, interests, and activities	Not discussed	• All-absorbing interest in a subject; manner of interest goes to extremes, excluding most other activities, and adhered to in a repetitive way • Relies on rote memory rather than on meaning and connection • Stereotyped way of trying to introduce and impose routines • Particular interest in all or almost all aspects of ordinary life	• Preoccupation with stereotyped and restricted patterns of interest, abnormal in intensity or focus • Apparently inflexible adherence to specific, nonfunctional routines or rituals • Stereotyped and repetitive motor mannerisms • Persistent preoccupation with parts of objects

Speech, communication, and cognition	• Odd speech • Repetitive speech patterns • Abnormalities in inflection, talks too much or too little • Lack of cohesion, idiosyncratic use of words	• Delayed language development compared with social language background • Superficially perfect expressive language; often formal and pedantic; flat, staccato-like prosody • Mild to moderately impaired language comprehension with concrete misinterpretations of spoken language, with much better expressive language skills • Impaired nonverbal communication	• No clinically significant general delay in language • No significant delay in cognitive development
Motor skills	• Gestures large and clumsy	• Motor clumsiness	• Motor delays or clumsiness during preschool period
Development or functioning	Not discussed	Not discussed	• No clinically significant delay in adaptive behavior other than in social interaction • No significant delay in curiosity about the environment in childhood • No significant delay in self-help skills • Significant impairment in social, occupational, or other areas of functioning • Criteria not met for pervasive developmental disorder or schizophrenia

Source: From Refs. 23, 24, and 44.

Common marked clumsiness is mentioned. ICD-10 criteria are somewhat more descriptive than algorithmic, compared with DSM-IV. The diagnostic criteria are "a lack of any clinically significant general delay in language or cognitive development plus, as with autism, the presence of qualitative deficiencies in reciprocal social interaction and restricted, repetitive, stereotyped patterns of behavior, interests, and activities. There may or may not be problems in communication similar to those associated with autism, but significant language retardation would rule out the diagnosis" (31).

One main difference between the ICD-10 and the DSM-IV criteria is the DSM-IV requirement for "a clinically significant decrease in viability occupationally, socially, or in other important areas of functioning." In one sense, this could be used to distinguish Asperger's syndrome (ICD-10) from "Asperger's disorder" (DSM-IV), in the sense that the word "syndrome" may not necessarily imply impact on social functioning, or may not necessarily imply psychopathology. Conversely, the word "disorder" implies psychopathology in the sense of pathology adversely impacting occupational or social functioning, following Sigmund Freud who originally defined psychopathology by its impairment on *"arbeiten und lieben,"* i.e., impairment on the capacity "to work and to love." In other words, the extent of psychopathology is defined by the extent to which "occupational or social functioning" is impaired. However, although DSM-IV versus ICD-10 could differentiate the disorder from the syndrome, one finds little of any such convention in the literature.

A second major difference between the ICD-10 and the DSM-IV criteria is found not in the DSM-IV Asperger's criteria, but in the DSM-IV autistic disorder (autism) criteria. The DSM-IV criteria exclude a diagnosis of Asperger's disorder if criteria are met for autism, as a pervasive developmental disorder. Conversely, the DSM-IV criteria permit a diagnosis of autistic disorder if there is "stereotyped and repetitive use of language or idiosyncratic language," as an indicator of "qualitative impairment in communication" (criterion 2 C). Although the literature is replete with observations of such speech abnormalities as a feature of Asperger's, as discussed below with our comparison to high-functioning autism (HFA), a strict interpretation of such speech as being a qualitative impairment in communication can result, under the current criteria, in all cases of Asperger's being diagnosed as autistic disorder instead. As will be seen below, interpretation of the criteria in this way results in a diagnostic nihilism for the case of Asperger's disorder, resulting in much confusion in the literature.

DIFFERENTIAL DIAGNOSIS OF ASPERGER'S DISORDER

The recognition of Asperger's disorder can be complicated by features that overlap with similar, but distinct, psychiatric disorders. There are similarities between Asperger's disorder and autistic disorder (32–37), schizophrenia (26,32,38–42), schizoid personality disorder (32,40,43), and schizotypal personality disorder (44–47). These make for distinct diagnostic challenges for making the

Asperger's diagnosis, especially in adults. Because of this, Asperger's individuals often receive one or more misdiagnoses before a proper diagnosis of Asperger's disorder is made (5,7).

Diagnostic distinctions between Asperger's disorder, autistic disorder, schizophrenia, schizoid personality disorder, and schizotypal personality disorder can be complicated by a number of the factors discussed further below. Adding to the complexity are differences in deficit patterns that can be specific to developmental level (13). The diagnostic criteria have been criticized for overweighting an age-specific emphasis, a childhood emphasis, such that the criteria may not translate well for distinction of clinically significant, relevant differences in functioning at later ages (48,49).

Asperger's Disorder Vs. HFA

There has been considerable debate over whether Asperger's disorder and HFA (IQ ≥ 70) are distinct conditions (50). Many writers consider Asperger's disorder to be one of the ASDs—sharing clinical features with autism, but without developmental delay in language acquisition. Some authors have advocated incorporation of autism and Asperger's disorder into one diagnostic category, distinguishing between the two only with severity modifiers (51).

As above, according to DSM-IV, Asperger's disorder is not diagnosed if the criteria for autistic disorder are met. For DSM-IV-TR criteria, the autism diagnosis always has priority over the Asperger's disorder. If a patient meets the DSM-IV criteria for autism, then the DSM-IV diagnosis of Asperger's disorder is ruled out (criterion F).

Whereas children with autism exhibit delays in social interaction, language, or play before age 3 years, those with Asperger's disorder do not manifest clinically significant delays in language, cognitive development, self-help skills, most adaptive behavior, or curiosity about the environment.

Autism presents with qualitative communication impairments, which can include uncompensated deficits in spoken language development, impairment in initiating or sustaining conversation, deficits in communication through play, as well as language stereotypies or idiosyncrasies. In contrast, notwithstanding the observation that Asperger's disorder commonly presents with stereotyped, repetitive, or idiosyncratic language (30), clinically significant general delays in language abilities are not observed in Asperger's disorder under DSM-IV (Fig. 1).

Asperger's and autistic disorders share the same criteria for qualitative impairment in social interaction. Both diagnoses require the presence of two or more of the following: marked nonverbal behavioral impairment; impaired peer relationships; lack of spontaneous sharing of enjoyment, interests, or achievements with others; and lack of social or emotional reciprocity (44). However, the DSM-IV-TR explains that unlike persons with autistic disorder, whose typical patterns of social interaction are characterized by "self-isolation or markedly rigid social approaches," persons with Asperger's disorder may be motivated to

DSM-IV Diagnostic Criteria

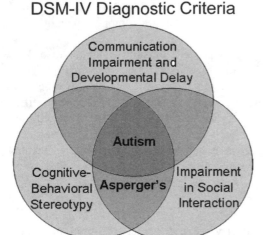

Figure 1 DSM-IV diagnostic criteria. Diagnostic distinctions between Asperger's disorder and autism are shown above.

approach others, "even though this may be done in a highly eccentric, one-sided, verbose, and insensitive manner."

Similarly, Asperger's and autistic disorders share criteria for restricted and stereotyped behavior and interests. To be a candidate for either diagnosis, an individual must show an encompassing, stereotyped, restricted, preoccupied pattern of interests; an inflexible adherence to nonfunctional routines or rituals; motor stereotypies; or persistent preoccupation with parts of objects (44). Again, the DSM-IV-TR describes differences in preoccupations that elaborate on differences in the diagnostic criteria between autism and Asperger's. The "restricted, repetitive, and stereotyped interests and activities" observed in autism are characterized by "motor mannerisms . . . rituals, and marked distress in change." Conversely, the preoccupations in Asperger's disorder (criterion B) tend to be marked simply by an "all-encompassing pursuit of a circumscribed interest involving a topic to which the individual devotes inordinate amounts of time."

Although the descriptive manifestations of these criteria tend to be somewhat different, the diagnostic criteria for impaired social interaction and stereotyped behavior and interests are identical for Asperger's disorder and autistic disorder. Regardless of these descriptive differences in criterion B, it is the presence or absence of developmental delay and communication impairment that is the main differentiator of autism and Asperger's under DSM-IV. However, several lines of evidence (52–54) suggest that the course of language development may be over-emphasized as a distinguishing feature between autism and Asperger's.

Mayes and colleagues have argued that a DSM-IV diagnosis of Asperger's disorder is unlikely if not impossible, since all Asperger's cases they examined had a "DSM-IV communication impairment" qualifying the subjects in their eyes for a diagnosis of autistic disorder and not Asperger's disorder (30). Half of that sample (IQ $\geq$ 80) had no significant developmental delay in single words and communicative phrases, as required for Asperger's disorder, but, since 96% had "stereotyped and repetitive or idiosyncratic language" and the remaining 4% had "impairment in the ability to initiate or sustain a conversation," all were considered autistic by their interpretation of DSM-IV.

The DSM-IV-TR describes the social interaction impairment in autism to be *markedly* abnormal or impaired, however, often to the point of a *markedly impaired awareness of others*. In addition, the Asperger's DSM-IV-TR indicates that although there are no clinically significant delays or deviance in language acquisition, more subtle aspects of social communication may be affected, and subsequent language may be unusual, preoccupied, difficult, and socially dysfunctional, may fail to appreciate conventional rules of conversation and nonverbal cues, and may have limited capacities for self-monitoring (44).

The Mayes' study identifies the importance of clinical judgment in application and understanding of the intent of the criteria, as elaborated in the text revision. A need to improve the language for future DSM revisions is also elucidated by the study. It is important to understand that "in DSM-IV there is no assumption that each category of mental disorder is a completely discreet entity" (44), as well as "that DSM-IV not be applied mechanically," but be intended rather as "guidelines to be informed by clinical judgment" (44).

Future Diagnostic Language

Future diagnostic language may better distinguish the markedly impaired social interaction of autism from that of Asperger's cases, where such is not present. In this case, the term "marked," could be elaborated to differentiate from the more subtle speech stereotypy, idiosyncrasy, or difficulties with conversation maintenance prior to age 3 years described in Asperger's. Difficulties with conversation maintenance may be arguably normal for most individuals younger than three years and so may also confound the interpretation of criterion D, needing strict anchors for the normal degree of conversation maintenance for a given age.

Analysis of speech and communication patterns, cognitive batteries, and WISC (Wechsler Intelligence Scale for Children) findings (55) support the DSM-IV-TR interpretation that Asperger's and autism are distinct diagnostically. However, as above, significant differences may not be found between children with and without a speech delay on a variety of variables analyzed, including autistic symptoms and expressive language. Such results suggest that early speech delay may be irrelevant to later functioning in children who have normal intelligence and clinical diagnoses of autism or Asperger's syndrome (48,49).

Differences in associated features between HFA and Asperger's are reviewed further below in the section on associated features. These features are not part of the current diagnostic criteria, but may inform the differential diagnosis and development of future diagnostic criteria.

Table 3 Comparison of DSM-IV-TR Features of Asperger's Disorder, Schizophrenia, Schizoid Personality Disorder, and Schizotypal Personality Disorder (*Continued*)

Feature	Asperger's disorder	Schizophrenia	Schizoid personality disorder	Schizotypal personality disorder
Behavioral stereotypies (mannerisms)	Restricted, repetitive, and stereotyped patterns of behavior and activities; inflexible adherence to specific, nonfunctional routines or rituals; stereotyped and repetitive motor mannerisms	Pacing, rocking; ritualistic, stereotyped behavior; odd mannerisms	Usually not significantly abnormal	Eccentric behavior; magic rituals; odd behavior, unusual mannerisms
Cognitive stereotypies (circumstantiality, overinclusive thinking)	Encompassing preoccupation with stereotyped patterns of interest	Delusions; disorganized speech, tangentiality	May prefer mechanical or abstract tasks; directionless, may drift in their goals	Stereotyped, overelaborate thinking and speech
Hallucinations	Absent	May be present	Absent	Absent
Delusions	Absent	May be present	Absent	Suspiciousness
Impairment	Significant functional impairment	Social and occupational dysfunction	Distress or impairment present	Distress or impairment present

Patients with schizophrenia demonstrate two different deficits of language comprehension: difficulty with understanding irony, which is associated with poor theory of mind (i.e., a difficulty with inferring other people's thoughts), as well as poor recognition of metaphors, consistent with concrete thinking and difficulties with abstraction. Theory-of-mind impairments in schizophrenia tend to be less severe than in autism, but are specific and not a reflection of general cognitive deficits (63). Both paranoid schizophrenics and Asperger's may perform poorly on theory-of-mind tasks compared with the controls (64). In contrast, the personality disorders tend to perform better on theory-of-mind measures than Asperger's or schizophrenic subjects (65).

Negative Symptom Schizotypy in the Personality Disorders

Differentiating between diagnoses of Asperger's syndrome and personality disorders is difficult because the developmental disorders, including Asperger's syndrome, are diagnosed in consideration of their time course, while personality disorders are cross-sectional entities, diagnosed not by developmental trajectory, but in real time compared with the control, or normative condition (46). Tantam has suggested that Asperger's syndrome is a distinct syndrome from either schizoid or schizotypal personality disorder, but may be a risk factor for the development of schizoid personality disorder (29). According to DSM-IV criteria, a personality disorder diagnosis of schizotypal personality disorder or schizoid personality disorder cannot be made if the symptoms present exclusively within the context of a pervasive developmental disorder. Consequently, a diagnosis of Asperger's disorder precludes a diagnosis of schizotypal personality disorder or schizoid personality disorder.

Schizoid Personality Disorder

A differential diagnosis of Asperger's disorder from that of schizoid personality disorder may be difficult, especially in adults, without benefit of childhood diagnostic observation. In general, the social difficulties in Asperger's disorder are more severe and of earlier onset (44). A thorough childhood developmental history is important for differential diagnosis, since a diagnosis of schizoid personality disorder should not be made if the patient meets criteria for Asperger's disorder, according to DSM-IV, since Asperger's disorder is exclusionary as a pervasive developmental disorder for a diagnosis of schizoid personality disorder.

Several investigators however have noted a close relationship between Asperger's disorder and schizoid personality disorder. Schizoid personality disorder is like Asperger's disorder in that it is marked by restricted emotional expression and decreased social interaction and relatedness. It has been asserted that "the clinical features of [children with schizoid personality disorder are] identical in all respects to those described by Asperger" (66). It has also been suggested that Asperger's disorder in children and schizoid personality disorder in adults are analogous (67). A similar concept is that of Tantam's, above, that

Asperger's disorder may be a "risk factor" for the "development" of schizoid personality disorder (29). Some have considered Asperger's disorder and schizoid personality in childhood as being the same in childhood and subsumed by the more general clinical picture psychiatrists have of schizoid personality in adult life (68).

The Table 3 comparison of DSM-IV diagnostic criteria between Asperger's and schizoid personality disorders suggests less overlap than that found for schizophrenia or schizotypal personality disorder.

The assertion that the features of children with schizoid personality disorder are identical to Asperger's (66) was based on the now-discounted belief that schizoid personality disorder presents with marked stereotypies. Stereotypies are less pronounced in schizoid personality disorder than Asperger's disorder, essentially absent in schizoid personality disorder for the most part in comparison with Asperger's. Schizoid personality disorder is different from Asperger's disorder in that marked behavioral and cognitive stereotypies are not featured in DSM-IV schizoid personality disorder. In schizoid personality disorder, cognitive stereotypy may be present as a preference for mechanical or abstract tasks. The preference for mechanical or abstract tasks in these individuals may however in some ways be similar to the pronounced stereotypies exhibited by persons with Asperger's disorder and schizophrenia.

According to DSM-IV, individuals with schizoid personality disorder may have a restricted range of emotional expression and flattened affectivity. This is similar to the impaired nonverbal social behaviors described for Asperger's disorder in DSM-IV-TR. The failure to develop peer relationships, unwillingness to share interests, and absence of social and emotional reciprocity noted in Asperger's disorder resembles the emotional coldness and detachment from relationships, the lack of desire or enjoyment of relationships, the lack of confidants, and preference for solitary activities seen in schizoid personality disorder. However, as noted above, persons with Asperger's disorder may be motivated to approach others, "even though this is then done in a highly eccentric, one-sided, verbose, and insensitive manner" (44).

Schizoid personality disorder presents differently from Asperger's in the capacity to imagine what goes on in the minds of other people (theory of mind). Schizoid children are not lacking in imaginative functions. They engage in make-believe play and typically have an active and unusual fantasy life. Sometimes they behave as if they cannot differentiate between their imagination and reality. They may appear not so much as being unable to imagine how other people feel and think, as they appear unable to mount reactions to meet the needs of others. Moreover, the onset of their social disabilities is not in early but in middle childhood, when the development of more public social skills normally begins (47). Schizoid subjects tend to look more at the other person and to make less self-stimulatory gestures than Asperger's subjects (69). However, parents of children on the autistic spectrum may present with features of schizoid personality disorder (70,71).

Schizotypal Personality Disorder

Although Asperger's disorder and schizotypal personality disorder are mutually exclusive but similar diagnoses (DSM-IV-TR), the criteria have similarities that also require attention for differential diagnosis. The speech, stereotypy, and social impairment seen with schizotypal personality disorder bear many similarities to that of Asperger's disorder (Table 3). According to DSM-IV-TR, it can be difficult to differentiate children with schizotypal personality disorder from "the heterogeneous group of solitary, odd children whose behavior is characterized by marked social isolation, eccentricity, or peculiarities of language" and whose diagnoses would include the milder forms of autistic disorder and Asperger's disorder.

Like persons with Asperger's disorder, those with schizotypal personality disorder exhibit a pervasive pattern of social and interpersonal impairments and expressive and receptive deficits of emotion processing (72–74). Because of this, questionnaires designed to characterize the presence of Asperger's symptoms and those designed to characterize the presence of schizotypal personality disorder correlate with each other. There is, however, a stronger correlation between the social-interpersonal questionnaire items of the two diagnoses than those between the communication-disorganization items (45).

Individuals with schizotypal personality disorder typically exhibit diminished eye contact and impaired, constricted, unresponsive, or inappropriate affect or facial expression. The lack of close friends or confidants, the reduced capacity for close relationships other than immediate family, the failure to develop peer relationships, and the absence of social and emotional reciprocity seen in schizotypal disorder resemble the social and interpersonal deficits noted in Asperger's disorder. However, the DSM-IV-TR states that persons with Asperger's disorder typically manifest "an even greater lack of social awareness and emotional reciprocity and stereotyped behaviors and interests" than those with schizotypal personality disorder.

Also, "odd, eccentric, or peculiar" behaviors characteristic of DSM-IV schizotypal personality disorder bear similarity to the impaired nonverbal social behaviors seen in Asperger's disorder. Behavioral and cognitive stereotypies characterize both disorders in DSM-IV. Stereotypy is less pronounced in schizotypal personality disorder than Asperger's disorder, however, and more pronounced in schizotypal personality than schizoid personality disorder (i.e., for stereotypy, Asperger's >schizotypal >schizoid). Stereotypy may manifest in schizotypal personality disorder potentially as idiosyncratic speech, magic rituals, odd behavior, or unusual mannerisms (44).

Schizotypal adults show normal recognition of metaphors, yet like schizophrenia, are significantly impaired in their ability to appreciate irony (75). Individuals with high schizotypal personality scores may not show impairment of social cognition. Although impaired in social function, they may not show some of the impairments found in Asperger's disorder. Schizotypal subjects may be without impairment in theory-of-mind tasks, emotion perception, verbal secondary memory, or executive functioning (76).

Obsessive-Compulsive Disorder and Obsessive-Compulsive Personality Disorder

Obsessive-compulsive behaviors are common and disabling across the ASDs. Some data suggest that obsessive-compulsive disorder (OCD) patients as a group may show the same frequency of obsessive-compulsive symptoms as Asperger's, although somatic obsessions and repeating rituals may be more common in the OCD group than in Asperger's or HFA (77).

Up to 50% of autistic spectrum individuals report at least moderate levels of interference from OC symptoms (77), although OCD patients typically have a higher severity of obsessive-compulsive symptoms than that of Asperger's or HFA. It is important to recognize that obsessive symptoms associated with Asperger's may be increased during an episode of depression, and episodes of depression in Asperger's carry a higher tendency for self-injury as well (78).

Unlike the case for schizoid or schizotypal personality disorder, a diagnosis of Asperger's disorder under DSM-IV does not preclude a concomitant diagnosis of OCD, where the obsessions or compulsions cause marked distress or impairment beyond distress or impairment explained by the Asperger's diagnosis alone.

DSM-IV also does not preclude a diagnosis of obsessive-compulsive personality disorder (OCPD), except that personality disorders (axis II diagnoses) are not to be made where the features occur solely within the course of an axis I disorder. Given the early onset, and enduring course of Asperger's, it is difficult then to imagine how both a diagnosis of Asperger's and OCPD would be appropriate, especially notwithstanding the fact that the OC symptoms of Asperger's are typically closer to OCD than are they like those described for OCPD.

ASPERGER'S ASSOCIATED FEATURES AND DIAGNOSTIC CLUES

A number of features associated with Asperger's disorder can be found in the literature, many of which are not included in the DSM-IV criteria. While it is necessary for a diagnosis of Asperger's to be made according to the criteria, i.e., necessary for an Asperger's individual to meet the criteria in order to have the diagnosis, a number of additional differential diagnostic clues may be gleaned from observations of such associated features. Below are reviewed cognitive, language, behavioral, perceptual, motor, sleep, and physical characteristics associated with Asperger's disorder that are discussed in the literature with pertinence to differential diagnostic distinction. The discriminative contribution of each may not necessarily differentiate diagnosis; in many cases, these features present on a spectrum of abnormality, not necessarily clearly demarcated in severity level for diagnostic purposes. However, a discussion of associated features is also important both for the diagnosis of associated conditions as well as for understanding the diagnosis' effect on various presenting signs, symptoms, and levels of impairment.

Speech and Communication

Discussed above, abnormalities of speech in Asperger's may confound the differential DSM-IV diagnosis from that of autism. Since the Asperger's literature is replete with reference to abnormalities of speech, it is interesting to note that abnormal speech is not mentioned in DSM-IV-TR diagnostic criteria for Asperger's disorder. Patients with Asperger's disorder frequently exhibit phonic tics in addition to other abnormalities of speech (79), including one-sided verbosity, restricted prosody and intonation, and pedantic speech (80).

Asperger's subjects are unlikely to have the marked speech abnormalities often characteristic of autism and HFA (81). Asperger's subjects may demonstrate better nonverbal communication than high-functioning autistic subjects (50), less echolalia and pronoun reversal (82), but more pedantic speech than autistic subjects (80). Pedantic speech may be common in Asperger's disorder, present in as many as three-quarters of subjects, and may help differentiate it from HFA (80).

Language and Verbal IQ

Some communicative difficulties in Asperger's subjects are largely similar to that of high-functioning autistic subjects (81). Both Asperger's disorder and high-functioning autistic subjects may show deficits in language comprehension (13). Asperger's subjects may have better language skills than high-functioning autistic subjects of equivalent IQ (83), with higher verbal IQ, higher vocabulary, and higher comprehension (50). Correlated with communication ability, there is evidence to suggest that a history of normal language acquisition in early childhood is predictive of better verbal ability in mid-childhood or later (50).

Cognition

Subjects with Asperger's disorder have tested with *higher* abstract-reasoning ability than *normal* individuals (2). Some individuals with Asperger's or HFA have mathematical giftedness, although the majority may have a significant but clinically modest math weakness (84).

Some demonstrate enhanced mental focus, excellent memory abilities, superior spatial skills, and an intuitive understanding of logical systems. They typically have an ability to focus intensely on areas of interest. They may show hypersensitivity or hyposensitivity to certain stimuli. However, to understand and manage the emotions and intentions of others, it is necessary to have an integrated perceptual assessment, language comprehension, communication ability, and executive problem-solving ability.

suggests that individuals with Asperger's disorder may lack an intuitive theory of mind, but may be able to acquire an explicit theory of mind. Although there is some controversy, it has been suggested that Asperger's individuals may do this through a "second-order theory of mind," i.e., they may not typically use mental state terms (101). Under this notion, they would typically solve theory-of-mind tasks not so much through empathic perception, or social/emotional intuition, but rather through a systematized set of observations and laws accounting for past experience, from attention to its parts rather than its whole.

Perception of Emotions and the Intentions of Others

In Asperger's disorder, there is thus a deficit in the capacity to imagine what goes on in the minds of other people, with difficulty observed in the interpretation of facial expressions and other social cues. Consequently, Asperger's subjects typically show disturbances in reciprocal social interaction with the potential for associated depression and anxiety (85). In addition to difficulty with perceiving emotions in others, they may have difficulty communicating their own emotions (alexithymia) (12).

When normal controls are asked to perform a theory-of-mind test (Faux Pas), positron emission tomography reveals increased activity in the left medial prefrontal cortex. Using the same paradigm in normal intellect patients with Asperger's disorder, there is no left medial prefrontal cortical activity found with a theory-of-mind task where they show deficits (102).

Neural Substrates of Emotion Perception

The amygdala is thought to play a role in the development of the circuitry mediating theory of mind; damage to the amygdala has been associated with a loss of at least some theory of mind functions (103). Subjects with bilateral amygdala damage show specific impairment in rating sad faces, but perform normally in rating happy faces (104).

A group of individuals with Asperger's syndrome exhibit a pattern of abnormality in differentially acquiring fear, which suggests that their fear responses are atypically modulated, modulated not only by conditioned but also by non-conditioned stimuli. This is consistent with an altered connectivity between the amygdala and functionally associated cortical areas (105). Brain imaging studies pinpoint a network that links medial prefrontal cortex and temporal cortex (overlying the amygdala) as the neural substrate of intuitive theory of mind. This network shows reduced activation and poor connectivity in Asperger's syndrome (12).

The typical enhancement of perception for emotionally arousing events is significantly reduced in Asperger's, suggesting a potential failure of the amygdala to amplify processing in cortex under such conditions, given its critical role in emotional modulation (106). Beneath temporal cortex, the amygdala processes emotional facial expressions encompassing multiple negative emotions, including fear and sadness. The amygdala is thought to play a role in the development of the circuitry-mediating theory of mind, as supported by observations of such functioning in individuals with amygdala damage (103).

Both Asperger's disorder and high-functioning autistic subjects may show outstanding deficits in facial recognition (13). Although normal in accuracy at distinguishing expressive faces and voices presented in isolation (107,108), Asperger's subjects may have difficulty distinguishing between congruent and incongruent expressive faces and voices (107). Similarly, Asperger's subjects may have difficulty recognizing emotions when faces are paired with mismatching words (108), demonstrating a bias toward words over faces and supportive of a compensatory verbal mediation strategy to process perceptions and recognition of facial emotion.

A lack of demonstrated empathy in Asperger's disorder is one of its more dysfunctional associated features (109). However, in comparison with those with HFA, Asperger's subjects may show better empathic ability (101), i.e., better ability to perceive emotion in others (110).

Motor Features Associated with Asperger's Disorder

Although motor deficits are not included in diagnostic criteria for Asperger's disorder coordination disorder (111) and gross motor, fine motor, and visuomotor deficits have frequently been described as an associated feature of Asperger's disorder (112). Patients with Asperger's syndrome frequently exhibit repetitive movements (stereotypies), motor and phonic tics, and self-stimulating ("stimming") behaviors, such as rocking back and forth and repetitive verbal utterances, among other motor abnormalities (79).

Clumsiness, deficits in motor coordination (13), and other motor signs have been widely reported both in individuals with autism and Asperger's disorder (113,114). Both autism and Asperger's disorder may show movement abnormalities comprising either simple motor stereotypies such as hand flapping, toe walking, whole-body movements, or complex motor stereotypies such as repetitive ritualistic/compulsive behaviors (79,85).

Quantitative motor differences between autism and Asperger's may have downstream effects on later stages of movement development, resulting in qualitative differences between the disorders, such as "motor clumsiness" in Asperger's disorder versus "abnormal posturing" in autism (115,116). Both groups may have abnormal arm posturing. Asperger's subjects may have more head and trunk posturing (117). An atypical deficit in *preparation* for motor response may be present in Asperger's disorder, compared with a *lack of anticipation* of movement in autism (118).

Gait abnormalities and motor signs have also been widely reported in individuals with autism and Asperger's disorder (113,114). The autistic group may show significantly increased stride-length variability versus Asperger's showing the significantly different head and trunk posturing during gait (113).

Tilting Test

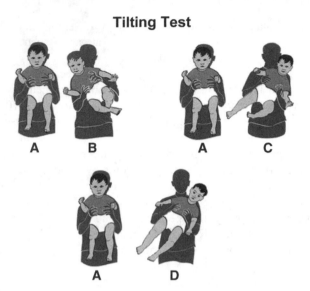

A   B   A   C

A   D

Teitelbaum, Osnat et al. (2004) Proc. Natl. Acad. Sci. USA 101, 11909-11914

Figure 3 The tilting test can be used as an early indicator for possible autism or Asperger's disorder. *Source*: From Ref. 119.

Some evidence suggests that Asperger's disorder can be detected in infancy and diagnosed very early, prior to indicators of language development. A simple test for using one such reflex of potential diagnostic value has been proposed for the early detection of a subgroup of children with Asperger's disorder or autism (119) (Fig. 3).

Sleep

Insomnia is a common and distressing symptom, which is frequently associated with coexistent behavior problems. Patients with Asperger's disorder may show decreased sleep time in the first two-thirds of the night, increased number of shifts into rapid eye movement (REM) sleep from a waking epoch, REM sleep disruption, significantly decreased EEG sleep spindles, and pathological index of periodic leg movements in sleep (120). Asperger's subjects have been found to have a relative insensitivity to circadian cues ("zeitgebers") (121). Identification and treatment of sleep problems should be a routine part of the treatment plan for those with Asperger's disorder (122).

Body Mass

Population-based body mass index (BMI) percentiles are useful for detecting associations between specific psychopathological syndromes and body weight.

An increased risk of being underweight during childhood and adolescence has been observed in male children and adolescents with schizoid personality disorder or Asperger's disorder (123). There is a risk for being underweight in association with disturbed eating behavior in patients with Asperger's disorder (124).

Ligamentous Laxity

Ligamentous laxity has been observed in some cases of Asperger's disorder, a Marfan-like disorder of connective tissue, speculatively related to an anomalous development of midline brain structures commensurate with social handicaps characteristic of Asperger's disorder (125).

Acrocyanosis

Acrocyanosis, blueness of the hands and feet, typically symmetrical, marked by a mottled blue or red discoloration of the skin of the fingers and wrists and the toes and ankles and by profuse sweating and coldness of the fingers and toes, may be more common in ASDs, including Asperger's disorder. Acrocyanosis is potentially related to the hyperserotonemia found in autism (126), although it is unknown whether or not Asperger's subjects have hyperserotonemia.

Neuro-ophthalmological Disturbances

Asperger's disorder may be associated with a variety of neuro-ophthalmological disturbances, including colobomatous defects involving the optic discs and peripapillary retina and abnormal ocular motility, described as an oculocephalic dyskinesia (127).

TOWARD A FUTURE DIAGNOSTIC UNDERSTANDING: BEHAVIORAL GENETIC DETERMINATES OF ENDOPHENOTYPES WITHIN DIAGNOSIS

Much work is underway to identify the genetic susceptibilities to various psychiatric disorders. These studies have deepened our understanding of the multivariant interactions between environment, experience, and polymorphisms of the genetic code as risk factors for the psychiatric disorders. In chapters 10–12, we discuss these interactions in depth.

Asperger's disorder is like the other psychiatric disorders studied to date in showing no simple mode of inheritance. It shows rather a more complex pattern of polygenetic heritability, one which may be potentially better advanced through the identification of behavioral endophenotypes within diagnosis, e.g., there may be heritable social endophenotypes, perhaps defined potentially from measures of face recognition, emotion perception, and theory of mind (128), as well stereotypy endophenotypes, setereotypies in cognition and behavior, i.e., restricted and repetitive interests and behaviors.

Notwithstanding the size and relevance of the emergent literature on potential etiologic candidate genes, the genetic literature is predominately parsed by *diagnosis* as the phenotype of study, reasonably so for its current stage. There is much less known about the genetic association to common, specific cross-diagnostic phenotypes. However, some research has already indicated that the endophenotypes comprising autistic-like traits, e.g., language ability, autistic-like social and communication traits, and restricted and repetitive behaviors and interests have specific, heterogeneous, genetic, and etiological determinants.

In a recent population-based sample of over 6000 twin pairs assessed prospectively through 2–8 years of age, specific genetic influences on early language were found which had a heritability discrete from other autistic-like traits (129). In that study, the Childhood Asperger Syndrome Test was used to measure autistic-like traits between twins in the general population. Social and communicative autistic-like traits were weakly correlated with language ability. In addition to specific genetic influences on early language that were not shared with other autistic-like traits, there were specific genetic influences on autistic-like traits that were not shared with earlier language performance supportive of discrete endophenotypes within diagnosis.

Perhaps more interesting, restricted, repetitive behaviors and interests were not correlated with language deficits (129). These results suggest that autistic-like language, autistic-like social and communication skills, and autistic-like restricted, repetitive behaviors and interests may have heterogeneous genetic diatheses. Supportive of this notion as well are family genetic studies indicating that autistic-like cognition may also characterize the "broader phenotype" among first-degree relatives not meeting criteria for an ASD diagnosis (130).

The contrasting similarities and differences in endophenotype are discussed above for the "negative symptom spectrum disorders," Asperger's disorder, autism, schizophrenia, schizoid personality disorder, and schizotypal personality disorder. The signs and symptoms defined in DSM-IV-TR, as reviewed above, suggest two broad categories of symptoms (Fig. 4). These negative symptoms may be categorized either as 1.) deficits in social competence, and 2.) stereotypy.

Deficits in social competence can be divided into 1.) afferent or perceptual deficits versus 2.) efferent or behavioral deficits. Afferent deficits would include deficits in emotion perception, social perception, and understanding the intention or perception of others. Efferent deficits include deficits in eye contact, facial expression, affect, relatedness, speech, and social interaction as well as other nonverbal social skills, including abnormalities in body language, posture, modulation of gestures, and social motivation.

The stereotypies can be divided into 1.) cognitive stereotypies versus 2.) motor or behavioral stereotypies. Cognitive stereotypies can include pre-occupations, overelaborate cognition, obsessions, or restricted interests. Delusional thinking, a positive symptom when presenting as delusions per se, may be construed as a severe form of cognitive stereotypy insofar as such cognition is repetitive, idiosyncratic, and usually obsessional. Where such thinking loses reality

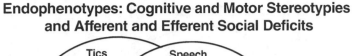

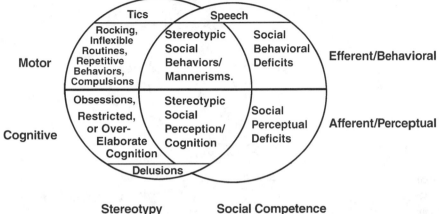

Figure 4 Endophenotypes: cognitive and motor stereotypies and afferent and efferent social deficits are symptomatically categorized.

testing, i.e., the ability to accept or reject the idea on the basis of plausibility and mutually perceptible evidence, it becomes classifiable as a delusion per se, a positive symptom.

Motor stereotypies can include 1.) complex or behavioral stereotypies versus 2.) simple motor stereotypies. Complex stereotypies comprise compulsions, inflexible routines, rituals, and repetitive behaviors. Simple motor stereotypies include mannerisms, motor tics, rocking, and posturing. A conceptual mapping of these endophenotypic sets is presented in Figure 4.

One consideration in mapping such phenotypes is whether deficits in social competence are really separate endophenotypes from that of the stereotypies. For example, one possibility would be that the stereotypies are causative of the deficits in social competence. Cognitive stereotypies could filter social perception by virtue of preoccupation or distraction from a repetitive interest, and limit social behavior into stereotypic behavioral sets. However, the above-noted study of autistic-like traits in twins from the general population suggests that deficits in social competence and stereotypic interests and behavior are separately inherited, supportive of the appropriateness of individual endophenotypes.

In Figure 5, we present endophenotype mapping across the five diagnoses considered within the negative symptom spectrum, those reviewed in Table 3. To do this, it is necessary to include the presence or absence of positive symptoms to distinguish schizophrenia from autism, Asperger's disorder, schizoid, and schizotypal personality disorder. Similarly, the presence or absence of developmental delay is needed to distinguish autism from the other four disorders.

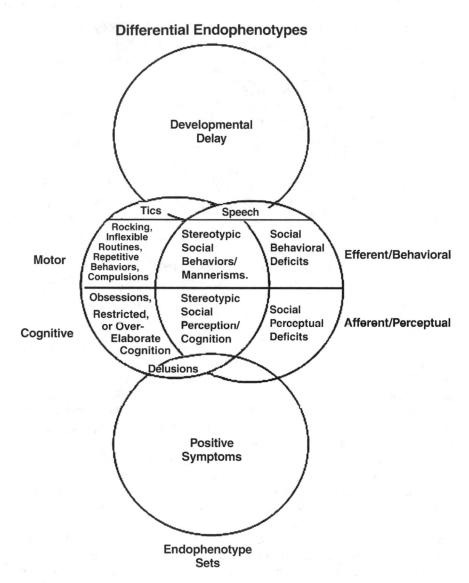

Figure 5 In addition to the social deficit and stereotypic negative symptoms, positive symptoms (delusions and hallucinations), and developmental delay, distinguish schizophrenia and autism, respectively, from Asperger's disorder, schizoid personality, and schizotypal personality disorder.

As can be seen in Figure 6, each disorder has its own "endophenomorphometry," to coin a term; each diagnosis has its own "endophenomorphic" pattern (Fig. 6). The exception is schizotypal personality disorder, which appears quite similar to that of Asperger's disorder, except for tics, a commonly associated feature of Asperger's, but not one ordinarily associated with schizotypal personality.

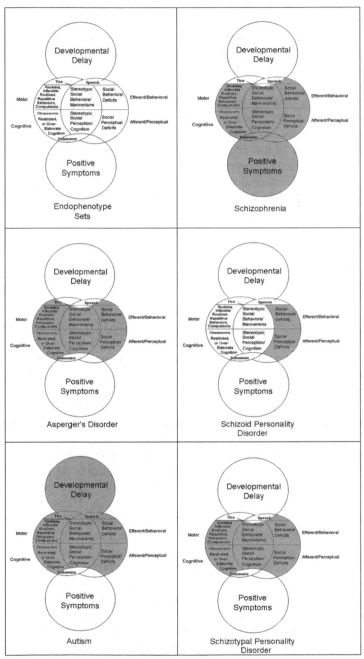

Endophenotype Patterns for Five Diagnoses

Figure 6 Endophenotype patterns for five diagnoses. Overlapping endophenotypes depicted for negative symptom spectrum disorders: Asperger's disorder, autism, schizophrenia, schizoid, and schizotypal personality disorder.

Genogram Comparisons for Markers Published to be in Significant LD for Autism, Schizophrenia, and Asperger's Disorder

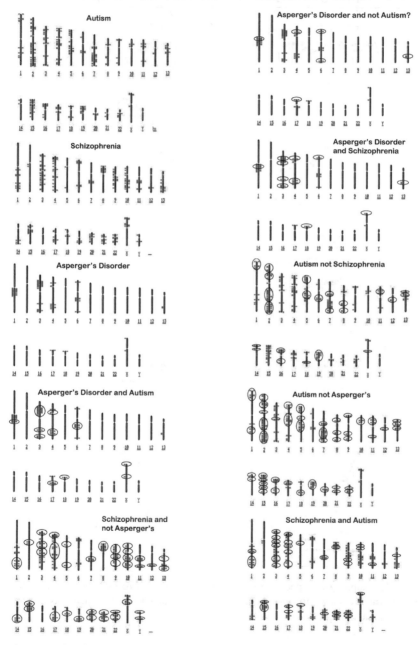

Figure 8 (...from next page).

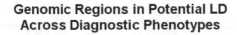

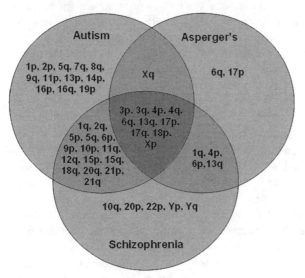

Figure 9 Genomic regions in potential LD across diagnostic phenotypes. Unique and overlapping genetic regions from Figure 8 are mapped above in diagnostic sets.

Figure 9 summarizes the chromosomal regions shown in Figure 8, organizing them into those found only so far in autism, only in Asperger's disorder, only in schizophrenia, only in autism *and* Asperger's disorder, only in autism *and* schizophrenia, only in Asperger's disorder *and* schizophrenia, as well as those regions in LD for all three diagnoses. Although some of these regions may turn out to be artifactual with more study, or subregions specific only to one diagnosis, and although there could be associated regions not yet identified, especially for the small numbers studied specifically for diagnosis of Asperger's, conceptually at least, we may note the similarity of the genotype-diagnosis sets with the endophenotype-diagnosis sets in Figure 7.

This endophenotype-genotype diagnosis analysis suggests the possibility that some of the genes may correspond to the endophenotype of negative symptoms, positive symptoms, developmental delay, or degree of disabling pathology. Although more work awaits the discovery of the precise genetic mechanisms at work, a number of interesting leads are now developing, as

←————————————————————————————————————

Figure 8 Genetic markers observed to be in significant LD in at least some published autism, schizophrenia, and Asperger's samples are comparatively mapped where ovals depict overlapping or discrete diagnostic sets. Notwithstanding caveats to date on the limits of our knowledge of specific genetic relationships, the above illustrates the potential for common and discriminate genetic diatheses, across diagnoses. *Abbreviation*: LD, linkage disequilibrium. *Source Tool*: From Ref. 132.

discussed in chapters 10–12, for a number of candidate genes and systems. The problem of more work needed is particularly acute for Asperger's disorder, as most genetic studies have lumped the Asperger's cases with the autistic subjects, studying ASD. This method helps to increase sample size, the convenience of which is served well by the argument that Asperger's disorder is the same as autism. However, until there is adequate, specific, genetic study of Asperger's disorder per se, the basis of its heritability will remain unclear.

CONCLUSION

Asperger's disorder is a commonly misunderstood and misinterpreted diagnosis with significant morbidity and mortality. Such limits in understanding contribute greatly not only to the challenges in clinical diagnosis but also to the challenge of researching and understanding the condition.

Studies demonstrating, for example, that all Asperger's cases that can be diagnosed as autistic are useful in pointing out where our common diagnostic criteria need improvement. For example, if Asperger's subjects typically have abnormal speech, one may well expect such speech abnormalities to emerge concurrent with emergence of speech. Consequently, more clarity is needed in the use of the present criteria to distinguish a lack of speech and communication from speech stereotypies (pedanticism, repetitive use of unusual speech, unusual prosody, vocal tics, etc.), which may begin with the development of speech, i.e., may have onset concurrent with the emergence of speech. Similarly, improvement is needed in distinguishing social interest limited by social awkwardness from the low a priori interest or motivation toward the social world found in autistic individuals.

In medicine, there are always two schools of thought: "lumpers" and the "splitters," those that focus on the coalescence of similarities and those that focus on the parsimony of distinctions. Both approaches are useful and necessary. However, we would argue that parsimony must precede coalescence, i.e., it is arguably necessary to understand how things are different before we can say how they are the same. For example, it is necessary to understand how daisies are different from roses before we can fully understand how each is a flower. To use another analogy, it is necessary to understand how white toy poodles are different from gray grand poodles before we can fully understand what makes them both poodles (e.g., not size or color evidently).

Thus, the Asperger's field suffers currently from this dilemma. So long as it is coalesced with autistic subjects in studies, we may remain with the current limitations in our knowledge of the subject, without the necessary research needed to better understand the condition.

From our analysis of the potential phenotype-genotype relationships, we may understand better that these diagnoses may be conceptualized as distinct clusters of cross-diagnostic endophenotypes. The importance of this is to move our diagnostic understanding beyond the rigid framework that drives diagnosis as sole phenotype, distinct from other diagnoses/phenotypes, the notion that the conditions should be as psychologically or biologically distinct as we make our diagnostic criteria distinct. The importance of advancing in the endophenotype direction can be exemplified within at least two dimensions.

One of these is the possibility that symptoms present in one diagnosis may respond to treatments effective for the same or similar symptoms of another diagnosis. We employed this notion in our trial of risperidone for the negative symptoms of Asperger's disorder (131), observing first that it had been reported to improve the negative symptoms of schizophrenia. A common problem in psychiatry currently is that pharmacotherapy is developed for diagnoses per se. Recognizing the possibility, or likelihood, that cross-diagnostic endophenotypes may bear greater biological parsimony than discrete diagnoses per se, our current diagnosis-driven system can complicate and slow the development of pharmacotherapy by greater time, effort, and expense needed to show that a pharmacological agent, or any treatment for that matter, may be effective for the same endophenotypes across diagnoses, given that current psychopharmacological development is diagnosis driven, requiring large studies for each endophenotypically similar diagnosis, rather than study therapeutic amelioration of discrete cross-diagnostic endophenotypic symptomatology.

The same problem is present in a second dimension as well as within research into the condition itself. In addition to that mentioned above, the problem that we cannot know more about Asperger's disorder until it is researched as a distinct condition is the fact that most research is, as would only be reasonable for its stage, conducted for diagnostic groups per se. Although we now have a number of large genetic studies into schizophrenia and autism, with many conflicting (and overlapping) findings, we do not yet have the necessary detail on the different endophenotypes within diagnosis. It is well possible that many of the conflicting findings in the genetic research may be resolved by understanding whether endophenotypic subgroups within a diagnosis could yield the needed parsimony to account for the usual pattern of results found in these studies: even when significant association is found, there is typically a sizable proportion of subjects with the diagnosis who do not have an implicated gene. The possibility that variations of endophenotypy within a diagnosis could potentially account for such variance seems straightforward.

Also, since most studies focus on a single diagnosis (rather than a single endophenotype), the methodologies have tendencies for stratification across diagnosis. For example, in comparing a study of schizophrenia in Costa Rica with a study of Asperger's in Finland, are we identifying gene differences between schizophrenics and Asperger's subjects, or are we identifying genetic differences between Costa Ricans and Finns?

Diagnostically stratified methodologies leave cross-diagnostic endophenotypic genetic associations uncertain. This is a dilemma indeed, since it is enough work, for example, for a group to scan the genome for schizophrenia, let alone do matching scans of similar-sized cohorts with autism, Asperger's, and negative schizotypy personality disorders, for example. However, as the methodologies become more standardized and certain in their identifications and data accrued from different global populations, our inferences across studies improve. Nonetheless, it appears at present, for psychiatric genetics, that the precision with which we can now genotype well exceeds the precision with which we currently now phenotype. It seems that much of the progress to be made at present may lie in the distillation of phenotype.

The future holds much promise for this area; not only will advances in endophenotypy come with advances in diagnostic distinction, but there is also great promise from the potential for advances with psychological and biological phenotyping, e.g., performance on theory-of-mind tasks and facial emotion recognition, coupled with studies of brain activation studied during such tasks. Such approaches hold promise for better definition and research utilization of phenotype beyond that of diagnosis per se as the sole phenotype.

The recognition of a variety of associated physical and neurological concomitants of these disorders, including Asperger's, could also serve well in this regard. The importance of meeting our challenges, with the proper recognition and understanding of Asperger's disorder, knowledge of the disability and morbidity often associated with it, combined with the research opportunities to answer many of today's questions make our need for the advancement of this knowledge all the more valuable. Advancement of our knowledge will serve toward improving an informed approach to those afflicted.

REFERENCES

1. Arshad M, Fitzgerald M. Did Michelangelo (1475–1564) have high-functioning autism? J Med Biogr 2004; 12(2):115–120.
2. Hayashi M, Kato M, Igarashi K, et al. Superior fluid intelligence in children with Asperger's disorder. Brain Cogn 2008; 66(3):306–310.
3. Popper CW, Gammon GD, West SA, et al. The American Psychiatric Publishing Textbook of Clinical Psychiatry. 4th ed. Washington, D.C.: American Psychiatric Pub, 2003.
4. Engstrom I, Ekstrom L, Emilsson B. Psychosocial functioning in a group of Swedish adults with Asperger syndrome or high-functioning autism. Autism 2003; 7(1): 99–110.
5. Tsatsanis KD. Outcome research in Asperger syndrome and autism. Child Adolesc Psychiatr Clin N Am 2003; 12(1):47–63.
6. Kasari C, Rotheram-Fuller E. Current trends in psychological research on children with high-functioning autism and Asperger disorder. Curr Opin Psychiatry 2005; 18(5):497–501.
7. Chen PS, Chen SJ, Yang YK, et al. Asperger's disorder: a case report of repeated stealing and the collecting behaviours of an adolescent patient. Acta Psychiatr Scand 2003; 107(1):73–75.
8. Rhoades RA, Scarpa A, Salley B. The importance of physician knowledge of autism spectrum disorder: results of a parent survey. BMC Pediatr 2007; 7(1):37.

9. Sanchez-Valle E, Posada M, Villaverde-Hueso A et al. Estimating the Burden of Disease for Autism Spectrum Disorders in Spain in 2003. J Autism Dev Disord 2008; 38(2):288–296.

10. Bankier B, Lenz G, Gutierrez K, et al. A case of Asperger's syndrome first diagnosed in adulthood. Psychopathology 1999; 32(1):43–46.

11. Fanous A, Gardner C, Walsh D, et al. Relationship between positive and negative symptoms of schizophrenia and schizotypal symptoms in nonpsychotic relatives. Arch Gen Psychiatry 2001; 58(7):669–673.

12. Frith U. Emanuel Miller lecture: confusions and controversies about Asperger syndrome. J Child Psychol Psychiatry 2004; 45(4):672–686.

13. Szatmari P, Tuff L, Finlayson MA, et al. Asperger's syndrome and autism: neurocognitive aspects. J Am Acad Child Adolesc Psychiatry 1990; 29(1):130–136.

14. Alonso Y, Miralles MC, Mulet B, et al. Asperger's disorder in adulthood: a case report. Actas Esp Psiquiatr 2007; 35(5):338–341.

15. Oslejskova H, Kontrova I, Foralova R, et al. The course of diagnosis in autistic patients: the delay between recognition of the first symptoms by parents and correct diagnosis. Neuro Endocrinol Lett 2007; 28(6):895–900.

16. Mandell DS, Novak MM, Zubritsky CD. Factors associated with age of diagnosis among children with autism spectrum disorders. Pediatrics 2005; 116(6):1480–1486.

17. Suzuki S. Diagnosis of Asperger syndrome in infancy and childhood. Nippon Rinsho 2007; 65(3):481–484.

18. Mikami K, Ohya A, Akasaka K, et al. Attempted suicide of youth with Asperger's disorder. Seishin Shinkeigaku Zasshi 2006; 108(6):587–596.

19. Abe T, Kato S. Environmental factors in Asperger syndrome. Nippon Rinsho 2007; 65(3):439–442.

20. Thede LL, Coolidge FL. Psychological and neurobehavioral comparisons of children with Asperger's Disorder versus High-Functioning Autism. J Autism Dev Disord 2007; 37(5):847–854.

21. Miller JN, Ozonoff S. Did Asperger's cases have Asperger disorder? A research note. J Child Psychol Psychiatry 1997; 38(2):247–251.

22. Hippler K, Klicpera C. A retrospective analysis of the clinical case records of 'autistic psychopaths' diagnosed by Hans Asperger and his team at the University Children's Hospital, Vienna. Philos Trans R Soc Lond B Biol Sci 2003; 358(1430): 291–301.

23. Szatmari P, Bremner R, Nagy J. Asperger's syndrome: a review of clinical features. Can J Psychiatry 1989; 34(6):554–560.

24. Gillberg IC, Gillberg C. Asperger syndrome—some epidemiological considerations: a research note. J Child Psychol Psychiatry 1989; 30(4):631–638.

25. Asperger H. Die 'Autisitic Psychopathen' im Kindesalter. Arch Psychiatr Nervenkr 1944; 117:76–136.

26. Wing L. Asperger's syndrome: a clinical account. Psychol Med 1981; 11(1): 115–129.

27. Wing L. The relationship between Asperger's syndrome and Kanner's autism. In: Frith U, ed. Autism and Asperger Syndrome. Cambridge: Cambridge University Press, 1991:93–122.

28. Tantam D. Asperger's syndrome. J Child Psychol Psychiatry 1988; 29(3):245–255.

29. Tantam D. Lifelong eccentricity and social isolation. II: Asperger's syndrome or schizoid personality disorder? Br J Psychiatry 1988; 153:783–791.

30. Mayes SD, Calhoun SL, Crites DL. Does DSM-IV Asperger's disorder exist? J Abnorm Child Psychol 2001; 29(3):263–271.
31. WHO. The ICD-10 Classification of Mental and Behavioural Disorders. 10th ed. Geneva, Switzerland: World Health Organization, 1992.
32. Kay P, Kolvin I. Childhood psychoses and their borderlands. Br Med Bull 1987; 43(3):570–586.
33. Klin A, Volkmar FR. Asperger syndrome: diagnosis and external validity. Child Adolesc Psychiatr Clin N Am 2003; 12(1):1–13.
34. Kerbeshian J, Burd L, Fisher W. Asperger's syndrome: to be or not to be? Br J Psychiatry 1990; 156:721–725.
35. Gillberg CL. The Emanuel Miller Memorial Lecture 1991. Autism and autistic-like conditions: subclasses among disorders of empathy. J Child Psychol Psychiatry 1992; 33(5):813–842.
36. Bowman EP. Asperger's syndrome and autism: the case for a connection. Br J Psychiatry 1988; 152:377–382.
37. Baron-Cohen S. An assessment of violence in a young man with Asperger's syndrome. J Child Psychol Psychiatry 1988; 29(3):351–360.
38. Silverstein SM, Palumbo DR. Nonverbal perceptual organization output disability and schizophrenia spectrum symptomatology. Psychiatry 1995; 58(1):66–81.
39. Rumsey JM, Andreasen NC, Rapoport JL. Thought, language, communication, and affective flattening in autistic adults. Arch Gen Psychiatry 1986; 43(8):771–777.
40. Klin A, Volkmar FR. Asperger's syndrome. In: Cohen DJ, Volkmar FR, eds. Handbook of Autism and Pervasive Developmental Disorders. 2nd ed. New York, NY: J. Wiley & Sons, Inc, 1997:94–122.
41. Frith CD, Frith U. Selective affinities in schizophrenia and childhood autism. In: Beggington PE, ed. Social Psychiatry: Theory, Methodology and Practice. New Brunswick, NJ: Transaction, 1991:65–88.
42. Ryan RM. Treatment resistant chronic mental illness: Is it Asperger syndrome? Hosp Community Psychiatry 1992; 43:807–811.
43. Wolff S, Chick J. Schizoid personality in childhood: a controlled follow-up study. Psychological Medicine 1980; 10:85–100.
44. Diagnostic and Statistical Manual of Mental Disorders-IV-TR. 4th text revision ed. Washington, D.C.: The American Psychiatric Association, 2000.
45. Hurst RM, Nelson-Gray RO, Mitchell JT, et al. The relationship of Asperger's characteristics and schizotypal personality traits in a non-clinical adult sample. J Autism Dev Disord 2007; 37(9):1711–1720.
46. Okajima Y. Personality disorder. Nippon Rinsho 2007; 65(3):502–505.
47. Wolff S. 'Schizoid' personality in childhood and adult life. I: the vagaries of diagnostic labelling. Br J Psychiatry 1991; 159:615.
48. Mayes SD, Calhoun SL. Non-significance of early speech delay in children with autism and normal intelligence and implications for DSM-IV Asperger's disorder. Autism 2001; 5(1):81–94.
49. Howlin P. Outcome in high-functioning adults with autism with and without early language delays: implications for the differentiation between autism and Asperger syndrome. J Autism Dev Disord 2003; 33(1):3–13.
50. Koyama T, Tachimori H, Osada H, et al. Cognitive and symptom profiles in Asperger's syndrome and high-functioning autism. Psychiatry Clin Neurosci 2007; 61(1):99–104.

51. Ariella RR, Ritvo ER, Guthrie D, et al. Clinical evidence that Asperger's disorder is a mild form of autism. Compr Psychiatry 2008; 49(1):1–5.
52. Eisenmajer R, Prior M, Leekam S, et al. Comparison of clinical symptoms in autism and Asperger's disorder. J Am Acad Child Adolesc Psychiatry 1996; 35(11): 1523–1531.
53. Eisenmajer R, Prior M, Leekam S, et al. Delayed language onset as a predictor of clinical symptoms in pervasive developmental disorders. J Autism Dev Disord 1998; 28(6):527–533.
54. Macintosh KE, Dissanayake C. Annotation: The similarities and differences between autistic disorder and Asperger's disorder: a review of the empirical evidence. J Child Psychol Psychiatry 2004; 45(3):421–434.
55. Ehlers S, Nyden A, Gillberg C, et al. Asperger syndrome, autism and attention disorders: a comparative study of the cognitive profiles of 120 children. J Child Psychol Psychiatry 1997; 38(2):207–217.
56. Fisman S, Steele M. Use of risperidone in pervasive developmental disorders: a case series. J Child Adolesc Psychopharmacol 1996; 6(3):177–190.
57. Weiser M, Noy S, Kaplan Z, et al. Generalized cognitive impairment in male adolescents with schizotypal personality disorder. Am J Med Genet B Neuropsychiatr Genet 2003; 116(1):36–40.
58. Torgersen S, Edvardsen J, Oien PA, et al. Schizotypal personality disorder inside and outside the schizophrenic spectrum. Schizophr Res 2002; 54(1–2):33–38.
59. Siever LJ, Koenigsberg HW, Harvey P, et al. Cognitive and brain function in schizotypal personality disorder. Schizophr Res 2002; 54(1-2):157–167.
60. Phillips KA, Yen S, Gunderson JG. Personality disorders. In: Hales RE, Yudofsky SC, eds. The American Psychiatric Publishing Textbook of Clinical Psychiatry. 4th ed. Washington, D.C.: American Psychiatric Publishing, 2003:803–832.
61. Cadenhead KS, Braff DL. Endophenotyping schizotypy: a prelude to genetic studies within the schizophrenia spectrum. Schizophr Res 2002; 54(1–2):47–57.
62. Bolte S, Poustka F. The recognition of facial affect in autistic and schizophrenic subjects and their first-degree relatives. Psychol Med 2003; 33(5):907–915.
63. Pickup GJ, Frith CD. Theory of mind impairments in schizophrenia: symptomatology, severity and specificity. Psychol Med 2001; 31(2):207–220.
64. Jaime S Craig, Christopher H, Fiona BC, et al. Persecutory beliefs, attributions and theory of mind: comparison of patients with paranoid delusions, Asperger's syndrome and healthy controls. Schizophrenia research 2004; 69(1):29–33.
65. Murphy D. Theory of mind in Asperger's syndrome, schizophrenia and personality disordered forensic patients. Cognit Neuropsychiatry 2006; 11(2):99–111.
66. Wolff S, Barlow A. Schizoid personality in childhood: a comparative study of schizoid, autistic and normal children. J Child Psychol Psychiatry 1979; 20(1):29–46.
67. Wolff S, Chick J. Schizoid personality in childhood: a controlled follow-up study. Psychol Med 1980; 10(1):85–100.
68. Cull A, Chick J, Wolff S. A consensual validation of schizoid personality in childhood and adult life. Br J Psychiatry 1984; 144:646–648.
69. Tantam D, Holmes D, Cordess C. Nonverbal expression in autism of Asperger type. J Autism Dev Disord 1993; 23(1):111–133.
70. Wolff S, Narayan S, Moyes B. Personality characteristics of parents of autistic children: a controlled study. J Child Psychol Psychiatry 1988; 29(2):143–153.

71. Narayan S, Moyes B, Wolff S. Family characteristics of autistic children: a further report. J Autism Dev Disord 1990; 20(4):523–535.
72. Mikhailova ES, Vladimirova TV, Iznak AF, et al. Abnormal recognition of facial expression of emotions in depressed patients with major depression disorder and schizotypal personality disorder. Biol Psychiatry 1996; 40(8):697–705.
73. Poreh AM, Whitman RD, Weber M, et al. Facial recognition in hypothetically schizotypic college students. The role of generalized poor performance. J Nerv Ment Dis 1994; 182(9):503–507.
74. Waldeck TL, Miller LS. Social skills deficits in schizotypal personality disorder. Psychiatry Res 2000; 93(3):237–246.
75. Langdon R, Coltheart M. Recognition of metaphor and irony in young adults: the impact of schizotypal personality traits. Psychiatry Res 2004; 125(1):9–20.
76. Jahshan CS, Sergi MJ. Theory of mind, neurocognition, and functional status in schizotypy. Schizophr Res 2007; 89(1–3):278–286.
77. Russell AJ, Mataix-Cols D, Anson M, et al. Obsessions and compulsions in Asperger syndrome and high-functioning autism. Br J Psychiatry 2005; 186:525–528.
78. Stewart ME, Barnard L, Pearson J, et al. Presentation of depression in autism and Asperger syndrome: a review. Autism 2006; 10(1):103–116.
79. Ringman JM, Jankovic J. Occurrence of tics in Asperger's syndrome and autistic disorder. J Child Neurol 2000; 15(6):394–400.
80. Ghaziuddin M, Gerstein L. Pedantic speaking style differentiates Asperger syndrome from high-functioning autism. J Autism Dev Disord 1996; 26(6):585–595.
81. Gilchrist A, Green J, Cox A, et al. Development and current functioning in adolescents with Asperger syndrome: a comparative study. J Child Psychol Psychiatry 2001; 42(2):227–240.
82. Szatmari P, Bartolucci G, Bremner R. Asperger's syndrome and autism: comparison of early history and outcome. Dev Med Child Neurol 1989; 31(6):709–720.
83. Szatmari P. Asperger's syndrome: diagnosis, treatment, and outcome. Psychiatr Clin North Am 1991; 14(1):81–93.
84. Chiang HM, Lin YH. Mathematical ability of students with Asperger syndrome and high-functioning autism: A review of literature. Autism 2007; 11(6):547–556.
85. Rinehart NJ, Bradshaw JL, Brereton AV, et al. A clinical and neurobehavioural review of high-functioning autism and Asperger's disorder. Aust N Z J Psychiatry 2002; 36(6):762–770.
86. Klin A. Autism and Asperger syndrome: an overview. Rev Bras Psiquiatr 2006; 28(suppl 1):S3–S11.
87. Channon S, Charman T, Heap J, et al. Real-life-type problem-solving in Asperger's syndrome. J Autism Dev Disord 2001; 31(5):461–469.
88. Delgado PL, Charney DS, Price LH, et al. Serotonin function and the mechanism of antidepressant action. Reversal of antidepressant-induced remission by rapid depletion of plasma tryptophan. Arch Gen Psychiatry 1990; 47:411–418.
89. Rinehart NJ, Bradshaw JL, Brereton AV, et al. Lateralization in individuals with high-functioning autism and Asperger's disorder: a frontostriatal model. J Autism Dev Disord 2002; 32(4):321–331.
90. Rinehart NJ, Bradshaw JL, Moss SA, et al. A deficit in shifting attention present in high-functioning autism but not Asperger's disorder. Autism 2001; 5(1):67–80.
91. Lim HK, Slaughter V. Brief Report: Human figure drawings by children with Asperger's syndrome. J Autism Dev Disord 2007. (Epub ahead of print).

92. McPartland J, Klin A. Asperger's syndrome. Adolesc Med Clin 2006; 17(3):771–788.
93. Macintosh K, Dissanayake C. A comparative study of the spontaneous social interactions of children with high-functioning autism and children with Asperger's disorder. Autism 2006; 10(2):199–220.
94. Khouzam HR, El-Gabalawi F, Pirwani N, et al. Asperger's disorder: a review of its diagnosis and treatment. Compr Psychiatry 2004; 45(3):184–191.
95. Prior M, Eisenmajer R, Leekam S, et al. Are there subgroups within the autistic spectrum? A cluster analysis of a group of children with autistic spectrum disorders. J Child Psychol Psychiatry 1998; 39(6):893–902.
96. Moore DG. Reassessing emotion recognition performance in people with mental retardation: a review. Am J Ment Retard 2001; 106(6):481–502.
97. Bowler DM. "Theory of mind" in Asperger's syndrome. J Child Psychol Psychiatry 1992; 33(5):877–893.
98. Duverger H, Dafonseca D, Bailly D, et al. Theory of mind in Asperger syndrome. Encephale 2007; 33(4 pt 1):592–597.
99. Ziatas K, Durkin K, Pratt C. Belief term development in children with autism, Asperger syndrome, specific language impairment, and normal development: links to theory of mind development. J Child Psychol Psychiatry 1998; 39(5):755–763.
100. Peterson CC, Slaughter VP, Paynter J. Social maturity and theory of mind in typically developing children and those on the autism spectrum. J Child Psychol Psychiatry 2007; 48(12):1243–1250.
101. Dyck MJ, Ferguson K, Shochet IM. Do autism spectrum disorders differ from each other and from non-spectrum disorders on emotion recognition tests? Eur Child Adolesc Psychiatry 2001; 10(2):105–116.
102. Happe F, Ehlers S, Fletcher P, et al. 'Theory of mind' in the brain. Evidence from a PET scan study of Asperger syndrome. Neuroreport 1996; 8(1):197–201.
103. Fine C, Lumsden J, Blair RJ. Dissociation between 'theory of mind' and executive functions in a patient with early left amygdala damage. Brain 2001; 124(pt 2):287–298.
104. Adolphs R, Tranel D. Impaired judgments of sadness but not happiness following bilateral amygdala damage. J Cogn Neurosci 2004; 16(3):453–462.
105. Gaigg SB, Bowler DM. Differential fear conditioning in Asperger's syndrome: implications for an amygdala theory of autism. Neuropsychologia 2007; 45(9): 2125–2134.
106. Corden B, Chilvers R, Skuse D. Emotional Modulation of Perception in Asperger's Syndrome. J Autism Dev Disord 2007. (Epub ahead of print).
107. O'Connor K. Brief report: impaired identification of discrepancies between expressive faces and voices in adults with Asperger's syndrome. J Autism Dev Disord 2007; 37(10):2008–2013.
108. Grossman JB, Klin A, Carter AS, et al. Verbal bias in recognition of facial emotions in children with Asperger syndrome. J Child Psychol Psychiatry 2000; 41(3):369–379.
109. Baskin JH, Sperber M, Price BH. Asperger syndrome revisited. Rev Neurol Dis 2006; 3(1):1–7.
110. Mazefsky CA, Oswald DP. Emotion perception in Asperger's syndrome and high-functioning autism: the importance of diagnostic criteria and cue intensity. J Autism Dev Disord 2007; 37(6):1086–1095.
111. Asai T, Sugiyam T. Impairment of social interaction, coordination disorder, and hypersensitivity in Asperger's syndrome. Nippon Rinsho 2007; 65(3):453–457.

112. Lopata C, Hamm EM, Volker MA, et al. Motor and visuomotor skills of children with Asperger's disorder: preliminary findings. Percept Mot Skills 2007; 104(3 pt 2): 1183–1192.

113. Rinehart NJ, Tonge BJ, Bradshaw JL, et al. Gait function in high-functioning autism and Asperger's disorder : evidence for basal-ganglia and cerebellar involvement? Eur Child Adolesc Psychiatry 2006; 15(5):256–264.

114. Jansiewicz EM, Goldberg MC, Newschaffer CJ, et al. Motor signs distinguish children with high functioning autism and Asperger's syndrome from controls. J Autism Dev Disord 2006; 36(5):613–621.

115. Rinehart NJ, Bellgrove MA, Tonge BJ, et al. An examination of movement kinematics in young people with high-functioning autism and Asperger's disorder: further evidence for a motor planning deficit. J Autism Dev Disord 2006; 36(6): 757–767.

116. Rinehart NJ, Bellgrove MA, Tonge BJ, et al. An examination of movement kinematics in young people with high-functioning autism and Asperger's disorder: further evidence for a motor planning deficit. J Autism Dev Disord 2006; 36(6):757–767.

117. Rinehart NJ, Tonge BJ, Bradshaw JL, et al. Gait function in high-functioning autism and Asperger's disorder : evidence for basal-ganglia and cerebellar involvement? Eur Child Adolesc Psychiatry 2006; 15(5):256–264.

118. Rinehart NJ, Bradshaw JL, Brereton AV, et al. Movement preparation in high-functioning autism and Asperger disorder: a serial choice reaction time task involving motor reprogramming. J Autism Dev Disord 2001; 31(1):79–88.

119. Teitelbaum O, Benton T, Shah PK, et al. Eshkol-Wachman movement notation in diagnosis: the early detection of Asperger's syndrome. Proc Natl Acad Sci U. S. A. 2004; 101(32):11909–11914.

120. Godbout R, Bergeron C, Limoges E, et al. A laboratory study of sleep in Asperger's syndrome. Neuroreport 2000; 11(1):127–130.

121. Hare DJ, Jones S, Evershed K. A comparative study of circadian rhythm functioning and sleep in people with Asperger syndrome. Autism 2006; 10(6):565–575.

122. Allik H, Larsson JO, Smedje H. Insomnia in school-age children with Asperger syndrome or high-functioning autism. BMC Psychiatry 2006; 6:18.

123. Hebebrand J, Henninghausen K, Nau S, et al. Low body weight in male children and adolescents with schizoid personality disorder or Asperger's disorder. Acta Psychiatr Scand 1997; 96(1):64–67.

124. Sobanski E, Marcus A, Hennighausen K, et al. Further evidence for a low body weight in male children and adolescents with Asperger's disorder. Eur Child Adolesc Psychiatry 1999; 8(4):312–314.

125. Tantam D, Evered C, Hersov L. Asperger's syndrome and ligamentous laxity. J Am Acad Child Adolesc Psychiatry 1990; 29(6):892–896.

126. Carpenter PK, Morris D. Association of acrocyanosis with Asperger's syndrome. J Ment Defic Res 1990; 34 (pt 1):87–90.

127. Brodsky MC, Barber LG, Lam BL, et al. Neuro-ophthalmologic findings in the Asperger disorder. J Neuroophthalmol 1996; 16(3):185–187.

128. Iarocci G, Yager J, Elfers T. What gene-environment interactions can tell us about social competence in typical and atypical populations. Brain Cogn 2007; 65(1): 112–127.

129. Dworzynski K, Ronald A, Hayiou-Thomas M, et al. Aetiological relationship between language performance and autistic-like traits in childhood: a twin study. Int J Lang Commun Disord 2007; 42(3):273–292.

130. Baron-Cohen S. Autism: research into causes and intervention. Pediatr Rehabil 2004; 7(2):73–78.

131. Rausch JL, Sirota E, Londino D, et al. Open-label risperidone for Asperger's disorder: Negative symptom spectrum response. J Clin Psychiatry 2005; 66(12):1592–1597.

132. NCBI. NCBI Map Viewer. National Center for Biotechnology Information, National Library of Medicine (NLM) www.ncbi.nlm.nih.gov/mapview/map_search .cgi?taxid=9606.

4

Asperger Syndrome—Mortality and Morbidity

Christopher Gillberg

Department of Child and Adolescent Psychiatry, Institute of Neuroscience and Physiology, Göteborg University, Göteborg, Sweden

INTRODUCTION

The systematic study of Asperger syndrome is still pretty much in its infancy even though it is now more than 80 years since Ssucharewa described the syndrome that Asperger referred to as "autistic psychopathy" in 1944 and Lorna Wing labeled "Asperger syndrome" more than a quarter of a century ago (1–3). It was not until 1989 that operationalized criteria for the condition were published (4,5), and the international classification manuals for psychiatric disorders did not acknowledge its existence until well into the 1990s (6–8).

Only a few hundred papers specifically on Asperger syndrome or Asperger's disorder are currently in the literature, and a very small fraction of these has had anything to say about mortality and morbidity (sometimes referred to as comorbidity). This chapter will draw on those papers as far as (and whenever) possible. Inevitably, however, given the relative dearth of systematic study in the field, I will sometimes also speculate on the basis of more than 30 years of clinical and research experience working with children and adults (and their families) with "autistic psychopathy" or Asperger syndrome.

It should be clear that Asperger syndrome is not considered—by me or by most people currently working in the field—to be conceptually completely different from autism or other so-called "autism spectrum disorders." Rather, at least in my book, it represents a condition sharing many, if not all, of the features of autistic disorder, and it is but one of the clinical presentations of "autism," which is seen as a spectrum of conditions ranging from autistic features in the general population, through autistic symptoms with impairment and atypical autism or pervasive developmental disorder not otherwise specified, to Asperger syndrome [as defined by Gillberg and Gillberg (4), later elaborated by Gillberg (9) or Szatmari (10), not by the ICD-10 or DSM-IV, whose definitions do not coincide with the real-life presentation of the syndrome that Asperger described] and autistic disorder (with its several subgroups, including those with low normal intelligence and those with profound mental retardation). Autistic disorder and Asperger syndrome are considered "subclasses of disorders of empathy" (11) with no clear boundary vis-à-vis other disorders or so-called "normality."

I should also make clear at this stage that much of what is known about mortality (very little) and morbidity (more) in Asperger syndrome pertains to males only. Very few studies have included sufficient details about any girls or women studied, and so conclusions in the following are mostly based on findings obtained in studies of boys or men. It is possible that girls or women have a different clinical presentation and a different outcome in terms of coexisting problems. Whenever there is data available on any possible differentiating features, I will do my best to outline these and discuss possible reasons for their presence.

MORTALITY

There have been less than a handful of studies documenting the prospective longitudinal course of Asperger syndrome (12,13). It is only from studies of this kind that one can make reasonable conclusions regarding mortality rates. The studies that have been published have only followed young people with Asperger syndrome from childhood to adolescence or young adult age (at the most). The longest follow-up study published to date (13) included 100 males with the syndrome followed to the age of 16 to 36 years. No deaths were reported in this group. There had, however, been one very serious suicide attempt. The author is aware of at least two clinical cases of young men (under age 30 years) with Asperger syndrome (one of whom also had bipolar disorder) who committed suicide (hanging and jumping from bridge) after no prior warning (and leaving no message). There have been no studies of girls with Asperger syndrome and their long-term outcome.

MORBIDITY

There have been a considerable number of reports documenting the co-occurrence ("comorbidity") of Asperger syndrome and physical and psychiatric disorders of various kinds.

Physical Disorders

There are a number of physical disorders that have been reported to be associated with Asperger syndrome in some cases. Even though it is, for the time being, unclear as to whether these are in any way linked to the ethiopathogenesis of Asperger syndrome—either directly or via transactional effects—I will review them here with the understanding that, for many of them, links reported may have been the effect of chance co-occurrences.

Genetic Conditions

Table 1 lists some of the genetic conditions that have been reported to occur in a proportion of cases (sometimes only in one or two individuals) with Asperger syndrome. Very few of these documented co-occurring conditions have been reported by more than one group of researchers or clinicians. It is difficult to assess the meaning, if any, of these possible associations. It is particularly problematic that many of the associated genetic conditions have been reported in tables in papers on autism *and* Asperger syndrome and in book chapters on autism spectrum disorders or genetic disorders. This means that it is not possible to judge the strength of any association on the basis of medical journal systematic review searches using Asperger syndrome as the main entry point.

The majority of the reported genetic conditions have been documented to be overrepresented also in classic cases of autism, and one should definitely not assume that any possible ethiopathogenic link would be specifically with Asperger syndrome, but rather that the genetic condition is in some way, directly or indirectly, generally associated with the broader phenotype of autism spectrum conditions (or with the cognitive dysfunction—albeit not at the level of intellectual disability—that has actually been present in the majority of the literature case reports on genetic conditions and Asperger syndrome).

There is no obvious common feature that links the various disorders that have been reported in certain cases of Asperger syndrome. However, numerical and structural abnormalities involving the sex chromosomes have been documented fairly often, even though, again, these chromosome abnormalities have also been reported relatively frequently in lower-functioning individuals with autistic disorder.

Only one study has been published looking at the relative rate of associated medical conditions in Asperger syndrome (14). In that study, 4% of males with Asperger syndrome had epilepsy and 17% in total had a diagnosable clinically important "physical" disorder.

Other Behavioral Phenotype Syndromes

A few independent studies have reported a high rate of Asperger syndrome (and other autism spectrum conditions) in children with fetal alcohol syndrome (30). These studies, in general, have not looked at the possible contribution of the

Table 1 Definitely and Probably Genetic Syndromes That
Have Been Reported in Cases of Asperger Syndrome

Genetic syndrome	Ref.
22q11 deletion syndrome	15
Benign partial epilepsy in infancy	16
Fragile X syndrome	17
Marfan-like syndrome	18
MRX23: X-linked mental retardation	19
Neuro-ophthalmologic disorders	20
Rubinstein-Taybi syndrome	21
SCNA1 epilepsy	22
Sotos syndrome	23
Steinert's myotonic dystrophy	24
Tuberous sclerosis	25
45X/46XY mosaicism	26
XXY syndrome?	27
XYY mosaicism	28
XYY syndrome	29

alcohol effects on the brain and their specific part, if any, in the pathogenesis of the autism spectrum disorder. However, in one study, there was a clear effect of the length of the period of fetal exposition to alcohol and the presence of neuropsychiatric disorder (including Asperger syndrome) in children aged 11 to 14 years. Nevertheless, genetic factors were not analyzed, the findings have not been replicated, and so, generalized conclusions cannot be drawn (30).

There is at least one case report in the literature documenting the co-occurrence of Asperger syndrome in a boy with congenital hypothyroidism (31). There are several leads in the literature regarding the possible association of hypothyroidism and autism spectrum disorders, including studies showing a high rate of maternal hypothyroidism in pregnancy and the preconception period, and congenital hypothyroidism in the child on the one hand and autistic disorder on the other (32).

Other Predisposing or Associated Conditions

Hans Asperger believed that "his" syndrome was associated with a high prevalence of complications around the time of birth (2). A few systematic studies have reported a high rate of autism spectrum disorders (including Asperger syndrome) in children who have survived extremes of prematurity (usually with birthweights under 1000 g). There is also a study from Australia documenting a high prevalence of autism spectrum disorders in children who have suffered severe asphyxia at birth. A Swedish study of 100 males with Asperger syndrome found high rates of prematurity (and postmaturity) in Asperger syndrome, and a high rate of nonoptimal factors around the time of the child's birth (14,21).

A sibling-controlled study from Australia looking at pre- and perinatal factors in autism, atypical autism, and Asperger syndrome found increased rates of a number of nonoptimal factors in the pre- and perinatal periods (as suggested already in the 1980s by our group (33)) but noticed that these were almost as common in siblings of children with these diagnoses, suggesting the effects of a genetic predisposition or the combined effect of a genetic disposition and negative environmental influences during pregnancy or the perinatal period (34).

Epilepsy

The rate of epilepsy in autism spectrum disorders is decidedly very high (35), affecting at least one in three individuals with classic autistic disorder at any one time during the first 30 years of life. Epilepsy is clearly much less prevalent in Asperger syndrome than in autistic disorder (14), but probably much overrepresented as compared with the general population. One study found 5 out of 100 males with Asperger syndrome aged 16 to 36 years had or had had epilepsy. This is about 10 times the expected rate in the general population. Given the normal to high IQ levels typical of the samples of individuals with Asperger syndrome and epilepsy reported in the literature, the association appears to be one which is more specific to the autism symptomatology than to the overall degree of intellectual impairment.

Cerebral Palsy and Other Neuromuscular Disorders

Cerebral palsy has been reported in a few cases with Asperger syndrome (36), and autism spectrum problems (including Asperger syndrome) appear to be much overrepresented in groups of children with cerebral palsy, particularly those with hemiplegias (37).

In a study of cerebral palsy ataxia, Ahsgren and coworkers reported that 2 out of 32 examined children (12 and 15 years old) had Asperger syndrome (38). Both of them were mildly affected by ataxia at the time of assessment for autism spectrum disorder but had had much more impairing motor symptoms when they were younger. One of these individuals had a very mild learning disability, but the other was of normal intelligence. Several other individuals in the ataxia cohort (population study) had "non-Asperger-syndrome" autism spectrum problems.

Developmental Coordination Disorder

According to the Gillberg criteria (9) for Asperger syndrome, motor clumsiness is one of the defining features of the disorder. However, other definitions do not require motor problems to be present, even though it is acknowledged that clumsiness is often present (8), and Hans Asperger himself certainly remarked on the consistency of motor clumsiness in the boys with autistic psychopathy that he saw.

The clumsiness in Asperger syndrome is sometimes very marked, and both gross and fine motor movements and visuomotor skills are affected (39). In some of these cases, it is clinically indicated to make a separate diagnosis of developmental coordination disorder (DCD), or, at least, refer the individual affected for physiotherapy or occupational therapy.

Psychiatric Disorders

Attention Deficit Hyperactivity Disorder

Attention deficit hyperactivity disorder (ADHD) is probably the most commonly suspected clinical comorbidity of Asperger syndrome (with the possible exception of tic disorders; see below). Several recent studies have shown extremely high rates of ADHD in clinical samples of children and adolescents diagnosed with Asperger syndrome, one of these documenting a rate of 78% ADHD in autism spectrum disorder (many of whom had Asperger syndrome) (40). One population study (41) of Asperger syndrome reported ADHD (mainly inattentive subtype or combined) in 80% of all clear or suspected Asperger syndrome cases in school age (7–16 years old).

Conversely, children diagnosed with attention disorders, including ADHD and deficits in attention, motor control, and perception (DAMP) have long been recognized as suffering from autism spectrum disorders in a significant proportion of cases (42–44). Given the much higher rate of diagnosed ADHD than of diagnosed Asperger syndrome (and other autism spectrum disorders), it should come as no surprise that only a minority of those with ADHD have concomitant Asperger syndrome. Nevertheless, the strong associations between attention disorders and autism spectrum disorders that have been documented regardless of diagnostic entry point argue convincingly for a "real" relationship between the two types of disorders or conditions.

It has yet to be determined whether or not the ADHD symptomatology encountered in Asperger syndrome is the same, similar, overlapping, slightly, or qualitatively different from ADHD symptomatology in the "garden variety" of the syndrome (in which there is no association with autistic symptoms). The Swedish studies (41,45,46) suggest that inattentive rather than hyperactive impulsive symptoms may be more strongly associated with an "autismlike/ Aspergerlike" phenotype, and that, if such symptoms co-occur with motor clumsiness or DCD, then the risk for Asperger syndrome or symptoms is very considerable (47). However, several studies have documented a very high rate of ADHD symptoms (including hyperactivity) in young children with autism (48–50). It is possible that this hyperactivity is "secondary" to the communication deficit and that appropriate interventions for the latter will help ameliorate or even alleviate the problems associated with the hyperactivity.

The interesting possibility that the link between ADHD and autism spectrum problems might be mediated by cerebellar dysfunction was recently raised

(51). Genetic leads for an underlying link between the two types of problems come from studies of possible susceptibility genes for autism and ADHD on chromosome 16p (52) and from the study of tuberous sclerosis (one variant of which is caused by a gene defect on chromosome 16p) in which autistic and ADHD symptoms co-occur in about half of all individuals affected by symptoms before age five years (25). Further, in the 22q11 deletion syndrome, there is a relatively high risk of co-occurring autism spectrum and ADHD symptoms (53–55). However, unlike in tuberous sclerosis, where both the autism spectrum problem and ADHD symptom pattern tend to be of the "classical" variants (with typical autistic disorder and combined severe ADHD), in 22q11 deletion syndrome, the symptoms are often more atypical.

Tics and Tourette Syndrome

Tics are very common throughout the autism spectrum. There have been a number of case reports (56) and at least one systematic population-based study (41) looking at the co-occurrence of tics and Asperger syndrome. In the latter study, 8 out of 10 cases with definite or probable Asperger syndrome had motor or vocal tics and 2 of the 10 met full criteria for Tourette syndrome. Studies of lower-functioning children with autism have found a lower, but yet substantial rate of tics and Tourette syndrome.

Some of the cases described in the literature with "comorbid" Asperger and Tourette syndrome or tic disorders have been associated with specific underlying factors such as fetal alcohol syndrome and fragile X syndrome (57). Zappella (58) has described a combination of symptoms or syndromes that he refers to as "dysmaturational autism," a condition in which the child develops normally for about 18 to 24 months, then regresses with appearance of autistic behaviors and tics—motor and vocal—and eventually progresses into a "high-functioning" state with few, if any, autistic symptoms, but with the persistence of tics over time. Zappella has argued that the coexistence of tics in autism spectrum disorder could be a marker for improvement and a good outcome in terms of the autistic symptomatology.

There have been a few studies looking at the coexistence of Asperger syndrome in individuals with tic disorders. Kadesjö and Gillberg (59) found a rate of about 15% of those with Tourette syndrome in a larger cohort meeting criteria for an autism spectrum disorder, usually Asperger syndrome. Almost two thirds of cases with Tourette syndrome had some degree of impairment from autistic type symptoms.

Obsessive-Compulsive Disorder

Obsessive-compulsive disorder (OCD) could be seen to be a portion of the clusters of symptoms that constitute the diagnosis of Asperger syndrome. The repetitive and ritualistic phenomena typical of (and required for) a diagnosis of Asperger syndrome are also part and parcel of the syndrome of OCD, at least as it appears "on paper," such as, for instance, in the DSM-IV. Adults with Asperger syndrome or high-functioning autism have the same level of obsessive-compulsive symptoms as those who have been diagnosed with OCD. However, the very typical symptoms of classic OCD (such as hand washing, contamination concerns, and various checking behaviors) are not characteristic of Asperger syndrome. When such problems do occur to an impairing degree in individuals with Asperger syndrome, a "separate" diagnosis of OCD is often warranted.

Depression and Anxiety

It is not uncommon for people with Asperger syndrome to develop symptoms of depression or, indeed, to be clinically depressed (60). In a study of 100 males with Asperger syndrome in late adolescence and early adult age, 3 of 76 individuals interviewed personally were diagnosed as suffering from impairing clinical depression (one of whom hade committed a very serious suicide attempt). Several more (9 of 76) had depressed mood (13) or had been treated with medication in the past for depression (11 of 96).

Bipolar Disorder

There have been several clinical reports documenting the co-occurrence of Asperger syndrome and bipolar disorder (61–63). De Long et al. (62) reported on the comorbidity of Asperger syndrome and bipolar disorder in a clinical setting, concluding that there is a strong link between bipolar disorder and autism spectrum conditions in a substantial minority of cases presenting with an autism spectrum condition. De Long has also suggested that there might be an important minority of individuals with Asperger syndrome or autism spectrum disorder with a family history of severe affective disorder, particularly of the bipolar type (64). Even though systematic large-scale studies of bipolar disorder in representative cases of Asperger syndrome have not been published to date, it is my clinical impression that De Long's observation applies in other than his own clinical cohorts.

Schizophrenia

There has long been a debate as to the distinction between certain variants of schizophrenia and high-functioning cases of autism or Asperger syndrome.

It does not appear to be possible to differentiate between adults with Asperger syndrome and schizophrenia on measures of theory of mind (65). However, adults with schizophrenia have more widespread, global functioning impairments.

In Scandinavia, individuals with "quiet" forms of "schizophrenia" (with few or no "active" symptoms such as hallucinations and delusions) have sometimes been diagnosed as suffering from "pseudoneurotic" schizophrenia

(Eberhard Nyman, personal communication). The clinical description of this category suggests a fairly typical presentation of Asperger syndrome.

Children with Asperger syndrome appear to have an increased rate of familial loading for schizophrenia compared with the general population (66). It is not currently possible to conclude whether this familial risk factor is at a level over and above that of other psychiatric disorders.

Other Psychoses

Many individuals with the typical presentation of Asperger syndrome develop transient symptoms of "psychosis" either in the absence of evident "triggers" or in connection with stress (67). The stressors triggering psychotic episodes are often perceived as nonconvincing or even "non-stressors" by people not affected by autism spectrum problems. It could be anything from promotion at work and request to change rooms through expectation of participation in social events to the "stress" of having to take time off for a holiday. Because of the often unperceived stressing quality of the changes that the person with Asperger syndrome would have to go through to accommodate the demands, expectation, and aspiration of well-meaning people in the environment, it usually comes as a complete shock when that person "breaks down." The person starts behaving in a child-like fashion, begins obsessing and ruminating, and finally complaining, crying, shouting, swearing, and behaving in a fashion that is associated in most people's minds with "psychosis" (violent, self-injurious, disruptive, and confused behaviors may dominate the clinical picture at this stage). A few days of "stress-relief" will often get things back to normal, but, unfortunately, it is not rare for the underlying autism spectrum condition to be missed, a diagnosis of psychosis to be made, neuroleptic treatment to be started, and a whole chain of unnecessary (largely iatrogenic) events to unravel.

Once in a blue moon, a person with Asperger syndrome does develop a "real" psychosis (including psychosis with bipolar mood swings and psychosis with a schizophreniform symptom pattern). It is unclear at the present time whether such psychoses are more common in Asperger syndrome than in the general population.

Features of catatonia (see below) are quite common and would, by some, be diagnosed under the more general heading of psychosis, or, indeed, as a variant of schizophrenia.

Catatonia and Catatonic Features

Lorna Wing and her group were probably first to highlight the co-occurrence of autism spectrum conditions (including Asperger syndrome) and catatonia (68). Our own group has since replicated their findings in several different studies of autism spectrum disorders (including autistic disorder and Asperger syndrome) and documented the prevalence of catatonia or severe catatonic features to be about 10% to 15% by adolescence or early adult age (13,69).

The catatonic symptoms may involve prolonged posturing, "frozen states," the inability to move, *signe d'oreiller*, "Houdini-type" interlocking limb positioning, stopping in the middle of an ongoing movement, and failure to move without a physical (more rarely verbal) prompt. Extreme motor slowness is common in this group, as is reduction of facial expression and overall degree of gesturing. A wide variety of treatments have been attempted, but catatonic symptoms in Asperger syndrome have proven hard to affect with medication.

Selective Mutism

My own group (70), a Norwegian group (71), and Wolff (72) have reported instances of comorbid selective mutism and Asperger syndrome (although Wolff's cases have sometimes been referred to as "schizoid"). In our own study, one (a girl) out of five children with "classic" selective mutism had Asperger syndrome.

Eating Disorders

Anorexia nervosa has been suggested to be strongly associated with autism spectrum disorders including Asperger syndrome (73). In 1983, I reported cases of concomitant anorexia nervosa and autism and of familial clustering of the two disorders. This observation, for many years, appeared to be out of keeping with clinical experience accumulated by other experts, particularly specialists from the field of eating disorders. Today, it has become more generally acknowledged that a considerable minority of adolescents (and adults) with eating disorders— perhaps especially the group with anorexia nervosa—have premorbid autistic features that sometimes amount to the full-blown clinical picture of the disorder described by Asperger (74,75).

Several papers have been published relating to body mass index (BMI), weight, thinness, and obesity in Asperger syndrome, but the balance of the evidence in these respects is equivocal. Some studies (76) have suggested a significantly reduced BMI, whereas others have found no differences compared with general population norms or selected control groups (77).

In a study of adults with severe eating disorders, including anorexia and bulimia nervosa, the rates of autism spectrum disorder (Asperger syndrome included), Tourette syndrome, and ADHD were all extremely elevated compared with general population norms (78).

Personality Disorders

The majority of individuals with a clinical diagnosis of Asperger syndrome would meet DSM-IV-TR diagnostic criteria for at least one personality disorder (79). The most clear-cut examples of personality disorder categories that would fit with the overall phenotype of Asperger syndrome are schizoid, obsessive-compulsive, and schizotypal personality disorder. It is clinically undisputed that most men with Asperger syndrome would qualify for one or several personality disorder diagnoses. However, it is doubtful whether anyone with a childhood condition in the autism spectrum would benefit from an adult diagnosis of "personality disorder." After all, a diagnosis is intended to help guide understanding, help, and intervention whenever a person has a major problem that he or she cannot cope with adequately without professional assessment. Personality disorder diagnoses are not likely to benefit anybody whose primary problems are—and have always been—in the field of autism spectrum problems. Whether or not women with Asperger syndrome are also misdiagnosed or "comorbidly" diagnosed as suffering from personality disorder is not known.

Forensic Psychiatric Problems

Autism spectrum disorders are clearly much more common than expected by chance in groups of individuals (particularly males) who have been incarcerated or admitted for forensic psychiatric evaluation because of violent crimes. Nevertheless, the vast majority of individuals with Asperger syndrome will never get involved in violent crime or any other form of criminal activity.

CLOSING REMARKS

The mortality of Asperger syndrome may or may not be increased compared with the standardized mortality ratio of the general population; there is currently no good evidence either way. Clinically, it does appear that the rate of suicide might be increased, but this has not, so far, been borne out by systematic empirical study.

The rate of "morbidity" in Asperger syndrome is clearly much increased as compared with general population expectations, but it is not known, in detail, whether or not the increased problem rates are due to specific disorders, diseases, or symptom clusters being overrepresented or to the kinds of problems that are generally more common than expected in any psychiatrically or behaviorally disturbed population.

Some guidelines for clinicians are provided here on the basis of the summary I have made of the very limited evidence hitherto published in the field of associated morbidity in Asperger syndrome.

First, whenever a diagnosis of Asperger syndrome is made, it is important to determine the level of intellectual functioning in that individual and whether or not there is, in addition to the autism spectrum condition, a diagnosable nonverbal learning disability. If there is—which would be likely in about half of all young children with an Asperger diagnosis and about one in five of adults diagnosed with the syndrome—the implications of living with a considerable verbal or nonverbal discrepancy should be discussed in some detail with the patient, parents, or both. Insight into the basis for the good or superior verbal skills in the face of severe problems in coping with the practicalities of life is often something of a "breakthrough" in the life of a person with an autism

13. Cederlund M, Hagberg B, Billstedt E, et al. Asperger syndrome and autism – A comparative longitudinal follow-up study more than 5 years after original diagnosis. J Autism Dev Disord 2008; 38:72–85.

14. Cederlund M, Gillberg C. One hundred males with Asperger Syndrome: a clinical study of background and associated factors. Dev Med Child Neurol 2004; 46:652–660.

15. Niklasson L, Rasmussen P, Óskardòttir S, et al. Autism, ADHD, learning disability, and behaviour problems in 100 individuals with 22q11 deletion syndrome. 2007 (submitted).

16. Okumura A, Watanabe K, Negoro T, et al. The clinical characterizations of benign partial epilepsy in infancy. Neuropediatrics 2006; 37:359–363.

17. Hagerman RJ, Hagerman PJ. The fragile X permutation: into the phenotypic fold. Curr Opin Genet Dev 2002; 12:278–283 (review).

18. Tantam D, Evered C, Hersov L. Asperger's syndrome and ligamentous laxity. J Am Acad Child Adolesc Psychiatry 1990; 29:892–896.

19. Searcy E, Burd L, Kerbeshian J, et al. Asperger's syndrome, X-linked mental retardation (MRX23), and chronic vocal tic disorder. J Child Neurol 2000; 15:699–702.

20. Brodsky MC, Barber LG, Lam BL, et al. Neuroophthalmologic findings in the Asperger disorder. Neuroophthalmolgy 1996; 16;185–187.

21. Gillberg C, Cederlund M. Asperger syndrome: familial and pre- and perinatal factors. J Autism Dev Disord 2005; 35:159–166.

22. Osaka H, Ogiwara I, Mazaki E, et al. Patients with a sodium channel alpha 1 gene mutation show wide phenotypic variation. Epilepsy Res 2007; 75:46–51.

23. Zappella M. Autistic features in children affected by cerebral gigantism. Brain Dysfunction 1990; 3:241–244.

24. Blondis TA, Cook E Jr., Koza-Taylor P, et al. Asperger syndrome associated with Steinert's myotonic dystrophy. Dev Med Child Neurol 1996; 38:840–847.

25. Gillberg IC, Gillberg C, Ahlsén G. Autistic behaviour and attention deficits in tuberous sclerosis: a population-based study. Dev Med Child Neurol 1994; 36:50–56.

26. Fontenelle LF, Mendlowicz MV, Bezerra de Menezes G et al. Asperger syndrome, absessive-compulsive disorder, and major depression in a patient with 45,X/46,XY mosaicism. Psychopathology 2004; 37:105–109.

27. Jha P, Sheth D, Ghaziuddin M. Autism spectrum disorder and Klinefelter syndrome. Eur Child Adolesc Psychiatry 2007; 16:305–308.

28. Gillberg C, Steffenburg S, Jakobsson G. Neurobiological findings in 20 relatively gifted children with Kanner-type autism or Asperger syndrome. Dev Med Child Neurol 1987; 29:641–649.

29. Hagerman RJ. Chromosomes, genes and autism. In: Gillberg C, ed. Diagnosis and Treatment of Autism. New York and London: Plenum Press, 1989:105–131.

30. Aronson M, Hagberg B, Gillberg C. Attention deficits and autistic spectrum problems in children exposed to alcohol during gestation: a follow-up study. Dev Med Child Neurol 1997; 39:583–587.

31. Gillberg IC, Gillberg C, Kopp S. Hypothyroidism and autism spectrum disorders. J Child Psychol Psychiatry 1992; 33:531–542.

32. Gillberg C, Coleman M. The Biology of the Autistic Syndromes. 3rd ed. London, UK: Cambridge University Press, 2000.

33. Gillberg C, Gillberg IC. Infantile autism: a total population study of reduced optimality in the pre-, peri-, and neonatal period. J Autism Dev Disord 1983; 13:153–166.

34. Glasson EJ, Bower C, Petterson B, et al. Perinatal factors and the development of autism: a population study. Arch Gen Psychiatry 2004; 61:618–627.
35. Danielsson S, Gillberg IC, Billstedt E, et al. Epilepsy in young adults with autism: a prospective population-based follow-up study of 120 individuals diagnosed in childhood. Epilepsia 2005; 46:918–923.
36. Gillberg C. Asperger syndrome in 23 Swedish children. Dev Med Child Neurol 1989; 31:520–531.
37. Neville B, Goodman R, eds. Congenital Hemiplegia. Cambridge, UK: MacKeith Press, 2001.
38. Åhsgren I, Gillberg C, Erikson A, et al. Ataxia, autism, and the cerebellum: a clinical study of 32 cases of congenital ataxia. Dev Med Child Neurol 2005; 47:193–198.
39. Lopata C, Hamm EM, Volker MA, et al. Motor and visuomotor skills of children with Asperger's disorder: preliminary findings. Percept Mot Skills 2007; 104:1183–1192.
40. Lee DO, Ousley OY. Attention-deficit hyperactivity disorder symptoms in a clinic sample of children and adolescents with pervasive developmental disorders. J Child Adolesc Psychopharmacol 2006; 16:737–746.
41. Ehlers S, Gillberg C. The epidemiology of Asperger syndrome: a total population study. J Child Psychol Psychiatry 1993; 34:1327–1350.
42. Gillberg C. Perceptual, motor and attentional deficits in Swedish primary school children: some child psychiatric aspects. J Child Psychol Psychiatry 1983; 24:377–403.
43. Clark T, Feehan C, Tinlne C, et al. Autistic symptoms in children with attention deficit-hyperactivity disorder. Eur Child Adolesc Psychiatry 1999; 8:50–55.
44. Reiersen AM, Constantino JN, Volk HE, et al. Autistic traits in a population-based ADHD twin sample. J Child Psychol Psychiatry 2007; 48:464–472.
45. Kadesjö B, Gillberg C. The comorbidity of ADHD in the general population of Swedish school-age children. J Child Psychol Psychiatry 2001; 42:487–492.
46. Sturm H, Fernell E, Gillberg C. Autism spectrum disorders in children with normal intellectual levels: associated impairments and subgroups. Dev Med Child Neurol 2004; 46:444–447.
47. Gillberg C, Kadesjö B. Why bother about clumsiness? The implications of having developmental coordination disorder (DCD). The clumsy child. Neural Plast; 2003; 10:59–68 (special issue).
48. DeMyer MK, Bryson CO, Churchill DW. The earliest indicators of pathological development: comparison of symptoms during infancy and early childhood in normal, subnormal, schizophrenic and autistic children. Res Publ Assoc Res Nerv Ment Dis 1973; 51:298–332.
49. Sinzig J, Morsch D, Lehmkuhl G. Do hyperactivity, impulsivity and inattention have an impact on the ability of facial affect recognition in children with autism and ADHD? Eur Child Adolesc Psychiatry 2007 (epub ahead of print).
50. Billstedt E, Gillberg IC, Gillberg C. Autism in adults: symptoms patterns and diagnostic categories. Use of the DISCO in a community sample followed from childhood. J Child Psychol Psychiatry 2007 (in press).
51. Schmahmann JD, Weilburg JB, Sherman JC. The neuropsychiatry of the cerebellum - insights from the clinic. Cerebellum 2007; 6:254–267.
52. Ogdie MN, Fisher SE, Yang M, et al. Attention deficit hyperactivity disorder: fine mapping supports linkage to 5p13, 6q12, 16p13, and 17p11. Am J Hum Genet 2004; 75:661–668.

5

Prevalence of Asperger Syndrome[a]

Carrie Allison and Simon Baron-Cohen

*Autism Research Centre, Department of Psychiatry,
University of Cambridge, Cambridge, U.K.*

ESTIMATES OF PREVALENCE

Accurate estimates of prevalence of Asperger syndrome (AS) are required in order to anticipate the number of individuals who have a clinical need for support and services. Moreover, prevalence estimates may begin to inform us about the causes of the condition.

Terminology

Before examining the published research regarding the prevalence of AS, it is important to consider some terminology. "Prevalence" is used to refer to the number of cases of a specified condition in a defined population at a particular moment in time. Prevalence is calculated by dividing the number of identified cases within the population under investigation by the total number of individuals within the entire population. It is common to then multiply this number by

---

[a]**Note on terminology**: While the official term in DSM and ICD is "Asperger disorder," we opt for the term "Asperger syndrome" since every brain is disordered in certain environments (like saltwater fish in freshwater, or vice versa) but in our view the term "disorder" should be reserved for individuals who cannot function well in *any* environment. Since people with Asperger syndrome can function well in predictable, systemizable environments and only become disabled in unpredictable social environments, we feel they deserve the respect of more neutral terminology that acknowledges their atypical neurological profile. We do not impose our terminology on others.

100 in order to express prevalence as a percentage, and often, when a condition is rare, to state this as a number per 10,000 people. This makes it simpler to translate into meaningful figures. For example, it is easier to state prevalence results as "32 per 10,000" rather than "0.0032."

It is important to distinguish between prevalence and incidence as these terms are often confused. "Incidence" can be defined as the number of *new* cases of a specified condition that are identified in a defined population at a particular moment in time. Incidence is calculated by dividing the number of new cases of a condition that are identified within the specified population at a given moment in time, by the total condition-free population. Figures relating to incidence are especially valuable to epidemiologists as they provide data concerning the risk of a condition, and therefore incidence can be thought of as a rate, while prevalence can be regarded as a proportion.

Case Definition

Neither AS nor any autism spectrum condition (ASC) can be detected through a biological test, so diagnostic definitions are based solely on behavioral descriptions. When individuals clearly meet diagnostic criteria, diagnosis is straightforward. However, it is difficult to find agreement among researchers and clinicians when individuals cross the border of behavior that is considered to be typical, into what is considered to be on the autistic spectrum. Prevalence estimates are influenced by the definition of the condition in question that is used to distinguish a "case" from the general population. One confound in the epidemiological data of AS is the variation in case definition that has been used across studies. There are ambiguous boundaries between AS and other Pervasive Developmental Disorders (PDD) according to the different diagnostic criteria that are employed.

There are currently four sets of diagnostic criteria for AS that are commonly used in prevalence research. Having four sets does complicate matters. These are ICD-10 (1), DSM-IV (2), Gillberg and Gillberg criteria (3), and Szatmari criteria (4). The ICD-10 and DSM-IV criteria are very similar, except for a few differences related to motor clumsiness and isolated skills (included in ICD-10 but not DSM-IV). Delay in language is not accepted under ICD-10 and DSM-IV criteria but is allowed in the Gillberg criteria (and not mentioned in the Szatmari criteria). In both the Gillberg and Szatmari criteria, odd speech and language are present, but not in ICD-10 or DSM-IV (5). In the Gillberg and Gillberg criteria, motor control difficulties must be present (6). In order to be able to properly evaluate prevalence studies of AS, diagnostic definitions of each variant within the autistic spectrum need to be honed, and consistency among researchers needs to be ensured by using standardized diagnostic screens, rather than using different screens and different diagnostic criteria.

A study by Woodbury-Smith et al. (7) highlights this point, whereby 23% of patients who had been clinically diagnosed with AS would be reassigned a diagnosis of childhood autism or autistic disorder (hereafter referred to as autism) according to either ICD-10 or DSM-IV, since this diagnosis takes precedence over AS in the diagnostic hierarchy. Another study found that 99% of individuals with an ASC met ICD-10 diagnostic criteria for childhood autism, and only 1% met criteria for AS. However, when the Gillberg criteria were applied, 45% met criteria for AS according to this diagnostic definition (8).

Debate surrounding the distinction between AS and high-functioning autism (HFA) has been contentious (9), although traditionally, HFA refers to an individual who meets diagnostic criteria for autism but who has no impairment in their cognitive ability. On some occasions, HFA and AS are used interchangeably, again complicating any systematic evaluation of prevalence data on AS. Similarly, the distinction between AS and Pervasive Developmental Disorder Not Otherwise Specified (PDD-NOS) also remains controversial (10,11), the debate regarding whether AS is qualitatively different from autism, rather than being at the milder end of the autistic spectrum, continues (12–14). ICD-10 continues to make the assumption that there is a "core" autism syndrome (15) where differential diagnosis is based on a categorical approach. If ASC lie on a continuum then we need a quantitative approach to diagnosis (16,17).

Results from the published prevalence studies of AS cannot simply be grouped and directly compared for several reasons. First, studies vary in the methodologies that have been employed, in terms of case-finding, sampling, and the diagnostic definitions used. Second, studies published to date have been conducted at different times and in different populations. When examining studies that have looked specifically at the prevalence of AS (and indeed any other psychiatric condition), it is important to question whether any differences or similarities found between studies are a reflection of the different methodologies used, or whether results reflect true variation in prevalence, both between and within the populations examined (18). One finding in reviewing the literature on this topic is that there are very few studies whose primary objective was to examine AS in isolation from other ASC. In fact, only two studies published to date have undertaken to do so, which are reported below (5,19). Numerous other studies have included AS in their estimates for the prevalence of ASC, some of which will be summarized later in this chapter. See Table 1 for a summary of all the prevalence studies cited in this chapter.

Ehlers and Gillberg (1993) Study (19)

The prevalence of AS was exclusively examined in an outer middle-class borough of Goteborg in Sweden (19). This population-based study screened 1519 children between the ages of 7 and 16 years, using the Autism Spectrum Screening Questionnaire (ASSQ) (20). This is a 27-item checklist assessing traits of AS or HFA in school-age children who are of normal intelligence. Teachers completed the ASSQ on each child. Those children ($N = 18$) who reached the cut-point of 5 were invited to take part in detailed assessments. Assessments included direct observation of the child, parental and teacher interviews, and

Table 1 Summary of Prevalence Estimates for Cited Studies

First author	Year	Country	Population	Age range	Prevalence (per 10,000)	Confidence interval	Diagnostic criteria	Sex ratio
Ehlers	1993	Sweden	1,519	7–16	28.5–71	0.6–56.5[a]	ICD-10, Gillberg	4:1[b], 2.3:1[c]
Sponheim	1998	Norway	65,688	3–14	0.3	Not given	ICD-10 and DSM-IV	Not given
Kadesjo	1999	Sweden	826	7	48	13–124	DSM-III-R/ICD-10, Gillberg	Not given[d]
Taylor	1999	UK	490,000	<16	1.4	Not given	ICD-10	Not given
Baird	2000	UK	40,818	7	3.08	Not given	ICD-10	Not given[e]
Chakrabarti	2001	UK	15,500	2.5–6.5	8.4	4.5–14.3	DSM-IV	5.5:1
Lauritsen	2004	Denmark	682,397	<10	3.7[f]	3.2–4.1	ICD-8 - ICD-10	15.76:1[g]
Chakrabarti	2005	UK	10,903	4–6	11	5.7–19.2	DSM-IV	Not given
Ellefsen	2006	Faroe Islands	7689	8–17	26	14–38	Gillberg	6:1
Baird	2006	UK	56,946	9–10	–	–	ICD-10	
Fombonne	2006	Canada	27,749	5–14+	10.1	6.7–14.6	DSM-IV	2.1:1
Gillberg	2006	Sweden	102,485	7–24	9.2	7.2–11.0	Gillberg	10.8:1
Mattila	2007	Finland	5,484	8	16–43	2.8–6.7[h]	DSM-IV, ICD-10, Gillberg and Szatmari	1.7:1

[a] For lowest estimate.
[b] Using Gillberg criteria.
[c] When suspected cases of AS were included.
[d] 4 cases of AS diagnosed in males, none female.
[e] 5 cases of AS diagnosed in males, none female.
[f] 4.7 when corrected.
[g] Author's calculation.
[h] According to any of the four sets of diagnostic criteria.

14 children and their families agreed to take part. Using ICD-10 criteria, these detailed assessments revealed that four children warranted a definite diagnosis of AS, yielding a prevalence estimate of 28.5 per 10,000 (95% CI, 0.6–56.5/ 10,000). However, when Gillberg and Gillberg (3) criteria for AS were applied, a higher prevalence estimate of 36 per 10,000 was generated. Further, if *possible* cases of AS were included, the prevalence estimate rose to 71 per 10,000. The male-to-female ratio was 4:1 using the Gillberg criteria, but dropped to 2.3:1 when the possible cases of AS were included.

While this was the first systematic epidemiological study that specifically examined AS, Fombonne and Tidmarsh (21) noted some weaknesses with the study methodology. First, the population screened was small, and there was no justification given for the school selection to be included in the study nor the geographical area targeted or the sampling procedures. Second, the confidence intervals on the prevalence estimate are wide and therefore little conviction can be placed on the estimates reported by the authors. Third, at the time of the screening, there was no information regarding the reliability or validity of the screening instrument applied, and consequently it is unknown whether any cases were missed by the screen. Similarly, the screening instrument aims to identify both children with AS as well as those with HFA, which may have inflated the prevalence estimates. A further weakness is that the study relies on teachers as the sole informant of the child, when it may have been more appropriate to make use of parents as informants at the screening stage. Lastly and most importantly, questions regarding case definition are raised due to the differing prevalence estimates according to which diagnostic criteria was used. This has implications when evaluating the overall validity of case determination as established by the authors of this study.

Mattila et al. (2007) Study (5)

This was a comprehensive study that examined AS in Finland. The ASSQ (20) was completed by parents and/or teachers on 4422 children at age 8, from a population of 5484. From this sample, 125 children were invited for follow-up assessment, 73 of which were screen positive (either teacher or parent rated) children. Diagnostic examinations included the Autism Diagnostic Interview-Revised (ADI-R) (22), the Autism Diagnostic Observation Schedule (ADOS) (23), as well as the Wechsler Intelligence Scale for Children-Third Revision. A number of children in the assessment sample ($N = 24$) were observed at school, and consensus diagnoses were also made. The Asperger Syndrome Diagnostic Interview (24) (ASDI) was completed on the basis of information already obtained from the other assessments. Four sets of diagnostic criteria were then applied to the data: DSM-IV, ICD-10, Gillberg and Gillberg (3), and Szatmari et al. (4).

Results indicated a prevalence estimate, according to DSM-IV criteria to be 25 per 10,000. According to ICD-10 criteria, the estimate was 29 per 10,000.

If Gillberg and Gillberg (3) criteria were applied, the prevalence estimate was 27 per 10,000, and if Szatmari et al. (4) criteria were applied, the prevalence estimate was 16 per 10,000. In total, 19 children were diagnosed as having AS on at least one of the diagnostic criteria, yielding an overall prevalence estimate of 43 per 10,000. Interestingly, 47% of those who were diagnosed with AS in this study had not been diagnosed prior to the start of the study. This implies that any study that relies on case identification through health records may be underestimating the prevalence of AS. The overall male-to-female ratio in this study was 1.7:1. Another interesting point to note in this study was that DSM-IV and ICD-10 criteria overlapped exactly in all but two cases. These two cases did not meet DSM-IV criteria as they did not have clinically significant impairments in any of the important areas of functioning. (This raises the question as to why they received a diagnosis at all, since in most areas of medicine, diagnosis is reserved for individuals who are experiencing impairment in everyday functioning.) Fifteen children who were screened and selected to take part in the diagnostic evaluation refused to take part at this stage. Two of these children already had a recorded diagnosis of AS, but since these were not verified they were not included in the prevalence estimate. Therefore, it is likely that the estimates presented in this study are underestimated.

Overall, this study highlights three important issues. First, there is a need to refine the diagnostic criteria for AS since by applying different diagnostic criteria, different prevalence estimates are yielded. Second, combined teacher and parent screening may be important in the diagnostic process, since some parents may have no other children to compare their child's behavior to. Third, there are undetected cases of AS in the population, highlighting the reality that any prevalence estimates generated through studies that used a case-register design should be regarded as a *minimum* figure. Finally, since parents of children with an ASC often exhibit the "broader autism phenotype" (25,26) (a term that is used to describe the genetic liability for autism, which may be expressed in non-autistic relatives in a phenotype that is milder but qualitatively similar to the defining features of autism), in principle this could introduce a bias in the way in which they as parents report their child's behavior. It is therefore useful to have data provided by teachers as well as parents on children in this age group.

Studies Citing Prevalence Estimates for Asperger Syndrome

A study conducted by Kadesjo et al. in Sweden (27) simultaneously examined the prevalence of AS and autism in children. This was a total population study of all seven-year-olds (age range 6.7–7.7 years) in a town in central Sweden. 826 children were included in the study (438 boys and 388 girls), of which 818 were attending mainstream school, and the other eight children were in special classes for children with learning disabilities. All children were screened for a diagnosis of ASC. The authors used a 50% sample approach, whereby they comprehensively examined exactly half of the sample of 818 children attending mainstream classes. They asserted that this was a representative sample of the child population in mainstream education in the town. Therefore, in total, 409 children were examined, and for each child in the sample, at least one parent or teacher interview was completed, as well as teacher-rated questionnaires. At the time of the individual assessment, each child was monitored for (*i*) indications of problems relating to social and emotional reciprocity, (*ii*) social avoidance, and (*iii*) difficulties in nonverbal behavior. A child who received a score of 0 was recorded to be showing no difficulties in each area, a score of 1 indicated some problems, and a score of 2 or above indicated major social interaction difficulties at the time of the examination. Teachers were given questionnaires to complete about each child in the sample, examining five problem areas. These were (*i*) attention, (*ii*) social interaction, (*iii*) learning, (*iv*) language, and (*v*) emotion. Again, a score ranging from 0 to 2 on each area could be assigned and scores were added to generate a "social dysfunction" score (range 0–10). For any child who had a score of 1 or 2 in the social interaction domain, their teacher was given three symptom checklists, which were the DSM-III-R (28) list of 16 symptoms of Autistic Disorder, Gillberg's (29) list of 20 symptoms of AS, and the Szatmari et al. (1989) list of 22 symptoms of AS. Forty-eight months following the initial examinations (4,29), the ASSQ (20) was sent to parents of the 370 children who still lived in the town. Five parents refused to take part in the questionnaire study that left 365 (89% of the original sample) participants.

All those children who were suspected of having an ASC were given an IQ test, and their parents took part in an ADI-R (22). Three diagnostic classifications were made. These were autistic disorder, autistic-like condition and AS. In total, 10 cases of ASC were found in this population, which equates to 1.21% of the population. Specifically, 4 cases of AS were identified, equating to 48 cases per 10,000. However, there are wide confidence intervals for this proportion, ranging from 13 cases to 124. While the sample size in this study was fairly small, this drawback is offset by the high proportion of individuals who were examined in depth, thus reducing measurement error. It is interesting to note that higher rates of AS were reported when using Szatmari (4) rather than Gillberg (29) criteria, again highlighting how different case definitions impact on prevalence estimates.

A study in Norway by Sponheim and Skjeldal (30) used a case-finding approach whereby parents of all children with a known diagnosis of autism were contacted to participate in the study. The target population consisted of 12 birth cohorts of children, ranging from 3 to 14 years ($N = 65,688$). Children were also referred by pediatricians from health clinics if a child was delayed or deviant in their social communication behavior. From this population, 65 children were referred and screened using a schedule designed for the purpose of the study. Two children were given a diagnosis of AS, according to ICD-10 diagnostic criteria, equating to a prevalence estimate of 0.3 per 10,000. The prevalence of other ASC diagnoses (according to ICD-10 diagnostic criteria) was 4.9 per 10,000, giving an overall prevalence estimate for all ASC to be 5.2 per 10,000.

This estimate is 100 times lower than the estimate reported by Ehlers and Gillberg (19), and the authors acknowledge that this may have been because screening was not conducted in mainstream schools, and therefore, cases of AS are likely to have been missed. Further, Mattila et al. (5) point out that prevalence estimates are higher when teachers are involved in the screening process. Also, AS was only just beginning to be known about at the start of the study, which may have led to clinical insensitivity. One of the major weaknesses of this study is the lack of a validated screening instrument, which questions the validity of the prevalence estimates reported.

U.K. Prevalence Estimates

A large epidemiological study conducted in the United Kingdom (31) examined the prevalence of pervasive developmental disorders (PDD) among four- to six-year-olds who were identified through National Health Service records. Over 10,000 children were included in the population sample and children were routinely screened by a health visitor at four time points (at 6 weeks, 6–9 months, 18–24 months, and 42 months). Any child who was referred from this routine screening process was put forward for an additional screen by the child development team. Following this screen, any child who was deemed to have moderate or severe developmental problems underwent a detailed developmental assessment. Any child who was then suspected of having a PDD was further assessed with standardized measures, including the Autism Diagnostic Interview-Revised (22). Diagnoses were made using DSM-IV criteria for all PDD after a full review of all the data. Overall, 64 children were confirmed with a diagnosis of a PDD, yielding an overall prevalence estimate of 58.7 per 10,000 (CI 45.2–74.9). Twelve cases of AS were found, resulting in a prevalence estimate of 11 per 10,000 (CI 5.7–19.2). The prevalence estimate for autistic disorder in this study was 22 per 10,000 (CI 14.1–32.7), and for all PDD not including autistic disorder it was 36.7 per 10,000 (CI 26.2–49.9).

The results from this study validate and replicate the results from an earlier study by the same authors that used the same design (32), using an earlier cohort in the same geographical region of the United Kingdom. In the earlier study, the prevalence estimate for AS was 8.4 per 10,000 (CI 4.5–14.3). The authors reported a male-to-female ratio of 5.5:1 in this study (not reported in the earlier study). There was no significant difference between the prevalence estimates for each subtype of PDD in each of the two studies, and therefore the prevalence estimates were combined to provide more defined and accurate estimates. Consequently, the prevalence estimate for AS was 9.5 per 10,000 (CI 6.1–14.0), and for all PDD it was 60.6 per 10,000 (CI 51.6–70.7).

Another study that used a case-register approach was conducted in the North Thames area of the United Kingdom (33). This study examined the incidence of ASC before and after the introduction of the measles, mumps, and rubella (MMR) vaccine in 1988, but reported prevalence estimates for AS and other ASC. Children, born after 1979, with a diagnosis of ASC were identified from special needs and disability registers. ICD-10 diagnostic criteria were applied to the information in each record to confirm the diagnosis. A prevalence estimate of 1.4 per 10,000 was noted for AS. However, only 38% of cases could be confirmed using ICD-10 diagnostic criteria from information recorded in the clinical notes, which may suggest that the prevalence estimate is an underestimate.

A study conducted by Baird et al. (33) used five methods of ascertainment of cases over a period of five years, including screening using the Checklist for Autism in Toddlers (CHAT) (34), the Checklist for Referral, and a medical records search. They reported a prevalence estimate for childhood autism and pervasive developmental disorders (including AS) to be 57.9 per 10,000. A total of 50 cases of childhood autism using ICD-10 diagnostic criteria were identified when the children were aged 42 months, 5 of who also warranted a diagnosis of AS, yielding a prevalence estimate of 3.08 per 10,000. The authors note that the severity of their presentation was sufficient for these individuals to meet full criteria for autism, yet a high proportion of children (60%) diagnosed with childhood autism had an IQ greater than 70, suggesting that there may be more of an overlap with AS than originally thought.

A recent prevalence study published in the United Kingdom was conducted in a population of 56,946 children in the South Thames region aged 9 to 10 years (35). All children who had a current clinical diagnosis of an ASC were screened ($N = 255$) using the Social Communication Questionnaire (a screening measure for all ASC based on the ADI-R (22), as well as those who were considered to be at risk of being a previously unobserved case ($N = 1515$). These "at-risk" individuals all had a statement of Special Educational Needs, which is a legal document in the United Kingdom that states the number of hours of additional classroom support a child needs who has significant emotional, behavioral or cognitive difficulties. The authors conducted a comprehensive diagnostic assessment on a stratified sample ($N = 255$) that included parental interview (ADI-R), clinical observation ADOS (23), as well as an assessment of language and cognitive ability. Initial diagnoses made by the research team were subjected to consensus clinical evaluation and used ICD-10 criteria when determining diagnostic status. Prevalence estimates were derived using a sample weighting procedure.

The total prevalence including childhood autism and other ASC was 116.1 per 10,000. In this sample, there were 77 cases (77.2 per 10,000) of a consensus diagnosis of an ASC other than childhood autism, of which 67 met ICD-10 criteria for atypical autism, 7 met criteria for an unspecified ASC, and 3 for "overactive disorder" associated with mental retardation and stereotyped movements. No child in this sample was documented to be diagnosed with AS, although the authors acknowledge that seven cases who received a diagnosis of childhood autism also met criteria for AS under ICD-10 criteria. Like their previous study, this was because of the absence of a delay in language or cognitive development prior to three years of age. Therefore, these cases also satisfied the criteria for childhood autism, which takes precedence over AS. Because of the methodology of this study, only those children who had a Statement of Special Educational Needs or who had an existing diagnosis of an ASC were selected to take part in the study. Therefore, it is likely that cases may have been missed, as only those children who had already been identified as having difficulties were screened and assessed.

This study highlights two points. First, the way in which the hierarchy in the diagnostic classifications work meant that no cases of AS were documented in the prevalence estimates. This again raises questions regarding the definition of this diagnosis within the accepted diagnostic manuals. It could be that AS does not constitute a distinct categorical diagnostic label. Current thinking may benefit from shifting away from a categorical conceptualization of ASC to a continuum approach (16,17) with AS lying on the more able end of the continuum that acts as the "bridge" between autism and normality. Second, when the number of children identified by the study team as a case was compared with the percentage of locally recorded diagnoses, it was found that just over a half of those identified as having autism and under a quarter of those identified as having an ASC already had a locally recorded diagnosis. Clearly, prospective screening in the at-risk population identified many more cases than had previously been recorded, suggesting that there may be more undetected cases in the unscreened population, particularly at the milder end of the autistic spectrum. Baird et al. (35) asserted that the prevalence figures reported in this study should be judged to be as a *minimum* figure. There is clearly a discrepancy between the prevalence estimates of all ASC between the two studies over a relatively short period of time. The Baird et al. (35) study is the largest epidemiological study published that used prospective, serial, and active case ascertainment methodology and is likely to have generated robust and more precise results than previous studies, as there is a greater probability of complete ascertainment. One point to note from this study is that by simply counting the number of locally recorded cases lead to a prevalence estimate that was nearly two thirds lower than the figure produced through the serial ascertainment methodology. A discussion of factors influencing the apparent rise in the estimation of prevalence follows later in this chapter.

PREVALENCE ESTIMATES AROUND THE WORLD

A study conducted in Montreal, Canada (36), reported a prevalence of 64.9 per 10,000 for all PDD in school children born between 1987 and 1998. Over 27,000 children were included in this study, and children with an already diagnosed PDD were identified by a special needs team, using their local case register system. This prevalence estimate was broken down into distinct diagnostic categories, and for AS it was 10.1 per 10,000 (CI 6.7–14.6). The male-to-female ratio was 4.8:1 for all PDD and for AS it was 2.1:1, which the authors note is lower than for the other subtypes on the autistic spectrum. While this prevalence estimate approximates other reported estimates, it is possible that they are in fact underestimates, since case identification methodology for this study relied exclusively on medical or educational records (37) rather than prospective case ascertainment. Further, special schools were not selected to take part in the study, which may have resulted in an underestimation of the true population prevalence. Conversely, diagnostic misclassification may have occurred in this study since diagnoses were not contemporaneously verified, leading to possible misclassification of all PDD and therefore an inflation of the prevalence estimates. Finally, the target population is a geographical region that is known for being inclusive and supportive of children and families with PDD, so it is possible that families may have migrated to that region specifically to receive clinical support. A further selection bias may have been introduced as the study focused on one district in Montreal that is English speaking and is therefore not representative of the general population in Quebec.

A study conducted in the Faroe Islands found a population prevalence for AS to be 26 per 10,000 (CI 14–31) in a total population of children born between 1985 and 1994 (38), aged 8 to 17. If an additional child had been included in the estimate who had received an AS diagnosis prior to the start of the study and whose parents did not want him or her to take part in the study, the prevalence estimate would have been 27 per 10,000. There were also an additional four children who were strongly suspected of having AS but who were not examined; if these children were included, the prevalence estimate would have been 33 per 10,000. Screening took place in three stages. First, case notes of all those children who attended special schools were examined to identify those who would be put forward for detailed assessment. Second, teachers screened children in mainstream schools, who were previously undiagnosed and raised teacher concern by completing the ASSQ (20). Lastly, a number of children were recommended for further assessment as concerns had been raised about them by other sources such as private psychologists, parents, and social services. The children were all assessed using the Diagnostic Interview for Social and Communication Disorders (DISCO) (39), and clinical and DISCO diagnoses were made. ICD-10 criteria were used for making childhood autism diagnoses and Gillberg (29) AS criteria. The authors assert that the reason they did not apply ICD-10 criteria for AS diagnoses is because in practice very few individuals rarely meet full criteria for this condition (8), as it is stipulated that normal language and intellectual development must be present prior to three years of age. The male-to-female ratio was 6:1 (unadjusted population rate, including the case that was diagnosed prior to the start of the study). One interesting feature of this study is that the population in the Faroe Islands is small and isolated. Therefore, a higher level of inbreeding might be expected than in other geographical regions. Considering that ASC are in part genetic (40–44), a higher prevalence may have been expected, yet the estimate from this study is similar to other estimates from more heterogeneous populations.

A study by Lauritsen et al. (45) examined both the incidence and prevalence of all ASC in children below the age of 10 years in Denmark between 1971 and 2000. This was a total population study that followed over two million children, and cases were ascertained through the Danish Psychiatric Central Register. This is a database that contains information regarding all diagnoses reported by psychiatric hospitals in Denmark. This study was the first to attempt to estimate incidence and prevalence across a whole country, and for AS the estimated prevalence was 3.7 per 10,000. When this figure was corrected (the summation of the incident cases in each age group and each calendar year) the prevalence estimate was 4.7 cases per 10,000. However, caution must be employed when considering these results. First, since this was a case-register study, it is possible that some children, who would meet clinical criteria for AS, were not included as they may not have had any contact with the psychiatric services due to low levels of behavioral problems. Second, the authors included only children with diagnoses up to the age of 10 years. Since previous research indicates that the average age of a diagnosis of AS may not be made until age 11 (46), the study may have missed these cases, again leading to an underestimated prevalence estimate. Finally a new clinic that specializes in the diagnosis of ASC was opened during the course of the research that did not report to the Danish Psychiatric Central Register, so all prevalence estimates may be miscalculated. Sex ratios were not directly reported in this study, but on the basis of the percentages given by the authors (94% of cases of AS were males), the sex ratio equates to 15.76 to 1, which is the highest reported sex ratio for AS to date.

IS THE NUMBER OF CASES OF ASPERGER SYNDROME ON THE RISE?

In 1966, Lotter (47) conducted the first epidemiological survey of autistic conditions and screened a population of children who were between the ages of 8 and 10 years. He found 35 "autistic" cases that equate to a prevalence estimate of 4.5 cases per 10,000. While this estimate does not specify AS (since that was unknown at that time) and only reports an estimate for autistic disorder, it is considerably lower than the most recent estimate for the same condition (35).

There has been much discussion as to whether there has been an increase in the number of cases of individuals with ASC over the past decade (9,48,49). It might be reasonable to assume that if there has been a true rise in the incidence of ASC, this increase may also apply to AS. However, incidence studies usually relate to age of onset that may be difficult to determine, and which is easily confused with age of recognition of the condition. The only way to properly assess time trends is by controlling which case definition is applied across studies, and keeping the same case ascertainment methodology. A related point is that the age range examined across studies is a source of variation, thus making any comparison between studies invalid. Powell et al. (50) suggest that the only way in which any increase over time in ASC (including AS) could be detected would be to follow a single population over time.

When comparing prevalence estimates over time, any detected increase may be an artifact of improved screening methodology and better awareness of the condition. As the number of those individuals who are missed by the screen decreases over time with improved screening techniques, prevalence estimates increase. Similarly, because of the changes over time in diagnostic criteria and indeed who might be considered as a "case," it may appear that the prevalence has increased even when the incidence of the condition in any given year has not. For example, when comparing ICD-10 (1) and DSM-IV (2) with Szatmari (4) and Gillberg and Gillberg (3) diagnostic criteria, as was noted earlier, one study found different prevalence estimates according to which definition was applied (5).

The prevalence studies described above used different ascertainment methods and produced different prevalence estimates; the Baird et al. (35) study used serial ascertainment, the Kadesjo et al. (27) study used a total population approach, while the Sponheim et al. (30) study used a case-register approach. It is almost impossible to assess whether there has been an increase in AS specifically, since not enough data have accrued due to the late arrival of the condition in the diagnostic criteria.

Fombonne (51) concluded in his review of epidemiological studies of autism and PDD that the apparent increase in the prevalence of all ASC cannot be directly attributed to an increase in the incidence. Instead, higher prevalence estimates may be related to other factors such as improved service provision, changes over time in diagnostic criteria, and greater recognition among parents and health professionals.

However, Chakrabarti and Fombonne (31) suggest a study that can be used to elucidate whether there has been an increase over time in the prevalence of ASC. The study was conducted by Wing and Gould in the late 1970's (52). The authors identified a group of children who had autistic disorder, but also included those who exhibited the triad of impairments as described by Wing and Gould in the paper. They found a baseline prevalence of this broader set of conditions (which would have included AS) to be 20 per 10,000. Considering the most recently published prevalence estimate for all ASC is 116.1 per 10,000 (35), this is nearly a sixfold increase over the course of almost 30 years.

A study that looked at whether the prevalence of ASC has increased over time was carried out in Goteborg, Sweden (53). The authors included in their sample all individuals who were born between 1977 and 1994 and who were living in the city of Goteborg at the end of the year 2001. All individuals with a diagnosis of ASC registered at the Child Neuropsychiatry Clinic were identified and their case notes were reviewed. All individuals' notes that were recorded on the register were screened for any reference to autism. All those identified by these methods were assigned a diagnosis based on their medical records according to DSM criteria, except for AS where Gillberg and Gillberg (3) criteria was used, due to the strict criteria of normal development in the first three years. The time frame for this study covered 18 years, and the authors decided to split the period up into three sections in order to be able to ascertain whether there was a linear increase in prevalence over time.

It was found that over the whole period, the prevalence estimate for all ASC was 53 per 10,000. When split into three cohorts of six years, the prevalence for the earliest cohort (those born between 1977 and 1982) was 26 cases per 10,000, the prevalence for the middle cohort (those born between 1983 and 1988) was 61 cases per 10,000, and the prevalence for the latest cohort (those born between 1989 and 1994) was 80 cases per 10,000. The prevalence of AS over the whole period was 9.2 per 10,000 (CI 7.2:11.0) and was highest (15.1 cases per 10,000) in the middle birth cohort. In particular, for this cohort the prevalence of AS in boys was 27 per 10,000. The male-to-female ratio was 10.8:1. There was a steady increase in cases in the first and middle cohorts but then tailed off after this. This may have been due to the lack of cases of AS in the last cohort as diagnosis of AS is often delayed until late childhood or even early adulthood (54,55). One study found that AS was not diagnosed until on average 11 years of age (46). This study also appears to show that there has been an increase in the prevalence of core autistic disorder; the prevalence estimate for the oldest cohort was 11 cases per 10,000, rising to 35 cases per 10,000 in the youngest cohort. The authors assert that findings from this study must be regarded as the minimum number of cases who require support, and that there are outstanding cases that have not yet been referred or diagnosed that should be included in the prevalence estimate. Therefore, a total of 0.5% cases who are clinically impaired should be considered to be the minimum rate of ASC. While this study does show that there has been an increase over time in the prevalence of AS and ASC overall, the findings should be treated with caution. Possibly, a higher prevalence was observed in this study due to the migration of families to the area as a consequence of the improved services in the Goteburg region.

Effects of Sex

Traditionally, it is thought that boys are more likely to receive a diagnosis of AS than girls. Some reports indicate that boys are three times more likely to be affected by this condition than girls (56), while others have asserted that the ratio of boys to girls who are referred for diagnosis is as high as 10:1 (57). Wing (58) noted in her clinical series of cases that there were 15 boys and 4 girls. She asserted that the girls were outwardly more sociable than the boys, but on close investigation they still exhibited difficulties in reciprocal social interactions that are characteristic of AS. In the United Kingdom, there are three times as many adult males who use services provided by the National Autistic Society as females (59). In a prevalence study that examined all ASC in Cambridgeshire in the United Kingdom, the male-to-female ratio was 8:1 (60). The study by Lauritsen et al. (45) found a male-to-female ratio of 15.76:1. However, the most thorough and rigorous paper that reported prevalence figures on AS to date cast doubt on the idea that more males are affected by this disorder than females. The Finnish prevalence study by Mattila et al. (5) found the male-to-female ratio to be between 0.8 and 2.1:1 depending on which diagnostic criteria had been used. It is possible that there was not enough statistical power in this study to be able to properly assess the male-to-female ratio, as the total number of cases was only 19 (7 females, 12 males). The ratios reported in this paper are much lower than those found in other epidemiological studies (19,27).

There are various possibilities that have been proposed to account for the disparity between reports of the sex ratio of cases of AS in the literature. First, not all girls with AS are referred for diagnosis (19,58,61). Second, Kopp and Gillberg (62) postulate that girls are instead given a variety of other labels such as obsessive-compulsive disorder, conduct disorder, paranoid disorder, or anorexia nervosa. Third, the behavioral phenotype may be slightly different for girls than for boys, although the core features of AS are as common in girls as in boys. Attwood (61) noted that boys with AS show an uneven profile of social behavior and are more likely to exhibit disruptive behaviors than girls, which may be a factor in the higher rate of referrals. Further, girls who have AS may be more socially able, and impairments in social interaction not noticed as often as for boys, since they are more able to imitate social behavior than boys.

SUMMARY

The prevalence estimates for AS yielded from the studies described above show inconsistent results. There is a wide range of estimates ranging from 0.3 per 10,000 (30) to 71 per 10,000 (19). There is clearly a need to refine and hone the diagnostic criteria for AS so that useful comparisons between studies as well as meaningful conclusions can be made. There appears to be no evidence that there has been a rise in the number of cases of AS over the past 20 years, and from the data available, it is not possible to get a sense whether this has become more prevalent. Further, it is not really possible to evaluate whether the prevalence of AS is same across the world for similar reasons of variable methodology. The male-to-female ratio across the studies cited in this chapter range from 1.7:1 to 15.76:1. Thorough prospective, serial case ascertainment methodology is needed in studies rather than using retrospective ascertainment. In a meta-analytic review of prevalence data for all ASC, Williams et al. (18) concluded that there were many factors that explained the variance in prevalence estimates across studies. These included the age of the children screened, the diagnostic criteria used, and the country studied, and some of these factors may be acting as a proxy for other influences on prevalence estimates, which need to be investigated.

CONCLUSIONS

Epidemiological surveys that have focused solely on AS are rare, making comparisons between studies difficult. Prevalence estimates from studies that included AS used heterogeneous methods, producing very different results. In order to ascertain a more precise estimate of this condition in the population, repeated, multicenter prevalence studies employing identical methodology are required, which will allow researchers to investigate variations both geographically and over time (18). Exploration of any true variation in prevalence of AS may help to move forward our knowledge regarding etiology and helpful interventions for this condition.

ACKNOWLEDGMENTS

CA and SBC were supported by the Big Lottery and the MRC during the period of this work. We are grateful to Carol Brayne, Jo Williams, and Fiona Matthews for valuable discussions.

REFERENCES

1. World Health Organisation. The ICD-10 Classification of Mental and Behavioural Disorders: Diagnostic Criteria for Research. Geneva: WHO, 1993.
2. American Psychiatric Association. Diagnostic and Statistical Manual of Mental Disorders (DSM-IV). 4th ed. Washington, DC: APA, 1994.
3. Gillberg IC, Gillberg C. Asperger syndrome—some epidemiological considerations: a research note. J Child Psychol Psychiatry 1989; 30(4):631–638.
4. Szatmari P, Bremner R, Nagy J. Asperger's syndrome: a review of clinical features. Can J Psychiatry 1989; 34(6):554–560.
5. Mattila ML, Kielinen M, Jussila K, et al. An epidemiological and diagnostic study of asperger syndrome according to four sets of diagnostic criteria. J Am Acad Child Adolesc Psychiatry 2007; 46(5):636–646.
6. Hippler K, Klicpera C. A retrospective analysis of the clinical case records of "autistic psychopaths" diagnosed by Hans Asperger and his team at the University Children's Hospital, Vienna. Philos Trans R Soc Lond B Biol Sci 2003; 358(1430): 291–301.
7. Woodbury-Smith M, Klin A, Volkmar F. Asperger's syndrome: a comparison of clinical diagnoses and those made according to the ICD-10 and DSM-IV. J Autism Dev Disord 2005; 35(2):235–240.
8. Leekam SR, Libby S, Wing L, et al. Comparison of ICD-10 and Gillberg's criteria for Asperger syndrome. Autism 2000; 4(1):11–28.
9. Wing L, Potter D. The epidemiology of autistic spectrum disorders: is the prevalence rising? Ment Retard Dev Disabil Res Rev 2002; 8(3):151–161.
10. Volkmar F, Klin A. Diagnostic issues in Asperger syndrome. In: Klin A, Volkmar F, Sparrow S, eds. Asperger syndrome. New York: Guilford Press, 2000:25–71.
11. Klin A, Pauls D, Schultz R, et al. Three diagnostic approaches to Asperger syndrome: implications for research. J Autism Dev Disord 2005; 35(2):221–234.
12. Schopler E. Are autism and Asperger syndrome (AS) different labels or different disabilities? J Autism Dev Disord 1996; 26(1):109–110.
13. Baskin JH, Sperber M, Price BH. Asperger syndrome revisited. Rev Neurol Dis 2006; 3(1):1–7.

14. Frith U. Emanuel Miller lecture: confusions and controversies about Asperger syndrome. J Child Psychol Psychiatry 2004; 45(4):672–686.
15. Webb E, Morey J, Thompsen W, et al. Prevalence of autistic spectrum disorder in children attending mainstream schools in a Welsh education authority. Dev Med Child Neurol 2003; 45(6):377–384.
16. Wing L. The continuum of autistic disorders. In: Schopler EM, Mesibov GM, eds. Diagnosis and Assessment in Autism. New York: Plenum Press, 1988:91–110.
17. Baron-Cohen S, Wheelwright S, Skinner R, et al. The autism-spectrum quotient (AQ): evidence from Asperger syndrome/high-functioning autism, males and females, scientists and mathematicians. J Autism Dev Disord 2001; 31(1):5–17.
18. Williams JG, Higgins JP, Brayne CE. Systematic review of prevalence studies of autism spectrum disorders. Arch Dis Child 2006; 91(1):8–15.
19. Ehlers S, Gillberg C. The epidemiology of Asperger syndrome. A total population study. J Child Psychol Psychiatry 1993; 34(8):1327–1350.
20. Ehlers S, Gillberg C, Wing L. A screening questionnaire for Asperger syndrome and other high-functioning autism spectrum disorders in school age children. J Autism Dev Disord 1999; 29(2):129–141.
21. Fombonne E, Tidmarsh L. Epidemiologic data on Asperger disorder. Child Adolesc Psychiatr Clin N Am 2003; 12(1):15–21, v–vi.
22. Lord C, Rutter M, Le Couteur A. Autism diagnostic interview-revised: a revised version of a diagnostic interview for caregivers of individuals with possible pervasive developmental disorders. J Autism Dev Disord 1994; 24(5):659–685.
23. Lord C, Risi S, Lambrecht L, et al. The autism diagnostic observation schedule-generic: a standard measure of social and communication deficits associated with the spectrum of autism. J Autism Dev Disord 2000; 30(3):205–223.
24. Gillberg C, Rastam M, Wentz E. The Asperger syndrome (and high-functioning autism) diagnostic interview (ASDI): a preliminary study of a new structured clinical interview. Autism 2001; 5(1):57–66.
25. Bailey A, Parr J. Implications of the broader phenotype for concepts of autism. Novartis Found Symp 2003; 251:26–35; discussion 6–47, 109–111, 281–297.
26. Piven J, Palmer P, Jacobi D, et al. Broader autism phenotype: evidence from a family history study of multiple-incidence autism families. Am J Psychiatry 1997; 154(2): 185–190.
27. Kadesjo B, Gillberg C, Hagberg B. Brief report: autism and Asperger syndrome in seven-year-old children: a total population study. J Autism Dev Disord 1999; 29(4): 327–331.
28. American Psychiatric Association. Diagnostic and statistical manual of mental disorders. Revised. 3rd ed. Washington (DC): American Psychiatric Association, 1987.
29. Gillberg C. Clinical and neurobiological aspects of Asperger syndrome in six family studies. In: Frith U, ed. Autism and Asperger Syndrome. Cambridge: Cambridge University Press, 1991:122–146.
30. Sponheim E, Skjeldal O. Autism and related disorders: epidemiological findings in a Norwegian study using ICD-10 diagnostic criteria. J Autism Dev Disord 1998; 28(3): 217–227.
31. Chakrabarti S, Fombonne E. Pervasive developmental disorders in preschool children: confirmation of high prevalence. Am J Psychiatry 2005; 162(6):1133–1141.
32. Chakrabarti S, Fombonne E. Pervasive developmental disorders in preschool children. JAMA 2001; 285(24):3093–3099.

33. Baird G, Charman T, Baron-Cohen S, et al. A screening instrument for autism at 18 months of age: a 6-year follow-up study. J Am Acad Child Adolesc Psychiatry 2000; 39(6):694–702.
34. Baron-Cohen S, Allen J, Gillberg C. Can autism be detected at 18 months? The needle, the haystack, and the CHAT. Br J Psychiatry 1992; 161:839–843.
35. Baird G, Simonoff E, Pickles A, et al. Prevalence of disorders of the autism spectrum in a population cohort of children in South Thames: the Special Needs and Autism Project (SNAP). Lancet 2006; 368(9531):210–215.
36. Fombonne E, Zakarian R, Bennett A, et al. Pervasive developmental disorders in Montreal, Quebec, Canada: prevalence and links with immunizations. Pediatrics 2006; 118(1):e139–e150.
37. Fombonne E. Epidemiology of autistic disorder and other pervasive developmental disorders. J Clin Psychiatry 2005; 66(suppl 10):3–8.
38. Ellefsen A, Kampmann H, Billstedt E, et al. Autism in the Faroe Islands: an epidemiological study. J Autism Dev Disord 2007; 37:437–444.
39. Leekam SR, Libby SJ, Wing L, et al. The diagnostic interview for social and communication disorders: algorithms for ICD-10 childhood autism and Wing and Gould autistic spectrum disorder. J Child Psychol Psychiatry 2002; 43(3):327–342.
40. Bailey A, Le Couteur A, Gottesman I, et al. Autism as a strongly genetic disorder: evidence from a British twin study. Psychol Med 1995; 25(1):63–77.
41. Folstein S, Rutter M. Genetic influences and infantile autism. Nature 1977; 265(5596): 726–728.
42. Rutter M, Bailey A, Simonoff E, et al. Genetic influences in autism. In: Cohen D, Volkmar F, eds. Handbook of Autism and Pervasive Developmental Disorders. New York: Wiley, 1997:370–387.
43. Szatmari P, Jones MB, Zwaigenbaum L, et al. Genetics of autism: overview and new directions. J Autism Dev Disord 1998; 28(5):351–368.
44. Volkmar FR, Lord C, Bailey A, et al. Autism and pervasive developmental disorders. J Child Psychol Psychiatry 2004; 45(1):135–170.
45. Lauritsen M, Pederson C, Mortensen P. The incidence and prevalence of pervasive developmental disorders: a Danish population-based study. Psychol Med 2004; 34:1339–1346.
46. Howlin P, Asgharian A. The diagnosis of autism and Asperger syndrome: findings from a survey of 770 families. Dev Med Child Neurol 1999; 41(12):834–839.
47. Lotter V. Epidemiology of autistic conditions in young children I. Prevalence. Soc Psychiatry 1966; 1:124–137.
48. Fombonne E. The prevalence of autism. JAMA 2003; 289(1):87–89.
49. Fombonne E. Epidemiological studies of pervasive developmental disorders. In: Volkmar F, Paul R, Klin A, et al., eds. Handbook of Autism and Pervasive Developmental Disorders. Hoboken, NJ: Wiley, 2005:42–69.
50. Powell JE, Edwards A, Edwards M, et al. Changes in the incidence of childhood autism and other autistic spectrum disorders in preschool children from two areas of the West Midlands, UK. Dev Med Child Neurol 2000; 42(9):624–628.
51. Fombonne E. Epidemiological surveys of autism and other pervasive developmental disorders: an update. J Autism Dev Disord 2003; 33(4):365–382.
52. Wing L, Gould J. Severe impairments of social interaction and associated abnormalities in children: epidemiology and classification. J Autism Child Schizophr 1979; 9:11–29.

53. Gillberg C, Cederlund M, Lamberg K, et al. Brief report: "the autism epidemic". The registered prevalence of autism in a Swedish urban area. J Autism Dev Disord 2006; 36(3):429–435.

54. Barnard J, Harvey V, Prior A, et al. Ignored or ineligible? The reality for adults with autistic spectrum disorders. London: National Autistic Society, 2001.

55. Howlin P, Moore A. Diagnosis in autism: a survey of over 1200 patients in the UK. Autism: Int J Res Pract 1997; 1:135–162.

56. Asperger Syndrome Fact Sheet. 2007. Available at: http://www.ninds.nih.gov/disorders/asperger/detail_asperger.htm. Accessed August 30, 2007.

57. Gillberg C. Asperger syndrome in 23 Swedish children. Dev Med Child Neurol 1989; 31(4):520–531.

58. Wing L. Asperger's syndrome: a clinical account. Psychol Med 1981; 11(1):115–129.

59. Why do more boys than girls develop autism? National Autistic Society, 2003. Available at: http://www.nas.org.uk/nas/jsp/polopoly.jsp?d=1049&a=3370. Accessed August 30, 2007.

60. Scott FJ, Baron-Cohen S, Bolton P, et al. Brief report: prevalence of autism spectrum conditions in children aged 5-11 years in Cambridgeshire, UK. Autism 2002; 6(3): 231–237.

61. Attwood T, 2000. Asperger syndrome: some common questions: do girls have a different expression of the syndrome? Available at: www.asperger.org/asperger/asperger_questions.htm#girls. Accessed August 30, 2007.

62. Kopp S, Gillberg C. Girls with social deficits and learning problems: autism, atypical Asperger syndrome or a variant of these conditions. Eur Child Adolesc Psychiatry 1992; 1(2):89–99.

6

Screening Instruments for Asperger Syndrome[a]

Carrie Allison and Simon Baron-Cohen
*Autism Research Centre, Department of Psychiatry,
University of Cambridge, Cambridge, U.K.*

INTRODUCTION

Chapter 5 in this book addressed studies that have attempted to estimate the prevalence of Asperger Syndrome (AS). Some studies (1) used service records as the basis for their screen, while others (2) used instruments designed specifically for detecting risk for AS. In the United Kingdom, routine developmental screening is not carried out, which contrasts to the United States, where this has been recommended. This includes identifying possible symptoms of Autism Spectrum Conditions (ASC) which may warrant further investigation (3). It is likely that prospective screening, rather than case-note finding of those already diagnosed with AS would generate higher prevalence estimates.

There are a number of screening instruments that specifically aim to detect AS, although these are generally for use with older children and adults. Primarily, they are used to differentiate AS from other language and developmental disorders as well as other ASC. Typically, screening tools for AS that are currently available focus on children from approximately four years of age and concentrate on social and communicative behavior, as well as repetitive behaviors and circumscribed

---

[a]See our other chapter in this volume for a note on the terminology of Asperger Syndrome vs. Asperger's Disorder.

interests since these behaviors do not often present until around age four to five (4). Campbell (5) provides a useful summary of screening tools for AS, a summary of which follows in this chapter. One drawback with many screening instruments is that by screening the whole population and not just those at risk may cause unnecessary anxiety in individuals, and conversely creating a false sense of security when in fact the individual is at risk. Therefore, it is important that the psychometric properties of each screening instrument are evaluated prior to the screen being implemented. These include the *sensitivity* (which refers to the number of children detected by the screen to be at risk from having the condition), the *specificity* (the number of children without the condition who are identified not to be at risk from having the condition), and the *positive predictive value* (the number of children who are identified to be at risk by the screen who do have the condition). Glascoe (6) recommended that a screen has acceptable properties if the sensitivity is higher than 0.80 and the specificity is between 0.80 and 0.90.

ASPERGER SYNDROME DIAGNOSTIC SCALE

The Asperger Syndrome Diagnostic Scale (ASDS) (7) is a 50-item dichotomous questionnaire that can be completed by a range of informants, including parents, teachers and, psychologists. It is aimed at individuals between the ages of 5 and 18 years and covers the following five areas of behavior, namely, cognitive, maladaptive, language, social, and sensorimotor skills. The authors report that the items were selected on the basis of the Diagnostic and Statistical Manual of Mental Disorders IV (DSM-IV) (8) criteria and a review of the literature. The utility of the questionnaire was assessed using a small sample of 115 individuals with a diagnosis of AS recruited through mailings to teachers and parents. Raw scores on each item are summed across each of the five domains of interest, yielding five subscale scores, and an overall Asperger Syndrome Quotient (ASQ) score is obtained by summing the scores from the entire scale. Data indicated that this is a reliable scale suggested by a high Cronbach's alpha (0.83) and inter-rater reliability (0.93).

In the validation phase, the authors report that the ASQ total score correctly classified 85% of children across different clinical groups, including AS, autistic disorder, attention-deficit hyperactivity disorder (ADHD), and learning disability. However, data have not been reported regarding the sensitivity, specificity and positive predictive value of this instrument, or the cognitive functioning of each subgroup.

In a review by Goldstein (9), several concerns were raised about this instrument. First, given that the instrument was largely based on DSM-IV criteria, suggesting that the questionnaire would merely confirm diagnosis rather than screen for it per se, and therefore negate the need for a screening questionnaire, since scores on a questionnaire that is based on diagnostic criteria would be high for an individual who has a diagnosis. Second, concerns regarding differential diagnosis were raised. Goldstein (9) argued that most of the symptoms examined on the ASDS are present not exclusively in AS, but also autistic disorder, and therefore the screen is not suitable for discriminating between the subtypes on the autistic spectrum. Third, no data on positive and negative predictive value have been presented which is crucial when reviewing the utility of a screen in clinical practice. Fourth, no confirmation of diagnosis was sought once the participants in the normative sample had been recruited, and therefore it is possible that these individuals may have met criteria for high-functioning autism or other disorders. Lastly, no information was given regarding the cognitive ability in the validation samples. The greatest difference between the groups was in the cognitive and language samples as 80% of children diagnosed with autism also have comorbid mental retardation (5). If the autism group displayed cognitive impairment then the utility of the ASDS in differentiating between AS and autism is diminished, since the two samples are not directly comparable.

AUTISM SPECTRUM-SCREENING QUESTIONNAIRE

The autism spectrum-screening questionnaire (ASSQ) (10) consists of 27 behavioral descriptions of symptoms that are characteristic of AS in children and adolescents with normal intelligence or mild mental retardation aged between 7 and 16 years. This screening tool is the one that has been used most frequently in non-case register prevalence studies of AS. Items were selected by the authors on the basis of clinical experience. The behaviors covered by the questionnaire include social interaction, communication, restricted and repetitive interests, and motor clumsiness. Each behavior is rated as being not present, somewhat present or definitely present, each rating scoring 0, 1, and 2, respectively. The items are summed to yield a total raw score, which ranges from 0 to 54. Reliability and validity were assessed in two samples within a clinical population, one of which consisted of 110 children who were referred to a clinic with a variety of autism spectrum diagnoses, attention-deficit disorder (ADD) and learning disability, and the other sample comprised 34 children who had a diagnosis of AS. This screening questionnaire was used in epidemiological studies by Ehlers and Gillberg (2) and Mattila et al. (11), discussed earlier in Chapter 5. Cutoffs for parent-rated and teacher-rated questionnaires are set at 19 and 22, respectively.

This test has been shown to have good test-retest reliability for total ASSQ score with an eight-month interval between test administrations in an epidemiological sample, and for parent and teacher ratings in the clinical samples (0.94 and 0.96, respectively). No data on internal consistency has been provided for this instrument. Scores on the questionnaire for each clinical group (ASD, ADHD, etc.) differed significantly, and mean scores from the AS group were reported to be similar to the mean scores from the ASD subsample, although no data were provided. The ASSQ showed good specificity for identifying cases other than AS (0.90 for parent report ASSQ and 0.91 for teacher report ASSQ), but poor sensitivity in correctly classifying the AS cases (0.62–0.82 across the main clinic sample and the AS validated sample for parent report ASSQ, and 0.65–0.70 for teacher report ASSQ). This screen does show promising psychometric properties, although both internal consistency and positive predictive value data are missing. However, as the authors of this paper note, the data do not indicate that this instrument is able to distinguish between AS and other high-functioning ASC (10). Further, to date no data have been reported on the test accuracy when applied to a general population sample.

CHILDHOOD ASPERGER SYNDROME TEST

The Childhood Asperger Syndrome Test (12) (CAST) is a 37-item parental self-completion questionnaire, designed specifically to screen for AS in primary school–age children (4–11). Behaviors are scored on a dichotomous scale, being present or absent, either of which 31 are concerned with behaviors characteristic of AS. There are six filler items that sample general developmental behavior and do not contribute to the total score. Items on the CAST were selected from reviewing DSM-IV (8) and ICD-10 (13) diagnostic manuals, items from the ASSQ (10) and the Pervasive Developmental Disorders Questionnaire (PDD-Q) (14), and choosing items that were characteristic features of the core autistic spectrum.

Initially, it was piloted with 13 children who had a diagnosis of AS as well as 37 typically developing children (12). All ($N = 13$) children with a diagnosis of AS scored above 15, which is the score that indicates that a child needs further evaluation, and typically developing children scored significantly lower than the group with AS. In the validation phase (15), 500 CAST questionnaires were received from a mainstream school population. Sensitivity was 100% and specificity was 97%, indicating excellent test properties. However, positive predictive value of this instrument was moderate at only 50% (although this is expected with a condition that has a low population prevalence) (15,16). No data regarding inter-rater reliability has been published, but the screen shows moderate to good test-retest reliability (17,18), indicated by correlations of 0.67 and 0.83, respectively (Spearman's Rho). Campbell (5) points out that it is not clear whether this instrument exclusively identifies AS or whether the original AS sample contained children with other diagnoses within the autistic spectrum. Further data have been collected in a larger sample with a more diverse population, but results have not yet been published.

GILLIAM ASPERGER SYNDROME SCALE

The Gilliam Asperger Syndrome Scale (GADS) (19) is a 32-item rating scale covering four domains of behavior that may be indicative of AS. The subscales include social interaction, restricted patterns of behavior, cognitive patterns, and pragmatic skills. Raw scores across each domain are summed to yield domain scaled scores, which are then added together to generate an ASQ, which indicates the probability of AS in the individual. There is also a parent interview form that enquires about the presence or absence of delays in cognitive and language development, curiosity about the environment and adaptive behavior, although this does not contribute to the ASQ. Items on the GADS were selected on the basis of reviews from the literature, the diagnostic manuals [DSM-IV-TR (20) and ICD-10 (13)], as well as other screening instruments including the ASSQ (10). The GADS was initially administered to over 350 individuals with a diagnosis of AS whose age range was between 3 and 22. Using this sample, Cronbach's alpha for the GADS total score was 0.87. Test-retest reliability was reported to range from 0.71–0.77 across each subscale. This screen was able to discriminate between AS and children diagnosed with other conditions, such as ADHD, mental retardation, and a group of children with autism. However, no data regarding the sensitivity, specificity nor positive predictive value have been reported. While this test holds promise, it has not been tested at a population level, and the diagnoses in the validation sample were not verified, therefore raising questions about using this group as a validation sample (21).

KRUG ASPERGER SYNDROME INDEX

The Krug Asperger Disorder Index (KADI) (22) is a 32-item questionnaire that enquires about the presence or absence of behaviors that may be indicative of AS. The questionnaire is in two parts, the first 11 questions are used as a screen for AS, while the remaining items contribute to the total KADI score. There are two versions of the questionnaire; the first version is appropriate for children between the ages of 6 and 11, while the second version is appropriate for individuals between the ages of 12 and 21. If an individual does not score above 18 on the initial 11 screening questions, the rest of the questionnaire is not completed. The KADI was initially tested on three groups. First, a group of 130 individuals diagnosed with AS. Second, a group of 162 individuals diagnosed with autism, and finally, a group of 194 typically developing individuals. Individual items were weighted depending on how related each item was to diagnostic status. Results from this validation sample indicated that Cronbach's alpha was 0.93 for the total KADI score, sensitivity and specificity were 0.78 and 0.94, respectively; and positive predictive value was 0.83. Further, the KADI was able to discriminate between all three groups. Again, this instrument holds promise and may warrant a prospective screening study to properly evaluate the test properties, but there are a number of limitations. First, no verification of diagnosis was sought in the validation sample. Second, the relationship between cognitive ability and score is unknown, which is particularly relevant when constructing a test that aims to distinguish AS from other ASC. Finally, the majority of informants in each group in the validation of this instrument were relatives, and no data are currently available regarding how effective this screen could be if completed by teachers or other informants (despite the manual suggesting that teachers were appropriate raters).

ADULT SCREENING FOR ASPERGER SYNDROME

Diagnosing AS is often delayed into late childhood, and sometimes early adulthood (23), because of the nature of the difficulties with diagnosis of this condition. The most widely used diagnostic instrument for AS is the Autism Diagnostic Interview-Revised (ADI-R), although there is currently no available algorithm for diagnosing AS specifically. The development of screening questionnaires for AS is important, since many individuals are missed by the relevant health service throughout childhood, and go on to experience additional difficulties, such as anxiety and depression (24,25). Since diagnostic interviews entail an extensive process not only involving the individual but also an informant, it is critical that only those who are highly suspected to have AS are put forward for this thorough assessment. Further, as outlined earlier in Chapter 5, AS was not added into diagnostic manuals until relatively recently, implying that there may be many adult cases of AS that have not been formally diagnosed.

Only two efforts at designing screening tools for adults with AS have been published to date. The first is the Australian Scale for Asperger Syndrome (ASAS) (26). This questionnaire is a 25-item questionnaire, designed to be rated by a clinician. One of the major drawbacks about this questionnaire is the lack of clear scoring criteria (27). Further, to date no research has reported the psychometric properties of this instrument. The other, the Autism Spectrum Quotient (AQ) [Baron-Cohen et al. (28)], is a 50-item forced choice self-report screening questionnaire for adults that aims to identify and quantify autistic traits. This questionnaire was designed with the notion of ASC being continuously distributed (29,30), and therefore it may be more appropriate to use a quantitative rather than a categorical approach to screening and eventual diagnosis. The questions assess five domains, namely social skills, attention switching, attention to detail, communication, and imagination. In a preliminary study, 80% of adults with AS scored above a critical minimum of 32, compared with 2% of control adults (28). Test-retest reliability and inter-rater reliability were high. Another study that used the AQ showed very similar results in Japan, indicating that it produces consistent results cross-culturally (31). Further, Bishop et al. (32) found that parents of a child with an autism spectrum condition scored higher on the AQ than controls on two of the subscales.

A study by Woodbury-Smith et al. (27) examined AQ scores from 100 referrals to a national clinic in the United Kingdom who had suspected AS, in order to be able to assess whether the AQ could distinguish between those who received a diagnosis, and those who did not. Results showed a highly significant difference in the scores of those who went on to receive a diagnosis of AS and those who did not. In fact, for this referred clinic sample, the authors recommend that a cut-point of 26 should be employed, as this led to 83% of patients being correctly classified. At this cut-point, the sensitivity is 0.95, specificity 0.52, and positive predictive value is 0.84. These results suggest that the AQ may be an important screening tool for AS in adults for the purposes of referral to clinics as well as being quick and reliable to administer.

It is important to point out that there may be individuals in the general population who have a high AQ score but who do not warrant any clinical support, and this may be dependent on environmental factors (job satisfaction, tolerance by a partner) rather than individual characteristics that need to be systematically evaluated (27). Of particular note in this study was that 75% of patients had been referred by their general practitioner (GP) to the clinic. With an increased awareness regarding AS, it is likely in the years to come that more GPs will be asked by their patients to refer them to a specialist, and the AQ may be a valuable tool for the GP in deciding who to refer onward.

SUMMARY

Several screening tools have been developed that aim to identify risk for Asperger syndrome in the population. Two instruments cited in this chapter (the ASSQ and the CAST) have been used in research estimating the prevalence of AS (2,11) and ASC[b] (33), while the rest (including the AQ that is specifically designed for use with adults) have not yet been validated in a general population sample.

CONCLUSIONS

There are a number of screening tools available for AS designed for use in the general population and in clinical practice settings. Charman and Baron-Cohen (34) raise the question of what criteria should be set for acceptable levels of sensitivity, specificity, and positive predictive value for a screening test. They suggest that indices of test accuracy are likely to be higher in a referred rather than a population sample. If such tools are used in studies that aim to estimate prevalence of AS, it is important that the cut-point is set accurately in order that they "catch" all potential cases, without identifying too many individuals as potential cases who do not have the condition. Currently, screening tools for AS may be most useful in clinical settings to determine the likelihood of any individual falling on the higher functioning end of the autistic spectrum who warrants further, more detailed, assessment. However, as we highlighted in our previous chapter, regardless of whether these are used in prevalence research or in clinical practice, there is a need for the diagnostic criteria for AS to be revised and delineated. As Howlin (25) points out, without satisfactory diagnostic criteria, any attempt to develop both screening and diagnostic tools for AS may be futile.

ACKNOWLEDGMENTS

CA and SBC were supported by the Big Lottery and the MRC during the period of this work. We are grateful to Carol Brayne, Jo Williams, and Fiona Matthews for valuable discussions.

---

[b]A study by Scott et al. (32) used the CAST to estimate the prevalence of ASC in a general population, but did not report prevalence estimates for AS.

REFERENCES

1. Taylor B, Miller E, Farrington CP, et al. Autism and measles, mumps, and rubella vaccine: no epidemiological evidence for a causal association. Lancet 1999; 353(9169): 2026–2029.
2. Ehlers S, Gillberg C. The epidemiology of Asperger syndrome. A total population study. J Child Psychol Psychiatry 1993; 34(8):1327–1350.
3. Filipek PA, Accardo PJ, Ashwal S, et al. Practice parameter: screening and diagnosis of autism: report of the Quality Standards Subcommittee of the American Academy of Neurology and the Child Neurology Society. Neurology 2000; 55(4):468–479.
4. Shao Y, Cuccaro ML, Hauser ER, et al. Fine mapping of autistic disorder to chromosome 15q11-q13 by use of phenotypic subtypes. Am J Hum Genet 2003; 72(3): 539–548.
5. Campbell JM. Diagnostic assessment of Asperger's disorder: a review of five third-party rating scales. J Autism Dev Disord 2005; 35(1):25–35.
6. Glascoe FP. Developmental screening: rationale, methods, and application. Infants Young Child 1991; 4:1–10.
7. Myles B, Bock S, Simpson R. Asperger Syndrome Diagnosis Scale. Los Angeles, California: Western Psychological Services, 2001.
8. American Psychiatric Association. Diagnostic and Statistical Manual of Mental Disorders (DSM-IV). 4th ed. Washington, DC: APA, 1994.
9. Goldstein S. Review of the Asperger Syndrome Diagnostic Scale. J Autism Dev Disord 2002; 32(6):611–614.
10. Ehlers S, Gillberg C, Wing L. A screening questionnaire for Asperger syndrome and other high-functioning autism spectrum disorders in school age children. J Autism Dev Disord 1999; 29(2):129–141.
11. Mattila ML, Kielinen M, Jussila K, et al. An epidemiological and diagnostic study of asperger syndrome according to four sets of diagnostic criteria. J Am Acad Child Adolesc Psychiatry 2007; 46(5):636–646.
12. Scott FJ, Baron-Cohen S, Bolton P, et al. The CAST (Childhood Asperger Syndrome Test): preliminary development of a UK screen for mainstream primary-school-age children. Autism 2002; 6(1):9–31.
13. World Health Organisation. The ICD-10 Classification of Mental and Behavioural Disorders: Diagnostic Criteria for Research. Geneva: WHO, 1993.
14. Baird G, Charman T, Baron-Cohen S, et al. A screening instrument for autism at 18 months of age: a 6-year follow-up study. J Am Acad Child Adolesc Psychiatry 2000; 39(6):694–702.
15. Williams J, Scott F, Stott C, et al. The CAST (Childhood Asperger Syndrome Test): test accuracy. Autism 2005; 9(1):45–68.
16. O'Toole BI. Screening for low prevalence disorders. Aust N Z J Psychiatry 2000; 34(suppl):S39–S46.
17. Allison C, Williams J, Scott F, et al. The Childhood Asperger Syndrome Test (CAST): test-retest reliability in a high scoring sample. Autism 2007; 11(2):173–185.
18. Williams J, Allison C, Scott F, et al. The Childhood Asperger Syndrome Test (CAST): test-retest reliability. Autism 2006; 10(4):415–427.
19. Gilliam J. Gilliam Asperger's Disorder Scale. Austin, Texas: Pro-Ed Inc, 2001.
20. American Psychiatric Association. Diagnostic and Statistical Manual of Mental Disorders (DSM-IV) -Text Revision. 4th ed. Washington, DC: APA, 2000:69–84.

21. Campbell J. Diagnostic Assessment of Asperger's Disorder: a review of five Third-Party Rating Scales. Jl Autism Dev Disord 2005; 35(1):25–35.
22. Krug D, Arick J. Krug's Asperger's Disorder Index. Austin, Texas: Pro-Ed Inc., 2003.
23. Barnard J, Harvey V, Prior A, et al. Ignored or ineligible? The reality for adults with autistic spectrum disorders. London: National Autistic Society, 2001.
24. Tonge B, Brereton A, Gray K, et al. Behavioural and emotional disturbance in high functioning autism and Asperger syndrome. Autism 1999; 3:117–130.
25. Howlin P. Assessment instruments for Asperger Syndrome. J Child Psychol Psychiatry Rev 2000; 5:120–129.
26. Garnett M, Attwood A. Australian Scale for Asperger's Syndrome. In: Attwood T, ed. Asperger's syndrome: a guide for parents and professionals. London: Jessica Kingsley, 1998:17–20.
27. Woodbury-Smith MR, Robinson J, Wheelwright S, et al. Screening adults for Asperger syndrome using the AQ: a preliminary study of its diagnostic validity in clinical practice. J Autism Dev Disord 2005; 35(3):331–335.
28. Baron-Cohen S, Wheelwright S, Skinner R, et al. The autism-spectrum quotient (AQ): evidence from Asperger syndrome/high-functioning autism, males and females, scientists and mathematicians. J Autism Dev Disord 2001; 31(1):5–17.
29. Constantino JN, Lajonchere C, Lutz M, et al. Autistic social impairment in the siblings of children with pervasive developmental disorders. Am J Psychiatry 2006; 163(2):294–296.
30. Constantino JN, Todd RD. Autistic traits in the general population: a twin study. Arch Gen Psychiatry 2003; 60(5):524–530.
31. Wakabayashi A, Baron-Cohen S, Wheelwright S, et al. The Autism-Spectrum Quotient (AQ) in Japan: a cross-cultural comparison. J Autism Dev Disord 2006; 36(2):263–270.
32. Bishop DVM, Maybery M, Maley A, et al. Using self-report to identify the broad phenotype in parents of children with autistic spectrum disorders: a study using the Autism-Spectrum Quotient. J Child Psychol Psychiatry 2004; 45(8):1431–1436.
33. Scott FJ, Baron-Cohen S, Bolton P, F. Brief report: prevalence of autism spectrum conditions in children aged 5–11 years in Cambridgeshire, UK. Autism 2002; 6(3): 231–237.
34. Charman T, Baron-Cohen S. Screening for autism spectrum disorders in populations: progress, challenges and questions for future research and practice. In: Charman T, Stone W, eds. Social-Communicative Development in Toddlers and Preschoolers with Autism Spectrum Disorders: Implications for Early Identification, Diagnosis, and Intervention. New York: Guilford Press, 2007.

7

Neuropsychology in Asperger's Disorder

L. Stephen Miller

Clinical Psychology Program; Bio-Imaging Research Center; and
Neuropsychology and Memory Assessment Laboratory,
Department of Psychology, University of Georgia, Athens, Georgia, U.S.A.

Fayeza S. Ahmed

Department of Psychology, University of Georgia, Athens, Georgia, U.S.A.

INTRODUCTION

The major symptoms of Asperger's Disorder per the *Diagnostic and Statistical Manual of Mental Disorders-Fourth Edition* (DSM-IV) are social difficulty and rigidity of behavior (1). This chapter will focus on the cognitive components of these symptoms. Topics discussed in this chapter are cognitive difficulties found in Asperger's disorder, how these relate to neurobiology, differential diagnosis based on cognition, and assessment.

COGNITIVE DEFICITS

Social Difficulty

Children with Asperger's disorder have a tendency to prefer solitary activities to engagement in social interactions with other children. This is thought to be due to their lack of understanding what other children think and want, thus making it difficult to successfully interact with them. By the time children with Asperger's disorder become teenagers, their social cognitive deficit becomes more problematic, as these years require a much more advanced understanding of peers (2).

One hurdle that impedes individuals with Asperger's disorder in successful social interaction is difficulty in interpreting faces (3). For example, Ashwin et al. (4) examined performance of participants with Asperger's disorder in an emotional Stroop task. A traditional Stroop task presents participants with a series of color words. Participants are asked to name the color that the word is printed in. In one condition, the color of the word and the actual word are the same, whereas in another condition the color and the word are incongruent. Participants demonstrate a longer response time to incongruent words. The emotional Stroop requires participants to identify the color while a neutral or emotional word is presented. Research indicates that most participants have a slower reaction time when nonneutral words are presented. Participants often show the greatest increase in reaction time when the stimulus is perceived as threatening or is perceived as germane to their lives. In the study by Ashwin et al. (4), there were three categories of stimuli: angry faces, neutral faces, and nonface stimuli. Controls demonstrated an expected attentional bias toward the threatening versus nonthreatening stimuli, while participants with Asperger's disorder demonstrated biases toward both threatening and neutral faces versus nonface stimuli. The results indicate that perhaps people with Asperger's disorder attend to faces in general as a result of greater difficulty interpreting them.

A major model of the social deficits found in Asperger's disorder is that they have deficient theory of mind capabilities (5), performing poorly on a variety of theory of mind tasks (6–10). While theory of mind was first introduced by a study on chimpanzees and their ability to understand purpose in an actor (11), the concept currently refers to the ability to infer mental states of another person. A traditional test of theory of mind is the Sally-and-Anne test in which participants view the following scenario. Anne hides an object and leaves the room and, while she is gone, Sally comes into the room and moves the hidden object to another location. Participants are asked where Anne will look for the object when she returns to the room. This requires an ability to infer Anne's mental state and conclude that Anne is unaware that Sally has moved the object (12). According to Baron-Cohen (13), theory of mind appears to be more of a cognitive domain than an affective domain because it involves more than simply recognizing an emotion in another person. Specifically, it requires one to make an inference not only about emotion but of thoughts and beliefs as well (13).

Flavell (14) reviewed several theories of the development of theory of mind. The simulation theory postulates that children develop theory of mind because they understand their own beliefs, desires, and thoughts; they then extend their understanding of their own mental realm to other people's mental states. The modularity theory proposes that theory of mind is systematically acquired as a result of neurological development. Children first develop a theory of body by age one year, in which they understand that others are driven to actions by *something*. Next (still during age 1 year), children develop theory of mind mechanism 1, which leads them to comprehend that people's actions are the result of fulfilling a need. Finally, theory of mind mechanism 2 occurs at age two years and allows children to understand that other people have their own attitudes (called "propositional attitudes"). Another theory of theory of mind (called the theory theory) postulates that it is a "framework" that is affected by the child's experiences (14).

Brüne and Brüne-Cohrs (12) described the developmental stages of theory of mind in further detail, in which theory of mind complexity increases with age. The first stage occurs during age one year, in which the infant develops joint attention, the ability to mentalize one's own perception, that of another person, and of an object. The second stage occurs between ages 14 and 18 months, when the child begins to understand that there is a connection with another person's mood and their goal (12). The next stage is referred to as decoupling (or pretend play), which occurs at ages 18 to 24 months (12,15). By ages four to six years, children are generally able to comprehend false beliefs (16), although there has been some conflicting evidence (17,18). By ages six to seven years, the child begins to comprehend irony. By ages 9 to 11 years, the child is able to understand the most complex of social interactions: the faux pas. A faux pas is when a person utters an inappropriate comment without understanding its inappropriateness. The ability to comprehend that a faux pas has occurred requires a person to infer the mental state of *two* individuals at the same time; namely, that of the person who utters the faux pas and of the person who feels hurt or upset by the inappropriate comment (12,19). As one can see, the development of theory of mind begins in the first year of life, with the construct of joint attention. At the arrival of each stage, it evolves, increasing in complexity, and finally resulting in the ability to infer multiple mental states in others.

It has been found that certain clinical populations lack theory of mind abilities. For example, children with autism spectrum disorders perform poorly in theory of mind tasks (6–10). Individuals with Asperger's disorder have also been found to perform poorly in tasks requiring the understanding of a faux pas (19). Theory of mind deficits have been associated with individuals with schizophrenia (12,20). Furthermore, preliminary studies have found deficits in individuals with dementia and bipolar disorder (12,21–23).

Theory of mind is important to evaluate because of its impact on a wide range of areas, particularly social interaction. Most of what one does has a social component, and every day one is faced with interacting with others. For example, in school students have to interact with their peers and with the instructor. The instructor, in turn, needs to effectively interact with the students. A common task, such as a group project, demands the mastery of social skills to be an effective member of the group. The person needs the ability to listen to ideas from other group members and compromise with them, and they need to understand the group members' desires, thoughts, and beliefs to compromise. Finding and maintaining friends and significant others also require the successful use of social skills. Employment is another social realm in which one has to interact well with others, such as coworkers and supervisors. Generally, for successful social interaction, a person needs to be able to take the perspective of the other person.

Rigidity

Rigidity is defined in the DSM-IV as, "Restricted repetitive and stereotyped patterns of behavior, interests and activities ..." (1). An area of rigidity, as it applies to cognition in Asperger's disorder, involves circumscribed interests. Individuals with Asperger's disorder often develop specific areas of interest. They may then devote a significant portion of time trying to master every aspect of that topic. Circumscribed interests are not limited to childhood. In fact, individuals with Asperger's disorder continue to focus on specific areas of interest all their lives, sometimes gaining a tremendous knowledge base about them (24). The rigidity of maintaining very specific areas of interest also affects socialization, as others may not be amenable to listening to the details surrounding an individual's circumscribed interests (25). However, circumscribed interests can also be helpful, for example when mastery of a specific topic leads to a successful career in a related field. Circumscribed interests also involve repetition of learned facts about the specific topic. It may be a method of reducing anxiety, as rehearsal of these facts tends to increase with an increased level of anxiety (26).

COGNITIVE ASPECTS AS RELATED TO NEUROBIOLOGY

Executive Function

It has been theorized that executive function deficits may account for autistic symptomology (5,27). Broadly, executive function refers to "those capacities that enable a person to engage successfully in purposive, self-serving behavior" (28).

The prefrontal cortex has long been implicated in the control of executive function (29). Study of the frontal lobes began in earnest in 1848 with Phineas Gage's infamous accident damaging the frontal lobes, resulting in an extreme change in behavior (30).

There is still a significant debate as to what constitutes all of the components of executive function, as there are several models describing the nature of executive function and the specific domains associated with it (31). However, the same underlying principle occurs in most models. Namely, that executive function comprises those processes necessary to completely solve and implement a task (32).

The memory literature was one of the first areas to develop a theory of what is essentially executive function. Baddeley (33) and Baddeley and Hitch (34) first challenged the accepted model of short-term memory by proposing a model for consisting of three components (phonological loop, visuospatial sketchpad, and the central executive), collectively called working memory. Working memory refers to the ability to maintain and manipulate information mentally and is thought to be a primary executive capacity.

According to Lezak et al. (28), executive function can be conceptualized as having *four* domains: volition, planning, purposive action, and effective performance. Volition represents an individual's ability to formulate and execute behavior with intent. Planning refers to the ability to decide which actions are necessary to reach a goal. To move from the planning stage to actually executing the steps is the domain of purposive action. Finally, while executing behavior, there is a need to make sure that one is correctly carrying out the steps. The responsibility of this function is in the domain of effective performance.

In a recent attempt to identify the domains of executive function, a factor-analytic study examining 104 participants with traumatic brain injury found three factors that explained 52.7% of the variance: cognitive flexibility and fluency, working memory, and inhibition (35).

The cognitive-process approach does not try to identify separate domains. Instead it identifies the various skills that are required to successfully implement what are considered traditional domains of executive function. Traditional executive function tests typically yield only one score, usually representing an aggregate of a complex set of components of executive function. The cognitive-process approach derives multiple scores assumed to represent component processes as well as a "primary" executive function. Delis et al. (36) have espoused this approach. Unlike traditional executive function measures, this approach, exemplified in the Delis-Kaplan Executive Function System (D-KEFS) (explanation below) breaks down the various skills measured. This provides evidence as to the reason why a participant may have performed poorly on a primary executive function task (37). Primary executive functions identified by Delis et al. (36) are (*i*) cognitive flexibility, (*ii*) verbal fluency, (*iii*) design fluency, (*iv*) inhibition, (*v*) problem solving, (*vi*) categorical processing, (*vii*) deductive reasoning, (*viii*) spatial planning, and (*ix*) verbal abstraction. Cognitive flexibility refers to the ability to quickly adapt to new rules and concepts. Both verbal fluency and design fluency refer to the ability to generate unique constructions in the verbal and visuospatial modalities. The definition of inhibition is the ability to hold back one's automatic response for the correct one. Problem solving refers to the ability to execute behavior to successfully complete a task. Categorical processing is defined as the ability to organize information in systematic ways. Deductive reasoning refers to the ability to use given clues to learn something new. The definition of spatial planning is the ability to organize the steps needed to solve a visuospatially presented problem. Finally, verbal abstraction refers to the ability to comprehend statements beyond literal meaning (36). The advantage of the approach by Delis et al. is that they take a conservative, atheoretical approach to executive function, as prescribing to a specific theoretical approach for this complex set of processes appears premature (37).

Executive Function Vs. Theory of Mind

Individuals with autism and Asperger's disorder demonstrate poor performance in a number of traditional executive function tasks: Trail Making test, Tower of Hanoi, and Wisconsin Card Sort, all of which test executive functions (38). It has been argued that it may be wiser to conceptualize autism as an executive function deficit rather than perceiving it on a more complex level of theory of mind. Specifically, tests that are aimed at measuring theory of mind abilities (see below) may be better described as measuring sets of executive function. For example, theory of mind tests require that participants maintain an instructional set. The theory of mind model can be broken down to core Executive Function deficits, since "action-monitoring requires self-monitoring, self-monitoring requires concept of self, and a *concept* of self requires a theory of mental life" (39). Just as theory of mind deficits have been found in individuals with Asperger's disorder (19), executive function deficits have also been exhibited. For example, Kleinhans et al. (38) conducted a study that suggests that individuals with Asperger's disorder show impairment in the areas of cognitive switching but not in inhibition (38).

Executive Function and Theory of Mind

According to Hodges (5), the executive function deficits that account for autistic symptomology are particularly related to poor performance on theory of mind tests. There have been several studies examining the relationship between executive function and theory of mind. Not all of these studies have found a link between the two (40–42).

Many other studies, however, *have* found a relationship. As previously noted, individuals with autism spectrum disorders have been found to be deficient in both theory of mind and executive function (6,43). In a review, Hughes and Graham (44) reported that not only do individuals with autism spectrum disorders have a deficit in both executive function and theory of mind but that the two constructs are related to each other. It is not surprising, therefore, that several additional studies have examined the relationship between executive function and theory of mind within the autism spectrum disorder population. For example, Fisher and Happé trained children with autism spectrum disorders in either theory of mind or executive functions. They found that the improvement of executive functions was positively associated with improvement in theory of mind (43). It, therefore, appears that there is a linear relationship between executive function and theory of mind. In yet another study with autistic children, researchers found that theory of mind performance was positively related to inhibition and working memory (45).

The relationship between executive function and theory of mind is not specific to children with autism spectrum disorders. It has been found in children with behavioral attentional problems, individuals with Parkinson's disease, and even cross-culturally in U.S. and Chinese normally developing preschoolers (46–49). Additionally, an age of onset for the association of the executive tasks of inhibition and working memory with theory of mind in normally developing children was found at over three years of age (50). While examining this association in normally developing children, multiple executive function components have been measured. However, which one of the executive function domains is the best predictor of theory of mind? There has been some research attempting to answer this question. Thus far, results indicate that inhibition may be the best predictor of theory of mind (51,52). Theoretically, the relationship between inhibition and theory of mind is a viable argument. For example, the definition of a faux pas is making an inappropriate comment without realizing the error. As previously stated, recognition of a faux pas requires theory of mind abilities. Thus, to prevent one from making countless faux pas, one is required to be able to both recognize the inappropriateness of a statement and *inhibit* its utterance. Given past literature, inhibition appears to be a predictor of theory of mind. Additionally, since cognitive flexibility refers to the ability to quickly adapt to new rules and concepts (36), it may be related to theory of mind because it requires an individual to maintain information about another person's thoughts, beliefs, and emotions (13). This means that a person would need to adapt to a different perspective than one's own viewpoint, which theoretically includes a cognitive flexibility component.

Studies examining the association between executive function and theory of mind in individuals with Asperger's disorder are lacking. This association has been found in the general autism spectrum disorder domain (44,45,53), and individuals with Asperger's disorder have shown deficits in both executive function and theory of mind (38). Therefore, it would appear that the executive function-theory of mind association would also be present in Asperger's disorder. Additional research on this topic is necessary to investigate this further.

DIFFERENTIAL DIAGNOSIS AS IT RELATES TO COGNITION

Differential diagnosis is difficult with Asperger's disorder. One of the major problems is that many children who are diagnosed with Asperger's disorder also meet criteria for autistic disorder (54). For example in a study by Tryon et al. (55), the researchers found that in a sample of children previously diagnosed with Asperger's disorder, the majority actually had a diagnosis of autistic disorder. The implication of this study is that clinicians may not be strictly adhering to the DSM-IV criteria when making a diagnosis of Asperger's disorder. The authors indicated that many clinicians diagnose Asperger's disorder if the child is presenting with symptoms of autism with the absence of cognitive and language developmental delays. However, the DSM-IV criteria do not define Asperger's disorder in this exact manner (1). Eisenmajer et al. (56) also stipulated that clinicians may be diagnosing Asperger's disorder on criteria that are not outlined in the DSM-IV. Specifically, factors such as desire for social interaction, lecture-style speech, and a *decreased* chance of a communicative developmental delay are associated with a diagnosis of Asperger's disorder. Sciutto and Cantwell (54) argue that the DSM-IV overlooks the fact that language delays can be present in individuals with Asperger's disorder. Furthermore, the DSM-IV symptom criteria state that both Asperger's and autistic disorder individuals have restrictive behavioral patterns. However, the type of pattern is different between Asperger's and autistic disorder. Specifically, individuals with Asperger's disorder have more circumscribed interests on a specific subject, whereas individuals with autistic disorder have interests that deal with a fixation with object manipulation. The DSM-IV also does not recognize a difference in social interaction deficits between autistic and Asperger's disorder; it merely states that there is a difficulty within this domain. However, individuals with Asperger's disorder tend to yearn for social involvement compared with those with autistic disorder. These differences have been addressed in the differential diagnosis section of the DSM-IV-TR (1), but the criteria themselves do not reflect this. Sciutto and Cantwell (54) found that when clinicians evaluate children who meet criteria for autistic disorder but are on the high-functioning end, they tend to focus not only on the DSM-IV criteria (e.g., presence of a developmental delay in language) but also on cognitive ability, social desire, and not necessarily if there is an absence of the language delay.

It can be seen from the above discussion that there is a dilemma on whether or not Asperger's disorder and those with high-functioning autism (HFA) actually differ (57). What is the difference between Asperger's disorder and HFA? They tend to be viewed as the same disorder; however, if they are two distinct disorders, then research on Asperger's disorder becomes vastly different. This is because several past studies have tended to group individuals with Asperger's disorder and HFA in the same group. If HFA and Asperger's disorder are different, then this creates sampling error in the research. One way to see if Asperger's disorder and HFA are truly different is to investigate if they have the same or different underlying, primary symptoms (57). However, there is some research indicating no difference (58). On the other hand, Verté et al. (27) state that a major distinction between individuals with Asperger's disorder and those with HFA is that language deficits are found in HFA but not in Asperger's disorder. However, the authors point out that although language development in HFA is delayed and normal in Asperger's disorder, individuals with Asperger's disorder still have a different language *style* when compared with nonclinical children. Specifically, they tend to have a pedantic style of speech. Additionally, individuals with HFA have more difficulty with the restrictive pattern of behavior, whereas those with Asperger's disorder's restrictiveness generally fall in the domain of circumscribed interests. Additionally, individuals with Asperger's disorder demonstrate better first- and second-order theory of mind abilities than those with HFA, but there is still disagreement about whether or not there is a difference between the two. Furthermore, it has been shown that individuals with Asperger's disorder have a higher Verbal IQ and lower Performance IQ compared with those with HFA. However, the results are varied about these nonspecific neuropsychological profiles. Verté et al. (27) studied the executive function profile of children with Asperger's disorder, HFA, and PDD-NOS. If there are true differences between Asperger's disorder and HFA, then their executive function profiles should have different patterns of deficit.

However, results indicated no difference between the executive function profiles of persons with Asperger's disorder or HFA.

The current literature does not have significantly concluding evidence on whether or not there are discrepant cognitive and neuropsychological contrasts between the two.

Thus, there is a need for further research into whether or not HFA and Asperger's disorder are truly different disorders.

ASSESSMENT TOOLS

Diagnostic Measures

Because there are behavioral similarities between autism and Asperger's disorder (59), and because autism should be ruled out if possible before providing a diagnosis of Asperger's disorder (60), it is important to understand autism diagnostic and screening measures. Chapter 6 reviews the Asperger Syndrome Diagnostic Scale (ASDS), the Asperger Spectrum Screening Questionnaire (ASSQ), and the Krug Asperger's Disorder Index (KADI). Further discussion of the Autism Diagnostic Interview—Revised (ADI-R) and the Childhood Autism Rating Scale (CARS) is provided herein.

Autism Diagnostic Interview—Revised

The ADI-R is revised from the ADI. It is a widely used, semistructured, standardized interview of caregivers aimed at assessing autism according to DSM-IV criteria. It measures three domains of symptoms: social deficits, repetitive and restrictive behaviors, and communicative deficiencies (61,62).

The ADI-R has demonstrated high interrater reliability across the majority of areas (with percentage agreement ranging 0.88–0.96) as well as good internal consistency ranging from 0.54 to 0.77. It has also been demonstrated that the ADI-R is consistent after a time delay. After two to three months of initial administration, a follow-up administration yielded results that were consistent 83% of the time (62).

The ADI-R also appears to be a valid measure for autism, as 25 out of 26 children who were previously diagnosed with autism met criteria for autism on the ADI-R (62). It has also correlated strongly with a measure of social responsiveness (61).

Currently, the ADI-R can only diagnose autistic disorder. However, researchers and clinicians are able to use it to gather information about the profile of deficits seen in their participant or client across the ADI-R's three domains (63). Studies examining the ability to diagnose Asperger's disorder using the ADI-R are limited. However, one study found that the ADI-R has poor sensitivity in diagnosing Asperger's disorder in toddlers (64). Thus, the limited amount of research and the lack of promise in current research indicate that the ADI-R may not be an appropriate assessment tool for Asperger's disorder.

Childhood Autism Rating Scale

The CARS is another frequently used assessment of autism based on observation and interaction of the individual. It assesses three domains: language and communication skills, socioeconomic and interactional skills, and response to sensory information (65). It comprises15 items that measure 15 components: activity level, intellectual inconsistency, general impression, verbal communication, nonverbal communication, visual response, auditory response, near-receptor response, anxiety, imitation, emotional response, body use, object use, relationships with people, and adaptation to change (66).

Although the CARS has demonstrated consistency with the ADI-R (65) as well as established the ability to screen for autism (66), it has not been found to be a sensitive measure for screening for Asperger's disorder (67,68). Similar to the ADI-R, research in the use of the CARS as a diagnostic tool for Asperger's disorder is limited, but preliminary studies (67,68) have found that it is unable to discriminate Asperger's disorder from other pervasive developmental disorders.

Executive Function Measures

Measurement of executive function is pertinent in an evaluation of Asperger's disorder because individuals with Asperger's disorder show deficits in specific Executive processes. However, they do not show an overall decreased executive capacity (38). To fully evaluate an individual with a question of Asperger's disorder, then, their executive function profiles should also be measured. Furthermore, because individuals with Asperger's disorder do not just display a general decrease in executive function (38), it is important to assess a profile rather than singular tests of executive function. For this reason, two comprehensive executive function batteries are highlighted in this section.

Delis-Kaplan Executive Function System

The D-KEFS is a comprehensive measure of executive function. The developers of the D-KEFS used traditional neuropsychological tests known to measure an executive function (most of which were developed in the 1940s), updated them, and normed them on a large, representative sample. As stated previously, The D-KEFS measures: (*i*) cognitive flexibility, (*ii*) verbal fluency, (*iii*) design fluency, (*iv*) inhibition, (*v*) categorization ability, (*vi*) deductive reasoning, (*vii*) spatial planning, and (*viii*) verbal abstraction (36) derived from nine specific subtests. These nine subtests yield multiple scores, allowing for the ability to examine basic underlying skills (e.g., color naming, reading, etc.) required to successfully complete a task requiring executive abilities.

The D-KEFS has both high ceilings and low floors to accommodate a large age range (8–89 years) (37). Furthermore, it is the first executive function battery to be normed on a large sample of 1750 children and adults who were matched to

U.S. demographics (37). The D-KEFS has demonstrated moderate reliability and validity. Internal consistency ranges from 0.33 to 0.90, while test-retest reliability ranges from 0.06 to 0.90. The D-KEFS validity has been supported primarily via intercorrelations among the D-KEFS subtests, ranging from -0.94 to 0.95 (36).

Because the D-KEFS is a comprehensive measure of executive function but includes theorized component processes (37), it is a promising method of assessing profile differences in individuals with Asperger's disorder (38). Research on the full executive function profile using the D-KEFS of individuals with Asperger's disorder is lacking. However, a promising study conducted by Dierst-Davies (69) examined the performance of individuals with Asperger's disorder on two subtests from the D-KEFS: the Sorting test and the Color-Word Interference test. Results indicated that individuals with Asperger's disorder had difficulty in inhibition and cognitive flexibility (69). While this is a promising study, a comprehensive examination of the executive function profile of Asperger's disorder needs to be used. Research is still lacking in this domain.

A Developmental Neuropsychological Assessment

Whereas the D-KEFS is an extensive assessment of executive function that can be used with people ages 8 to 89 years (37), the NEPSY is a measure of neuropsychological development, specifically in children. The age range is 3 to 12 years (70,71). It measures five areas of neuropsychological development: (*i*) attention/ executive functions, (*ii*) language, (*iii*) sensorimotor functions, (*iv*) visuospatial processing, and (*v*) memory and learning (70). Because the NEPSY was designed for children, it takes a developmental perspective in neuropsychological assessment. Namely, it assesses the degree to which children's performance adheres to normative neuropsychological development for their age (72).

The NEPSY was modeled after Luria's theory of cognition. This theory postulates that cognition is based on building blocks of various cognitive functions. Specifically, complex functions comprise basic subcomponents of cognitive functions. Therefore, any deficit in a basic function will be detrimental to its corresponding higher-order functions. The NEPSY measures both basic and complex functions, asserting that the success of one function is a result of the assistance of multiple domains.

A major strength about the NEPSY is that it is standardized on a single sample of 1000 children that had equal numbers of males and females and was ethnically representative of the United States from the 1995 census. Split-half reliabilities were calculated, with the exception of subtests in which this reliability calculation was not logical, in which case test-retest reliability was calculated. Reliability of the five domains ranged from 0.79 to 0.91. Interrater reliability ranged from 0.97 to 0.99. There is a need for further validity studies, as there have been moderate correlations between the NEPSY and other neuropsychological tests (72). A study conducted by Schmitt and Worich (73) examined three groups of children: group 1 had neurological disorders, group 2 had school-related difficulties, and group 3 were normal controls. They found group differences even with IQ controlled. However, differences were not always present at the subtest level. Researchers, therefore, concluded that the data suggest that the NEPSY appears to have the ability to differentiate among these groups and would, therefore, be appropriate to use when assessing neurological disorders and school-related difficulties.

Similar to the D-KEFS, research examining the NEPSY's relationship to Asperger's disorder is very limited. However, a study conducted by Matson (74) has examined NEPSY neuropsychological profiles of children with Asperger's disorder. The children exhibited decreased scores across all five core domains [i.e., (*i*) attention/executive functions, (*ii*) language, (*iii*) sensorimotor functions, (*iv*) visuospatial processing, and (*v*) memory and learning] relative to normal controls. In the attention/executive function domain, they exhibited particular difficulty in tasks that required sustained attention and also demonstrated difficulty in shifting attentional sets. Furthermore, tasks that included planning also were problematic for these children. The language domain, although decreased relative to matched controls, was still in the normative range. In the sensorimotor domain, children with Asperger's disorder showed marked difficulty in tasks that required fine motor skills (e.g., imitating hand gestures). In the visuospatial domain, the Asperger's group obtained scores lower than any group in the study, to which the author contributed to past information that children with Asperger's disorder obtain lower performance IQ scores compared with their Verbal IQ. Finally in the memory and learning domain, the children showed particular difficulty in tasks that required list learning and repetition, to which the author attributed to a decreased attentional capacity (74).

In one of the very few studies to do so, Matson also compared the performance of children with Asperger's disorder with those with HFA. Children in the HFA group came from the standardization method for the NEPSY (70,74). A full-scale IQ score of 80 was necessary to consider these children high functioning. The Asperger's disorder group was identified through a pediatric clinic, in which the children had already been diagnosed with Asperger's disorder by a "standard clinical examination" (74). Additionally, the children from this group were assessed for autism by adhering to the DSM-IV criteria for Asperger's disorder (74). As can be seen, there are potential pitfalls to the method of group assignment in this study, as it is not clear who and specifically how children with Asperger's disorder were diagnosed and differentiated from having autism. Results suggested a few subtests that differentiated the two groups, namely, "measures that had high demands for executive function (i.e., Verbal Fluency and Tower, both favoring AS)" (74). Thus, Matson's study shows promise regarding the potential use of the NEPSY in differentiating Asperger's disorder from HFA, as they were found to have different neuropsychological profiles. However, there is still a need for further investigation of the neuropsychological profiles of children with Asperger's disorder using the NEPSY.

Theory of Mind Measures

As previously discussed, theory of mind is the ability of an individual to infer the mental state of another, thus enabling the individual to understand the thoughts, beliefs, and actions of that other individual (12). Persons with Asperger's disorder have been consistently found to have deficits in theory of mind (6). Additionally, it is important to evaluate to what degree an individual has a theory of mind deficiency, as individuals with Asperger's disorder generally pass gross measures of theory of mind but not advanced measures (7,8). The following section explains four theory of mind tests, beginning with a basic measure of theory of mind to the most complex form of theory of mind test.

Sally-and-Anne Test

In a Sally-and-Anne test, participants observe two dolls (Sally and Anne). Sally puts a marble in a basket, and, after leaving, Anne hides the marble in a box. Participants are asked several control questions (i.e., correctly naming the dolls, where the marble is now hidden). They are also asked a crucial false belief question about where Sally will look for the marble upon her return. In a seminal article by Baron-Cohen et al. (6), children with autism were unable to infer the mental state of Sally. This is a very basic measure of theory of mind, and it has been found that individuals with Asperger's disorder can pass a basic measure such as this, thus potentially differentiating them from individuals with autism (8).

Strange Stories Test

The Strange Stories test was developed to be an advanced theory of mind test (8,75). An "advanced" test refers to a change from the traditional theory of mind tests, such as the Sally-and-Anne test, but continuing to measure the general idea of infering the mental state of another. The Strange Stories test was developed to be sensitive enough for those who pass gross measures of theory of mind but may still exhibit deficit. The original Strange Stories test consisted of 24 short stories that test the following areas: (*i*) contrary emotions, (*ii*) double bluff, (*iii*) sarcasm, (*iv*) white lie, (*v*) lie, (*vi*) pretend, (*vii*) joke, (*viii*) misunderstanding, (*ix*) appearance or reality, (*x*) persuade, (*xi*) forget, and (*xii*) figure of speech. In addition to these 24 stories, there are also six control stories, called "physical stories." In the physical stories, the participant does not have to infer a mental state in the character in the story. Each outcome in these control stories are the result of a physical cause. It was found that children and adolescents with Asperger's disorder with normal intelligence are able to correctly infer the physical states but perform poorly on inferring mental states relative to controls (8). This test has been used with children and adolescents. In addition to this, a revised version with fewer stories has also been found to be a sensitive measure of theory of mind in adults (8,75–78).

The various sets of the Strange Stories test have been shown to have good psychometric qualities. Interrater reliability for the scoring of participants' responses has been used in previous studies, and a strong interrater reliability has been found at 87% (76). The Strange Stories have demonstrated good validity as well. Since people with autism and autism spectrum disorders have been shown to have theory of mind deficits, differences in the Strange Stories scores should be seen between those with and without autism. These gross differences have been found in addition to subtle differences among autism participants. Specifically, differences have been found in severely autistic participants who normally fail first-order theory of mind tests and higher-functioning autistic participants who pass first order but fail second order (i.e., a more complex version of the Sally-and-Anne test). This shows a differences in the degree of ability to infer mental states of others (varying degrees of theory of mind) (8–10). The Strange Stories test thus may be useful in diffeentiating indivisuals with autism versus those with Asperger's disorder, as autistic individuals consistently perform worse than those with Asperger's disorder (75).

Reading the Mind in the Eyes Test

The Reading the Mind in the Eyes test (7) is conceptualized as a sensitive measure of theory of mind ability. Like the Strange Stories test, the Reading of the Mind in the Eyes test has also been developed as an advanced measure of theory of mind. It is noted for its ability to detect theory of mind deficits in high-functioning adults and those with HFA or Asperger's disorder (7). The test consists of 36 pictures of actors' eyes (Fig. 1). Next, the participant has to choose out of four possible answers the word that best reflects the mental state of the person in the picture. Each page has one picture of a set of eyes, and participants have to choose one of four answers that describes the person's emotion or thoughts. Participants are provided with a vocabulary list of all of the multiple-choice answers (3).

The revised version has better psychometric qualities than the original version. For example, normal performance is below ceiling after the revision. Therefore, there is a greater ability to differentiate HFA participants from normal

jealous   panicked

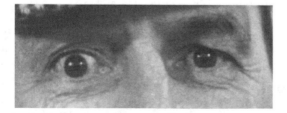

arrogant   hateful

Figure 1   Example from the Reading the Mind in the Eyes test.

Table 1 Example Item from the Faux Pas Test

"Jill had just moved into a new apartment. Jill went shopping and bought some new curtains for her bedroom. When she had finished decorating the apartment, her best friend, Lisa, came over. Jill gave her a tour of the apartment and asked, 'How do you like my bedroom?" "Those curtains are horrible," Lisa said. "I hope you're going to get some new ones!"

Source: From Ref. 79.

controls compared with the original. The validity of the Reading the Mind in the Eyes test is solid. Scores on the autism quotient and the Reading the Mind in the Eyes test were inversely correlated on the revised version ($r = -0.53$, $p = 0.004$), indicating greater severity of autism associated with poorer scores. This revised version was also designed for both normal adults and adults with HFA, thus making it a potential measure for subtle theory of mind deficits (3).

Faux Pas Test

The Faux Pas test (21,79) was also developed to be a sensitive measure of theory of mind deficits. Again, a faux pas occurs when a person says something that was not supposed to be said (based on social norms), thus resulting in hurt feelings (79). In the Faux Pas test, participants read a series of stories, half of which contain a faux pas. At the end of each story, participants have to answer if any character in the story said something inappropriate (Table 1). This test requires that a person recognize the occurrence of a faux pas, understand the mental state of the character who made the faux pas (i.e., that the character does not realize he/she made a faux pas), and recognize the mental state of the other character who may feel upset (21). Because of the complex nature of the construct being measured, good interrater reliability needs to be demonstrated. In a previous study, an interrater reliability of 0.98 was found (21). Furthermore, the Faux Pas test has shown good correlation with other theory of mind tests ($r = 0.76$) (21). The Faux Pas test, then, may be useful for evaluation of an individual with Asperger's disorder, given their relative difficulty in comprehension of a faux pas compared with peers (19).

CONCLUSION

Asperger's disorder remains a complex, misunderstood disorder. Part of the complexity arises from difficulty in determining appropriate differential diagnostic criteria between Asperger's disorder and HFA. There are several assessment tools, but the field of neuropsychology is still lacking in an appropriate measure for the assessment and diagnosis of Asperger's disorder. Overall, the field of Asperger's disorder will benefit from further research to arrive at consistent, conclusive profiles of individuals with Asperger's disorder.

In the meantime, results from promising research can be used to help clinicians understand the neuropsychological nature of difficulties found in individuals with Asperger's disorder. As previously stated, individuals with Asperger's disorder tend to pass first-order theory of mind tests, but not higher-order ones (8–10). Therefore, administering higher-order theory of mind tests (such as the Strange Stories test and Faux Pas test) along with tests that are considered sensitive measures of theory of mind deficits (such as the Reading the Mind in the Eyes test) may be beneficial as a potential clue to whether the individual is in the high-functioning end of the autism spectrum. Assessment of executive function deficits is yet another domain that should be examined. Thus far, a difficulty in cognitive switching has been implicated in individuals with HFA or Asperger's disorder. Furthermore, research has indicated that people with Asperger's disorder do not have general decreased executive functions (38). Therefore, it is helpful to examine their neuropsychological profile with measures such as the D-KEFS and NEPSY. There is limited research on the neuropsychological profiles specific to people with Asperger's disorder, but preliminary research indicates that tasks requiring inhibition, cognitive flexibility, sustained attention, planning, fine motor control, list learning, and construction received poorer performance in children with Asperger's disorder (69,74).

Differentiating between HFA and Asperger's disorder remains problematic (27,54,56–58). Nevertheless, there has been promising preliminary research with the NEPSY that suggests greater executive function performance in Asperger's disorder relative to HFA (i.e., Verbal Fluency and Tower, both favoring AS) (74).

Thus, a neuropsychological perspective of Asperger's disorder should include assessment of theory of mind and executive function. Taken individually, one is unlikely to be able to diagnose a person with Asperger's disorder. Collectively, however, assessment of all of these areas is helpful in understanding the nature of the presenting problems and to provide greater differential data.

REFERENCES

1. American Psychiatric Association. Diagnostic and Statistical Manual of Mental Disorders. 4th ed. Washington, DC: Author, 2000 (revision).
2. Ritvo ER. Understanding the nature of autism and Asperger's disorder. London, UK: Jessica Kingsley Publishers, 2006.
3. Baron-Cohen S, Wheelwright S, Hill J, et al. The "reading the mind in the eyes" test revised version: a study with normal adults, and adults with Asperger syndrome or high-functioning autism. J Child Psychol Psychiatry 2001; 42:241–251.
4. Ashwin C, Wheelwright S, Baron-Cohen S. Attention bias in faces in Asperger syndrome: a pictorial emotion stroop study. Psychoil Med 2006; 1–9.
5. Hodges S. A psychological perspective on theories of Asperger's syndrome. In: Rhode M, Klauber T, eds. The Many Faces of Asperger's Syndrome. London, UK: Karnac Books, 2004:39–53.
6. Baron-Cohen S, Leslie AM, Frith U. Does the autistic child have a "theory of mind"? Cognition 1985; 21:37–46.

7. Baron-Cohen S, Jolliffe T, Mortimore C, et al. Another advanced test of theory of mind: Evidence from very high functioning adults with autism or Asperger syndrome. J Child Psychol Psychiatry 1997; 38:813–822.
8. Happé FG. An advanced test of theory of mind: Understanding of story characters' thoughts and feelings by able autistic, mentally handicapped, and normal children and adults. J Autism Dev Disord 1994; 24:129–154.
9. Kaland N, Moller-Nielsen A, Callesen K, et al. A new 'advanced' test of theory of mind: evidence from children and adolescents with Asperger syndrome. J Child Psychol Psychiatry 2002; 43:517–528.
10. Gottlieb D. The strange stories test: A replication of children and adolescents with Asperger syndrome. Eur Child Adolesc Psychiatry 2005; 14:73–82.
11. Premack D, Woodruff G. Does the chimpanzee have a theory of mind? Behav Brain Sci 1978; 4:515–526.
12. Brüne M, Brüne-Cohrs U. Theory of mind- evolution, ontogeny, brain mechanisms and psychopathology. Neurosci Behav Rev, xx, 2005; 1–19.
13. Baron-Cohen S. Social and pragmatic deficits in autism: Cognitive or affective? J Autism Dev Disord 1988; 18:379–402.
14. Flavell JH. Cognitive development: Children's knowledge about the mind. Annu Rev Psychol 1999; 50:21–45.
15. Leslie AM. Pretense and representation: the origins of "theory of mind." Psychol Rev 1987; 94:412–426.
16. Wimmer H, Perner J. Beliefs about beliefs: Representation and constraining function of wrong beliefs in young children's understanding of deception. Cognition 1983; 13:103–128.
17. Cutting AL, Dunn J. Theory of mind, emotion understanding, language, and family background: Individual differenes and interrelations. Child Dev 1999; 70:853–865.
18. Moses LJ, Flavell JH. Inferring false beliefs from actions and reactions. Child Dev 1990; 61:929–945.
19. Baron-Cohen S, O'Riordan M, Stone V, et al. Recognition of faux pas by normally developing children and children with Asperger syndrome or high-functioning autism. J Autism Dev Disord 1999; 29:407–418.
20. Frith CD. The Cognitive Neuropsychology of Schizophrenia. Hove, UK: Lawrence Erlbaum Associates, 1992.
21. Gregory C, Lough S, Stone V, et al. Theory of mind in patients with frontal variant frontotemporal dementia and alzheimer's disease: theoretical and practical implications. Brain 2002; 125:752–764.
22. Inuoe Y, Tonooka Y, Yamada K, et al. Deficiency of theory of mind in patients with remitted mood disorder. J Affect Disord 2004; 82:403–409.
23. Kerr N, Dunbar RIM, Bentall RP. Theory of mind deficits in bipolar affective disorder. J Affect Disord 2003; 73:253–259.
24. Volkmar FR, Klin A. Diagnostic issues in Asperger syndrome. In: Klin A, Volkmar FR, Sparrow SS, eds. Asperger Syndrome. 2000:25–71.
25. Klin A, Volkmar FR. Treatment and intervention guidelines for individuals with Asperger syndrome. In: Klin A, Volkmar FR, Sparrow SS, eds. Asperger Syndrome. 2000:340–365.
26. Tantam D. Adolescence and adulthood of individuals with Asperger syndrome. In: Klin A, Volkmar FR, Sparrow SS, eds. Asperger Syndrome. 2000:367–399.

27. Verté S, Geurts HM, Roeyers H, et al. Executive functioning in children with an autism spectrum disorder: Can we differentiate within the spectrum? J Autism Dev Disord 2006; 36:351–372.
28. Lezak MD, Howieson DB, Loring DW. Neuropsychological Assessment. 4th ed. New York: Oxford University Press, 2004.
29. Royall DR, Lauterbach EC, Cummings JL, et al. Executive control function: A review of its promise and challenges for clinical research. J Neuropsychiatry Clin Neurosci 2002; 14:377–405.
30. Raichle ME Foreword. In: Stuss DT, Knight RT, eds. Principles of Frontal Lobe Function. New York: Oxford University Press, 2002:vii–xii.
31. Stuss DT, Knight RT. Introduction. In: Stuss DT, Knight RT, eds. Principles of Frontal Lobe Function. New York: Oxford University Press, 2002:1–7.
32. Zelazo PD, Frye D. Cognitive complexity and control: II. The development of executive function in childhood. Am Psychol Soc 1998; 7:121–125.
33. Baddeley A. Fractioning the central executive. In: Stuss DT, Knight RT, eds. Principles of Frontal Lobe Function. New York: Oxford University Press, 2002.
34. Baddeley AD, Hitch GJ. Working memory. In: Bower GAed. The Psychology of Learning and Motivation. Vol 8. New York: Academic Press, 1974.
35. Busch RM, McBride A, Curtiss G, et al. The components of executive function in traumatic brain injury. J Clin Exp Neuropsychol 2005; 27:1022–1032.
36. Delis DC, Kaplan E, Kramer JH. Delis-Kaplan Executive Function System Examiner's Manual. San Antonio, TX: The Psychological Corporation, 2001.
37. Homack S, Lee D, Riccio CA. Test review: Delis-Kaplan executive function system. J Clin Exp Neuropsychol 2005; 27:599–609.
38. Kleinhans N, Akshoomoff N, Delis D. Executive functions in autism and Asperger's disorder: flexibility, fluency, and inhibition. Dev Neuropsychol 2005; 27:379–401.
39. Russell J. How executive disorders can bring about an inadequate 'theory of mind.' In: Russell J, ed. Autism as an Executive Disorder. Oxford, UK: Oxford University Press, 1997:256–304.
40. Rowe AD, Bullock PR, Polkey CE, et al. "Theory of mind' impairments and their relationship to executive functioning following frontal lobe excisions. Brain 2001; 124:600–616.
41. Bach LJ, Happé F, Fleminger S, et al. Theory of mind: independence of executive function and the role of the frontal cortex in acquired brain injury. Cognit Neuropsychiatry, 2005; 5:175–192.
42. Fine C, Lumsden J, Blair RJR. Dissociation between 'theory of mind' and executive functions in a patient with early left amygdala damage. Brain 2001; 124:287–298.
43. Lopez BR, Lincoln AJ, Ozonoff S, et al. Examining the relationship between executive functions and restricted, repetitive symptoms of autistic disorder. J Autism Dev Disord 2005; 35:445–460.
44. Hughes C, Graham A. Measuring executive functions in childhood: problems and solutions? Child Adolesc Mental Health 2002; 7:131–142.
45. Joseph RM, Tager-Flusberg H. The relationship of theory of mind and executive functions to symptom type and severity in children with autism. Dev Psychopathol 2004; 16:137–155.
46. Cole K, Mitchell P. Siblings in the development of executive control and a theory of mind. Br J Dev Psychol 2000; 18:279–295.

47. Fahie CM, Symons DK. Executive functioning and theory of mind in children clinically referred for attention and behavior problems. J Appl Dev Psychol 2003; 24:51–73.

48. Sabbagh MA, Xu F, Carlson SM, et al. The development of executive functioning and theory of mind: a comparison of Chinese and U.S. preschoolers. Psychol Sci 2006; 17:74–81.

49. Saltzman J, Strauss E, Hunter M, et al. Theory of mind and executive functions in normal aging and Parkinson's disease. J Int Neuropsychol Soc 1999; 6:781–788.

50. Carlson SM, Mandell DJ, Williams L. Execitive function and theory of mind: Stability and prediction from ages 2 to 3. Dev Psychol 2004; 40:1105–1122.

51. Carlson SM, Moses LJ, Breton C. How specific is the relation between executive function and theory of mind? Contributions of inhibitory control and working memory. Infant Child Dev 2002; 11:73–92.

52. Carlson SM, Moses LJ, Claxton LJ. Individual differences in executive functioning and theory of mind: An investigation of inhibitory control and planning ability. J Exp Child Psychol 2004; 87:299–319.

53. Fisher N, Happé F. A training study of theory of mind and executive function in children with autistic spectrum disorders. J Autism Dev Disord 2005; 35:757–771.

54. Sciutto MJ, Cantwell C. Factors influencing the differential diagnosis of Asperger's disorder and high-functioning autism. J Dev Phys Disabil 2005; 17:345–359.

55. Tryon PA, Mayes SD, Rhodes RL, et al. Can Asperger's disorder be differentiated from autism using DSM-IV criteria? Focus Autism Other Dev Disabil 2006; 21:2–6.

56. Eisenmajer R, Prior M, Leekam S, et al. Comparison of clinical symptoms in autism and Asperger's disorder. J Am Acad Child Adolesc Psychiatry 1996; 35:1523–1531.

57. Ozonoff S, Griffith EM. Neuropsychological function and the external validity of Asperger syndrome. In: Klin A, Volkmar FR, Sparrow SS, eds. Asperger Syndrome. New York: The Guilford Press, 2000:72–96.

58. Ozonoff S, Goodlin-Jones B, Solomon M. Evidence-based assessment of autism spectrum disorders in children and adolescents. J Clin Child Adolesc Psychol 2005; 34:523–540.

59. Ehlers S, Gillberg C, Wing L. A screening questionnaire for Asperger syndrome and other high-functioning autism spectrum disorders in school age children. J Autism Dev Disord 1999; 29:129–141.

60. Goldstein S. Review of the Asperger syndrome diagnostic scale. J Autism Dev Disord 2002; 32:611–614.

61. Constantino JN, Davis SA, Todd R, et al. Validation of a brief quantitative measure of autistic traits: Comparison of the social responsiveness scale with the autism diagnostic interview-revised. J Autism Dev Disord 2003; 33:427–433.

62. Lord C, Rutter M, Le Couteur AL. Autism diagnostic interview-revised: A revised version of a diagnostic interview for caregivers of individuals with possible pervasive developmental disorders. J Autism Dev Disord 1994; 24:659–685.

63. Green D, Baird G, Barnett AL, et al. The severity and nature of motor impairment in Asperger's syndrome: A comparison with specific developmental disorder of motor function. J Child Psychol Psychiatry 2002; 43:655–668.

64. Cox A, Charman T, Baron-Cohen S, et al. Autism spectrum disorders at 20 and 42 months of age: stability of clinical and ADI-R diagnosis. J Child Psyhol Psychiatry 1999; 40:719–732.

65. Pilowsky T, Yirmiya N, Shulman C, et al. The autism diagnostic interview-revised and the childhood autism rating scale: Differences between diagnostic systems and comparison between genders, 1998.

66. Perry A, Condillac RA, Freeman NL, et al. Multi-site study of the childhood autism rating scale (CARS) in five clinical groups of young children. J Autism Dev Disord 2005; 35:625–633.

67. Sponheim E. Changing criteria of autistic disorders: A comparison of the ICD-10 research criteria and DSM-IV with DSM-III-R, CARS, and ABC. J Autism Dev Disord 1996; 26:513–524.

68. Tachimori H, Osada H, Kurita H. Childhood autism rating scale-Tokyo version for screening pervasive developmental disorders. Psychiat Clin Neurosci 2003; 57: 113–118.

69. Dierst-Davies C. Executive funciton of adolescents with Asperger's disorder. Unpublished doctoral dissertation, Pacific Graduate School of Psychology, 2005.

70. Korkman M, Kirk U, Kemp S. A Developmental Neuropsychological Assessment Manual. San Antonio, TX: The Psychological Corporation, 1998.

71. Riddle R, Morton A, Sampson JD, et al. Performance on the NEPSY among children with spina bifida. Arch Clin Neuropsychol 2005; 20:243–248.

72. Ahmad SA, Warriner EM. Review of the NEPSY: A developmental neuro-psychological assessment. Clin Neuropsychol 2001; 15:240–249.

73. Schmitt AJ, Wodrich DL. Validation of a developmental neuropsychological assessment (NEPSY) through comparison of neurological, scholastic concerns, and control groups. Arch Clin Neuropsychol 2004; 19:1077–1093.

74. Matson MA. Neuropsychological performance in high-functioning autism, Asperger syndrome, and developmental language disorder on a developmental neuro-psychological assessment (NEPSY). Unpublished doctoral dissertation, University of Tulsa, 2003.

75. Jolliffe T, Baron-Cohen S. The strange stories test: A replication with high-functioning adults with autism or Asperger syndrome. J Autism Dev Disord, 1999; 29:395–404.

76. Happé FGE, Winner E, Brownell H. The getting of wisdom: Theory of mind in old age. Dev Psychol 1998; 34:358–362.

77. Maylor E, Moulson JM, Muncer A, et al. Does performance of theory of mind tasks decline in old age? Br J Psychol 2002; 93:465–485.

78. Sullivan S, Ruffman T. Social understanding: How does it fare with advancing years? Br J Psychol 2004; 95:1–18.

79. Stone VE, Baron-Cohen S, Knight RT. Frontal lobe contributions to theory of mind. J Cogn Neurosci 1998; 10:640–656.

8

Studies of Brain Morphology, Chemistry, and Function in Asperger's Disorder

Seth D. Friedman

*Department of Radiology, University of Washington,
Seattle, Washington, U.S.A.*

Natalia M. Kleinhans

*Department of Radiology and Autism Center, University of Washington,
Seattle, Washington, U.S.A.*

Jeff Munson

Autism Center, University of Washington, Seattle, Washington, U.S.A.

Sara J. Webb

*Autism Center; Department of Psychiatry and Behavioral Sciences;
and Center on Human Development and Disability,
University of Washington, Seattle, Washington, U.S.A.*

INTRODUCTION

Magnetic resonance (MR) has become a ubiquitous tool for noninvasive investigation of brain changes in individuals suffering from psychiatric disease. However, it was only a short time ago that such studies became possible. The crucial discovery of how to make images from MR occurred in early 1970s (1,2), with the first human head scanned in 1978, requiring several hours to make a single image (3). By the middle of the 1980s, technical advances in computing, scanner hardware, and acquisition methodologies, made rapid imaging of the whole brain feasible. By the late 1980s, the use of magnetic resonance imaging (MRI) as a clinical and research tool had become widespread for measuring structure volumes, tissue relaxation (described below), and brain chemistry. In the 1990s, blood oxygenation level-dependent (BOLD) imaging was developed to measure brain activation (4), a phenomenon known to occur since the turn of the century [for review see (5)]. Though oxygenation changes could previously be measured by single photon emission computed tomography (SPECT) or positron emission tomography (PET) using radioactive tracers (6), the noninvasive nature of BOLD MRI greatly facilitated the ability to make noninvasive examination about the "thinking" brain, leading to widespread studies of cognition in health and disease. In parallel with these improved data acquisition methods, analytic methods have also made dramatic improvements. Whereas early structural imaging studies were largely limited to tracing slice-by-slice areas using a digitizer, multidimensional assessment of many sophisticated image parameters can be rapidly obtained with modern computing and methods (e.g., regional cortical volumes, metrics of shape, cortical thickness, activation locations to a performed task, etc.).

An evolution of diagnostic specificity has also occurred over the last 25 years. Though Leo Kanner described autism in 1943 (7) and Hans Asperger, the syndrome now called Asperger's disorder (ASP) in 1944 (8), only autism was included in the diagnostic and statistical manual (DSM) in the 1980s. In 1994, ASP was added to the DSM, and criteria for both syndromes have been continually refined to the present day. The MRI literature parallels these diagnostic timelines, with fewer studies having investigated individuals diagnosed with ASP compared with those describing autism. The wider spectrum of the disorder, which may include autism and Asperger's are often referred to as autism spectrum disorders (ASD). In autism samples, subjects are often divided into low-functioning autism (LFA) and high-functioning autism (HFA) groups based on their intelligence quotient (IQ), although IQ is not always consistently defined in terms of domain (verbal/nonverbal/composite IQ) or threshold (e.g., >70, 75, or 80). Since few studies with rigidly defined ASP participants are available, and far more likely integrate ASP into the diagnosis of HFA, it is challenging to summarize the literature. To strike a balance between specificity (narrow ASP diagnosis) and greater generalizability (studies of HFA that may or may not include subjects with ASP, referred to as HFA/ASP), this review reports both samples, while operationalizing HFA as requiring IQ scores of 75 or above. Where ASP alone has been specifically studied, this is indicated. In a few situations, studies using lower IQ cutoffs are included for context; these are identified where mentioned. Following a brief overview of MR, summaries of the HFA/ASP literature to date are provided, divided into the three major categories of MRI, which measures volumes of brain structures, magnetic resonance spectroscopy (MRS), which measures chemistry in brain tissues, and functional magnetic resonance imaging (fMRI), which measures brain activation in response to specific cognitive tasks. For all sections, differences are in comparison to a healthy comparison subject group, or "controls." A broader discussion concludes the review, which focuses on drawing conclusions from the

MR studies to date, identifying what questions require further study, and suggesting future directions for MR studies of HFA/ASP.

OVERVIEW OF MAGNETIC RESONANCE

Atomic nuclei that have a magnetic moment and spin quantum number 1/2, such as hydrogen (^{1}H) or phosphorus (^{31}P), can be readily investigated by MR. When placed in a strong magnetic field, these nuclei line up like bar magnets in two opposing directions: one aligned with the magnetic field (low-energy state) and one opposite the magnetic field (high-energy state). Slightly more nuclei are present in the low-energy state, so at rest, the combination of all nuclei, or net magnetization, can be described as a single vector aligned with the magnetic field. To make MR measurements, it is necessary to alter this baseline state. This is achieved by an application of radiofrequency (RF) energy, or radio waves tuned to the nucleus of interest. Simply put, RF energy causes nuclei in one state to transition to the other state. If the RF is applied for a sufficient duration, it is possible to tip the baseline magnetization vector 90°, into what is called the transverse plane. A loop of tuned wire can then measure the excited signal. With the application of gradients (electric currents) in three directions, it is possible to reconstruct an image, the pioneering discovery of Lauterbur (1).

Because the MR magnet is always on, after a short time (seconds), the excited signal returns to the baseline magnetization state. This is primarily the result of two kinds of relaxation: one that occurs in the transverse plane (T_2), reflecting the tipped vector becoming less coherent, and the other that occurs along the magnet axis (T_1), that reflects the excited vector returning to the baseline magnetization state. Brain components (gray matter, white matter, cerebrospinal fluid, and blood) have different relaxation properties, so sampling the signal at different times can provide pictures with enhancement of one tissue type or another. To obtain whole brain spatial coverage with sufficient signal quality, MRI sequences replay many repeated excitations, which are then combined to form a final data set. By varying the properties of excitation and reception, it is possible to make measurements sensitive to a wide range of brain properties, the results of which in HFA/ASP are described for MRI, MRS, and fMRI below.

MAGNETIC RESONANCE IMAGING

Brain Volume

One of the most consistent findings in ASD samples including both low- and high-functioning subjects has been an increase in total brain volume compared with healthy control subjects (9), with recent reports suggesting that the increase in total brain volume or head circumference may occur in early childhood (10–12). Two reports suggest increased intracranial volumes in HFA/ASP adolescents and adults compared with healthy controls (13,14). However, five reports have not observed significant differences [(ASP children-adolescents (15,16), HFA/ASP children-adults (17,18), ASP adults (19)].

Another way of investigating macroscopic aspects of the brain is to investigate whether normal progression of volume changes occur across age. In a cross-sectional sample of individuals with ASP, McAlonan (15) demonstrated that normal decreases in volume were not present with age, suggesting altered developmental factors in the absence of overt volume changes.

Gray Matter

Dividing up the cerebrum into very small units of analysis can help us better understand the specific ways the brain may be built or function differently in HFA/ASP. A common way to parcel the cortex into tissue type is either gray (cell bodies) or white matter (axons). When investigating volumes of gray matter, results have been quite variable. One study has observed volume increases in HFA/ASP compared with control children-adolescents (20). In a study by Lotspeich (21), gray matter volumes in LFA or HFA subjects were increased as compared with healthy control group; ASP subjects had values that were not dissimilar from the healthy control group, though they could not be discriminated from autism samples split by IQ. One further study observed no differences in gray matter volumes in HFA/ASP compared with controls (22). In contrast, two studies have measured gray matter volume decreases in HFA/ASP compared with control groups [absolute volume decreases (23), proportionately smaller (13)]. Some of the variability in these results likely stems from the contribution of developmental factors. These developmental effects are inferred from cross-sectional studies investigating samples across an age range; no study to date has evaluated longitudinal changes in subjects across the life span. It is important to note that the presence of both volume decreases and increases in specific areas of cortex may be obscured when combined in a total or overall brain volume. Investigating regional changes, decreases in gray matter density (volume) have been observed in the frontal lobes, including regions of the left inferior frontal gyrus (Broca's area, a motor center for speech), right inferior paracingulate gyrus (24), right inferior frontal gyrus (25), cingulate (15,26), and dorsolateral prefrontal cortex (27). A further HFA/ASP study demonstrated thinning in the pars opercularis (28), a region related to imitating or mirroring the behavior of others. Temporal regions have also observed decreases including the left superior temporal sulcus (STS) (25), right inferior temporal cortex, entorhinal cortex and fusiform gyrus (29), and the latter region involved in face processing. Alternatively, some gray matter regions appear to demonstrate increased volumes, including orbital frontal cortex (30), right inferior temporal gyrus (24), left superior temporal gyrus, left medial temporal gyrus, left/right post-central regions (25), and the lateral occipitotemporal sulcus (27). Many of these regions activate to tasks that tap core symptoms in HFA/ASP, domains that are described in more detail in the fMRI section to follow.

White Matter

In children with HFA/ASP, general white matter volume increases have been found in one study (13), but not in another (23). Similar to gray matter, it is possible that only regional areas of white matter are affected in the disease, impairing detection when total volumes are measured. This notion is supported by Herbert et al. (22), who demonstrated that only the total radiate compartment (intra-hemispheric fibers) of white matter was larger in individuals with HFA/ASP as compared with controls, and that the frontal lobe was affected to the greatest degree. Using voxel-based analytic techniques, further regional changes in white matter have been described. In a sample of children with HFA/ASP, two white matter clusters showing volume reductions were identified, including a 19% reduction in the left internal capsule (axonal connections between the cerebral cortex and medulla) and 21% reduction in the bilateral fornices (axonal connections between the hippocampus and mammillary bodies and septal nuclei) (23). In adults, white matter deficits in ASP have been found in clusters extending fronto-temporally from frontal to the occipital lobe in the left hemisphere, a band that includes the inferior and superior longitudinal fasciculi and occipitotemporal fasciculus, the pons, and the left cerebellum (15).

These white matter changes may be related to impairment in connectivity between the two hemispheres, and idea that has been indirectly examined in a number of studies assessing the area of the corpus callosum. In adolescents and young adults with HFA/ASP, Chung et al. (31) observed marked white matter decreases in the genu, rostrum, and splenium. The latter result was also observed by Waiter et al. (32). Small callosal areas have also been observed in another HFA/ASP sample (33). Another study showed specific age-related regional increases in white matter only in the genu of HFA/ASP adolescents, suggesting atypical maturational scaling in other subregions (31).

Cerebellum

Cerebellar abnormalities, both at the cellular and systems level, are well documented in ASD (34). The cerebellum has many functions, some of which include the timing and coordination of movements, learning of motor skills, evaluating the match between intention and action, attention, and behavioral response inhibition. Cellular abnormalities in the cerebellum are one of the most reliable neuropathological findings in ASD (34), however MRI findings have been more variable for mixed HFA/ASP groups. It is possible that cerebellum gray matter is increased for HFA/ASP, as suggested in two studies [children and adolescents (27) and adolescents and adults (24)]. Measuring cerebellar subregions in a sample of HFA/ASP subjects (IQs > 70) demonstrated significantly smaller vermal lobes areas I–V and VI–VII than healthy control subjects (35). In contrast, in a slightly older HFA/ASP cohort studied by Holttum et al. (36), no significant differences in specific lobes of the vermis were observed.

Temporal Lobe Nuclei: Amygdala and Hippocampus

The amygdala, located in the medial temporal lobe has a primary role in the processing of emotional salience, most specifically to fear. While two studies have shown no differences in amygdala volume within a sample of HFA/ASP children and adolescents (16), and a sample of HFA/ASP across the age range (18), two reports in adult samples have demonstrated enlarged amygdala volumes (14,24). Studies examining age relationships have suggested that amygdalar enlargement decreases toward adulthood (16), a point that has been indirectly supported by adult study findings (37,38). In another report, lack of positive correlation between amygdala volume and intracranial volume (19), implicates atypical volume scaling for this region HFA/ASP, an idea supported by our results in a young sample of ASD children (39).

The hippocampus is also located in the medial temporal lobe and has extensive involvement in memory functions. In HFA/ASP children and adolescents, hippocampal volumes have been observed to be larger than controls (+10%) (40). Other studies, including those with a large age range spanning children to adults, have not observed volume alterations (18,41). When HFA/ASP adult samples are examined, decreased hippocampus volumes are more commonly observed, shown in three studies to date (13,14,38). Atypical scaling of the hippocampus and cortical volume reductions in the hippocampal and parahippocampal gyri have been observed in one study (14); further evidence for considering developmental course on structure volumes.

Striatum and Thalamus Nuclei

The striatum (composed of the caudate, putamen, and globus pallidus nuclei) and thalamus are involved in many functions including implicit sequence learning, motor function, and executive performance (cognitive abilities that control and regulate other abilities). In a HFA/ASP sample, Haznedar et al. (42) found volume increases in the right caudate nucleus. Caudate enlargement has also been observed in a study by Sears (43) with volume increases related to the degree of obsessional behaviors. Consistent with other regions, evidence for lack of age-related decreases in caudate volume within HFA/ASP subjects has been demonstrated (15).

In the thalamus, no absolute volumetric differences have been demonstrated in ASP (42) or HFA/ASP (44) samples. However, a similar absence of scaling to brain volume was observed (44), and volumes fail to scale normally with increasing age (17).

Summary

While there are too few reports to make strong conclusions about volumetric differences in HFA/ASP compared with healthy control subjects, several commonalities do emerge. First, widespread patterns of volumetric differences are present, with far more regions demonstrating volume decreases than increases. The regional pattern of changes parallels many systems implicated in the fMRI literature; a conceptualization of the value/challenges of integrating these measures follows in the general discussion. For many regions, a reversal of asymmetry or atypical scaling to whole brain volume is suggested. Volumetric differences may exist during different developmental periods, with regions being larger or smaller depending on the sample age. From the available literature, it does not seem possible to differentiate ASP and HFA using these measures. Since ASP and HFA do appear to differ from lower functioning subjects (who tend to show larger brain volumes), perhaps a starting point would be to understand what features differ between subjects stratified only by IQ. Further studies with increasingly narrow age ranges and clinical homogeneity will be useful to extend and refine these observations.

Persistent questions from the volumetric literature are "What do enlarged or decreased regional volumes signify in ASP/HFA?" and "Are larger volumes composed of more units (greater number of cells), different units (neuron/glial ratios, disorganized minicolumns (45), or larger units [bigger cells (46)]? Though it is not possible to answer these questions directly with MR, some characterization of the composition of tissues may be obtained using MR spectroscopy.

MAGNETIC RESONANCE SPECTROSCOPY

Instead of creating images, where the density of protons corresponds to pixel intensity, it is possible to acquire the MR signal in the absence of gradients as a free-induction decay (FID). After Fourier transformation, the time decaying signals may be displayed as a frequency spectrum, where the position of each resonance peak is determined by the precise magnetic field strength felt by that chemical. Figure 1 shows spectra from normal human brain acquired using hydrogen (^{1}H) and phosphorus (^{31}P) MRS, the two nuclei that have been evaluated to date in HFA/ASP studies.

In ^{1}H-MRS, signals can be measured if chemicals are in the millimolar range. By contrast, water is in the molar range and requires suppression during acquisition, and other chemicals, such as dopamine, in the micromolar range remain below the threshold for detection. The largest signals in the ^{1}H spectrum come from *N*-acetylaspartate (NAA), creatine (Cre) and phosphocreatine (PCr), choline-containing compounds (Cho), myoinositol (mI), glutamate, glutamine, and to a lesser degree, gamma-amino butyric acid (GABA), the major inhibitory neurotransmitter, and lactate. High concentrations of NAA are mainly found in neuron cell bodies, axons and dendrites within the brain, though other cell types such as oligodendrocytes, also express a small fraction of NAA (47). NAA is produced in neurons within mitochondria and microsomes (48), but like glutamate, it must be released before being broken down in astrocytes (49). NAA is involved in critical cell functions, including osmotic regulation, as an acetyl donor, a storage molecule for aspartate, a breakdown product of *N*-acetyl-aspartyl-glutamate, and a possible reservoir for glutamate (50,51). In diseases having active damaging processes, such as traumatic brain injury (52), NAA decreases correspond both to injury severity and behavioral dysfunction (52,53).

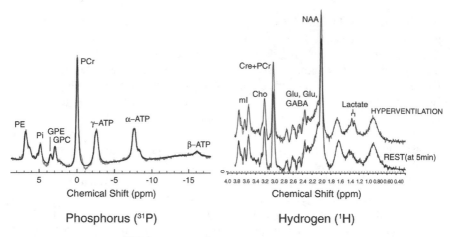

Figure 1 Phosphorus (^{31}P) and proton (^{1}H) spectra are shown from an individual subject. The jagged lines are the raw data, whereas the smooth lines correspond to line fitting. In the ^{31}P spectrum, PE, Pi, GPE, GPC, PCr, and adenosine triphosphate (γ,α,β) are observed. pH can be computed from the shift between PCr and Pi. ^{1}H labels correspond to mI, Cho, creatine + phosphocreatine (Cre + PCr), Glu, Gln, GABA, NAA, and lactate, observed during a hyperventilation challenge. *Abbreviations*: PE, phosphorylethanolamine; Pi, inorganic phosphate; GPE, glycerophosphorylethanolamine; GPC, glycerophosphorylcholine; PCr, phosphocreatine; mI, myoinositol; Cho, choline-containing compounds; Glu, glutamate; Gln, glutamine; GABA, gamma-amino butyric acid; NAA, *N*-acetylaspartate. *Source*: From Ref. 102.

Some amount of NAA decline may be reversible after injury (54), it remains unknown whether marked increases can occur with treatment. Postmortem studies demonstrate relationships between NAA and neuron number (55,56), although it is recognized that in studies of other pathological tissues, such as the epileptic hippocampus, cellular densities, do not directly always directly correlate with NAA (57). Cho-containing compounds in the ^{1}H-MRS spectrum stem from membranes and myelin components, and are observed as a single peak, or singlet. At least four major chemicals contribute to the ^{1}H-MRS Cho signal, including phosphorylethanolamine (PE) and phosphorylcholine (PC) as the primary components, with lesser contributions from glycerophosphorylethanolamine (GPE) and glycerophosphorylcholine (GPC) (58). These chemicals are observable at higher magnetic field strengths (3–4 T), or using proton decoupling (transmitting ^{1}H while acquiring ^{31}P that removes phosphorus chemicals with ^{1}H bonds). For the one study that will be described without decoupling, these four chemicals combine into two peaks, phosphomonoesters (PME) and phosphodiesters (PDE).

Cho-containing compounds are elevated following tissue breakdown from trauma, and with conditions characterized by inflammation, though Cho alterations in the absence of active disease processes have also been observed in HFA/ASP, perhaps related to reduced membrane/myelin precursors, membrane visibility, or both [(see review of changes in disease (59)]. Lactate, present at low levels in normal tissues, plays an essential role as a cellular energy source (60). Levels can be markedly elevated with ischemic or hypoxic conditions, or in conditions characterized by mitochondrial encephalopathy 59). One ASD study has suggested elevated lactate in brain tissue (61); this result has not been confirmed in other studies to date (e.g., 62).

Myoinositol, is thought to be an important regulator of brain osmotic balance, as well as a precursor to the phosphoinositides involved in the cellular membrane–based second messenger system (59). Some concordance between mI and Cho changes has been demonstrated, for example, in chronic hypernatremia, both mI and GPC are elevated (56). Other ^{1}H-MRS-visible compounds include glutamate, glutamine, and GABA. Glutamate, the major excitatory transmitter in brain, is released with neuronal activation, and then broken down by glial cells to glutamine. Glutamine is then transferred back to the neuron where it is made into glutamate. This cycle occurs continuously. Similarly, GABA, the major inhibitory neurotransmitter is produced in related steps. These three chemicals are challenging to measure unambiguously because they overlap in frequency, and each chemical has a multipeak shape making unambiguous line fitting difficult. For this reason, much of the literature refers to the sum as glutamate + glutamine (Glx) (with GABA at a much lower concentration, unreliable for analysis). Detailed measurement of these resonances can be obtained with specific editing acquisition sequences, though this has not been performed in ASD studies to date. With emerging interest in glutamatergic genetics in ASD, these chemicals will be important targets for studies in future.

Instead of acquiring data using ^{1}H, it is also possible to get signals from the brain from chemicals containing ^{31}P. ^{31}P provides a wealth of information about intracellular energy metabolism via measurement of adenosine tri-phosphate (ATP), PCr, and inorganic phosphate (Pi). pH can be reliably calculated from the shift between PCr and Pi, and as described above, Cho components can be sampled with less ambiguity. One technical advantage of ^{31}P-MRS over ^{1}H-MRS is that it may be acquired without solvent (water) suppression since ^{31}P-MRS does not detect protons. On the other hand, the signal strength of ^{31}P-MRS is one to two orders of magnitude weaker than that of ^{1}H-MRS, so longer signal averaging times or larger voxels are required to obtain data for measurement.

The majority of MRS studies in the literature have investigated ASD subjects having a wide range of cognitive dysfunction using either single voxel (cube) or chemical shift imaging (CSI) (matrix of cubes) approaches (46). Both of these techniques provide fairly equivalent data, though trade-off in the accuracy of spatial localization, how much signal is obtained per unit time, chemical resolution (how many points along each peak are sampled), or brain coverage remains limitations. Only two studies published to date have specifically examined subjects diagnosed as HFA and one with subjects diagnosed as ASP. To add to this literature, and provide a possibly useful developmental context for interpreting these three studies that focused on older children/adults, we reanalyzed a previous published subject sample of children studied using CSI at a very young age (3–4 years) (46,62), stratifying subjects by IQ [(high verbal IQ ≥ 75 (77–108), $N = 8$ (all male), age = 46.75 ± 5.18); low verbal IQ < 75 (18–73), $N = 37$ (30 males, 7 females, age 47.54 ± 4.05) compared with healthy control subjects ($N = 10$ (8 males, 2 females), age 46.6 ± 4.53)]. For the combined ASD sample (having a range of IQ scores), neurochemical decreases were observed in widespread nuclei, lobular regions of interest (62), and cortical gray matter (46). These significant anatomical loci were used as a priori hypotheses for the groups stratified by verbal IQ. Results from this reanalysis are shown in Tables 1 and 2.

Table 1 Regional Spectroscopy Data for ASD Subjects Stratified by IQ (High, Verbal IQ ≤ 75; Low, Verbal IQ < 75)

		ASD (vIQ < 75)			ASD (vIQ ≥ 75)			Control		
		N	Mean	Std	N	Mean	Std	N	Mean	Std
White matter	NAA	37	8.84	0.43	8	9.10	0.74	9	9.37	0.60
	MI	37	3.46	0.56	8	3.29	0.57	9	3.81	0.35
Gray matter	Cho	37	2.17	0.19	8	2.12	0.25	9	2.59	0.18
	Cre	37	8.15	0.55	8	7.89	0.57	9	8.69	1.05
	NAA	37	10.60	0.35	8	10.52	0.46	9	11.11	1.18
	MI	37	4.49	0.46	8	4.32	0.55	9	4.91	0.56
	Cho_T2r (%)	37	14.27	12.86	8	15.69	12.38	9	1.68	14.75
	R frontal WM	36	8.09	1.35	8	8.60	2.42	8	10.58	2.98
	R ant cing	37	10.33	1.86	8	10.28	2.32	7	12.51	2.52
NAA	L ant cing	37	10.19	1.51	8	10.83	2.52	7	12.79	3.08
	L thalamus	36	10.66	1.64	8	11.12	1.59	9	12.30	1.56
	L STG	36	10.42	1.58	8	10.51	2.04	9	11.78	1.30
	L parietal WM	37	9.33	1.00	8	9.36	0.60	9	10.71	2.19
	R frontal WM	35	6.40	0.95	8	6.45	1.35	7	7.96	1.62
	R thalamus	36	7.10	1.08	8	7.32	1.17	9	8.12	0.85
Cre	R insula	37	7.08	0.91	8	7.40	0.85	9	8.24	1.13
	Anterior CC	37	7.52	1.33	8	6.99	1.36	6	9.06	1.73
	R parietal WM	37	6.17	0.99	8	5.79	0.92	9	7.28	1.25
	R thalamus	36	2.91	0.51	8	3.06	0.50	9	3.40	0.45
Cho	L STG	34	2.25	0.41	7	2.19	0.38	9	2.60	0.40
	L MTL	36	2.77	0.28	8	2.68	0.42	9	3.13	0.31
	R caudate	35	3.50	0.72	8	4.19	0.92	9	4.59	1.33
	L caudate	31	3.43	0.74	8	3.10	0.77	8	4.37	1.07
mI	L insula	37	3.83	0.66	8	3.78	1.04	9	4.98	0.85
	Anterior CC	36	4.96	0.99	8	4.28	1.32	8	6.12	1.04
	R parietal WM	37	4.00	0.84	8	3.46	0.72	9	4.66	0.82
	Occiput	33	4.86	1.06	8	4.97	1.61	9	6.15	1.84

Abbreviations: ASD, autism spectrum disorders; vIQ, Verbal IQ; Std, standard deviation; NAA, *N*-acetylaspartate; R, right; WM, white matter; ant cing, anterior cingulate; L, left; STG, superior temporal gyrus; CC, corpus callosum; MTL, medial temporal lobe.

Table 2 Statistical Summaries for High-Functioning Autism (HFA) and Low-Functioning Autism (LFA) ASD Samples Compared With Healthy Control Subjects.

		Statistics		Post hoc		Post hoc	ASD-low vs. ASD-high	
		F	P	vIQ < 75	Change (%)[a]	vIQ ≥ 75	ASD-high	Change (%)
White matter	NAA	4.122	0.022	0.021	5.65	0.512	0.426	2.96
	mI	2.308	0.110	0.181	9.34	0.114	0.691	13.82
Gray matter	Cho	18.609	<0 001	<0 001	16.39	<0 001	0.779	18.38
	Cre	3.526	0.037	0.076	6.27	0.040	0.579	9.23
	NAA	3.118	0.053	0.057	4.56	0.099	0.926	5.32
	mI	3.609	0.034	0.061	8.64	0.042	0.651	12.09
	Cho_T2r (%)	3.633	0.033	0.033	14.27	0.081	0.958	15.69
	R frontal WM	5.943	0.005	0.003	23.52	0.092	0.761	18.70
	R ant cing	3.525	0.037	0.032	17.40	0.096	0.998	17.78
NAA	L ant cing	5.360	0.008	0.006	20.32	0.133	0.678	15.35
	L thalamus	3.700	0.032	0.024	13.34	0.299	0.754	9.63
	L STG	2.599	0.084	0.071	11.54	0.245	0.99	10.82
	L parietal WM	4.736	0.013	0.010	12.95	0.070	0.998	12.65
	R frontal WM	5.767	0.006	0.004	19.66	0.033	0.99	18.92
	R thalamus	3.335	0.044	0.034	12.61	0.274	0.858	9.90
Cre	R insula	5.481	0.007	0.005	14.00	0.171	0.662	10.13
	Anterior CC	4.218	0.021	0.037	17.03	0.021	0.594	22.83
	R parietal WM	5.455	0.007	0.014	15.26	0.011	0.601	20.56
	R thalamus	3.627	0.034	0.026	14.58	0.328	0.727	10.22
Cho	L STG	3.045	0.057	0.060	13.55	0.120	0.941	15.68
	L MTL	5.686	0.006	0.009	11.27	0.012	0.73	14.18
	R caudate	6.425	0.003	0.005	23.72	0.620	0.124	8.73
	L caudate	5.701	0.006	0.015	21.36	0.008	0.556	28.95
MI	L insula	8.932	<0 001	0.000	23.11	0.005	0.984	24.13
	Anterior CC	6.379	0.003	0.019	18.96	0.003	0.239	29.98
	R parietal WM	4.599	0.015	0.086	14.25	0.011	0.224	25.80
	Occiput	3.493	0.039	0.031	21.08	0.162	0.976	19.31

The reduced pattern of differences likely reflects statistical power; regions demonstrate similar mean changes comparing HFA and LFA groups.
[a]$p < 05, p < 10$.
Abbreviations: NAA, *N*-acetylaspartate; R, right; WM, white matter; ant cing, anterior cingulated; L, left; mI, myo-inositol.

A similar direction and magnitude of metabolite decreases were observed for the HFA and LFA groups compared with healthy control subjects. Though fewer statistically significant loci were observed in the HFA group, this pattern likely reflects statistical power (fewer subjects to analyze) as compared with real differences between HFA and LFA groups. This point is echoed by post hoc tests directly comparing HFA/ASP subgroups that revealed no statistically significant group effects (all $p > .1$, analyses not shown). Though decidedly exploratory, these results suggest that at age three to four years, higher functioning subjects with verbal IQ > 75 have brain chemistry that is similar to ASD subjects on the lower end of the verbal IQ spectrum. These findings provide evidence that membrane precursors and cellular integrity may be abnormal in HFA subjects early in development, factors to consider when conceptualizing overlap between chemical and histological features in the HFA/ASP brain.

The only ^{31}P study in the literature examined frontal lobe metabolites in 11 male HFA/ASP adolescent and adult subjects (IQ > 70) compared with 11 age, gender, and IQ-matched control subjects (63). In the HFA/ASP group, significantly reduced levels in PCr (10%) and ATP components (8.6%, alpha ATP + dinucleotides + uridine diphosphosugars) were observed compared with the matched control group. Note, in contrast to the proton spectrum that measures Cre + PCr, the ^{31}P spectrum only measures PCr, a metabolite that may be more clinically pertinent to evaluating changes in metabolism. These reductions were significantly associated with IQ and cognitive test performance (Wisconsin Card Sorting Task, California Verbal Learning Task) for HFA/ASP subjects (lower levels = poorer performance). Although not statistically different from the control group, HFA/ASP levels of PME and PDE were also correlated to the cognitive performance, with PME showing a similar direction as PCr, whereas higher PDE was related to worse performance. In total, these results provide intriguing further evidence that bioenergetics and membrane markers are altered in HFA/ASP.

Two additional studies have been published using proton spectroscopy to examine HFA/ASP and ASP samples. The first examined were 22 school-age children across a similar age range as the ^{31}P study compared with 20 healthy controls using a multi-voxel CSI technique (64). In left sided regions, NAA decreases were demonstrated (frontal white matter 15%, parietal white matter 15%, caudate 13%). Cre, the combination of Cre + PCr in the proton spectrum, was reduced in two regions in the HFA/ASP group (right occiput 23%; left caudate nucleus 25%) and increased within the right caudate nucleus (17%). Although frontal cortex metabolites did not differ statistically by group, the anterior cingulate, a region that may overlap with the surface coil approach used above, demonstrated reduced Cho. In parallel with increased Cre in right caudate nucleus, Cho was similarly increased in this region. When combined, these results suggest metabolite alterations in widespread regions in brain within HFA/ASP subjects across a later childhood range. Importantly, and perhaps paralleling the volumetric literature, several regions of increased chemistry in this older sample may hint at developmental progression of MRS changes.

In the one study investigating 14 adults with ASP compared with 18 healthy control subjects, single-voxel MRS was employed to sample the right medial frontal lobe and the right parietal lobe (white matter) (65). In the ASP group, increases in Cho (32%), Cre (15.5%), and NAA (18.8%) were observed in the right frontal lobe region, whereas no differences were observed in the parietal lobe. NAA levels were correlated to obsessionality, as measured by the Yale-Brown Obsessive Compulsive Scale, and Cho the degree of communication impairment [as measured by the autism diagnostic interview (ADI-R) (66)].

MRI/MRS/fMRI Summary

Though difficult to integrate these findings into a substantive whole, several interesting points warrant discussion. At the least, these data hint at a developmental time-course to brain chemistry not dissimilar from the volumetric findings, with early decreases in neurochemistry perhaps transitioning to increases in certain brain regions across adolescence/early adulthood. Since adolescence is characterized by a dramatic refinement of cellular synapses, numerous mechanisms could be suggested to underlie such a change. At the least, these data hint at several important avenues for further work, namely further careful description of what spectroscopy alterations really mean, and careful attention to the longitudinal time-course of changes. For example, since Cho can be broken up into constituent chemicals using ^{31}P-MRS at high-field, such an investigation would be invaluable to both replicate 31P findings to date, and reveal what specific component(s) of Cho is altered in the HFA/ASP brain. The convergence of MRI and MRS data suggest that volume and composition are altered in the HFA/ASP brain, with future studies needed to evaluate regional overlap within individual subjects (e.g., are large caudate nuclei characterized by low- or high-neurochemical concentrations). While the overlap between volumetric and chemical measures may inform how the HFA/ASP brain is constructed, they do not directly inform what pathways, circuits, or aspects of cognition are impaired.

For this type of inquiry, fMRI provides a fitting tool.

FUNCTIONAL MAGNETIC RESONANCE IMAGING

Using fMRI, it is possible to evaluate cognitive domains ranging from basic sensory processing to high-level tasks, often termed "executive functioning." Most studies have focused on delineating the neural correlates social cognition and its component processes, using studies of varying complexity to understand at what level of the system the alterations occur.

Several studies have investigated the abnormal response to faces in HFA/ASP. To evaluate whether basic sensory processing was impaired, Hadjikhani et al. (67) studied retinotopic maps in eight individuals with HFA/ASP. No difference in the quality or organization of the primary visual cortex was found in HFA/ASP compared with controls, indicating that behavioral deficits in perceptual face processing could not be accounted for by fundamental sensory impairment. At higher levels of face processing, several studies have demonstrated regional alterations in HFA/ASP within the fusiform gyrus, a region in the inferior temporal lobe that is part of the ventral visual processing stream associated with object identification. Typically developing individuals exhibit increased activation to faces compared with other classes of objects in the lateral fusiform gyrus, suggesting that face processing is mediated by this highly face-specialized brain region, termed the fusiform face area (FFA). Abnormal development of the FFA was initially proposed as a critical component of face-processing abnormalities in high-functioning HFA/ASP following several reports of reduced and/or absent activation to faces in this brain region (68–71). However, subsequent studies have failed to find differences in FFA activation (72–74), or found that FFA activation differences were mediated by task demands (75,76), familiarity (77), or amount of time spent fixating on the eyes (71). Thus, current evidence suggests that abnormal fusiform activation to faces in HFA/ASP may not be associated with primary neuroanatomical deficit in this brain region.

Emotional face–processing studies suggest that limbic system abnormalities, particularly in the amygdala, may underlie social deficits in HFA/ASP. Abnormal amygdala activation has been reported in response to emotional face processing (78,79), emotional discrimination (71), and emotional attribution (75). Functional abnormalities in the amygdala include abnormally increased activation (Dalton, et al. 2005), decreased activation (78–80), and reduction of expected task-related modulation (75,79,81) in HFA/ASP. For example, in the Wang et al. study (75), children with HFA/ASP were instructed to match the emotion on the target face to either other emotional faces or a verbal label. While no significant between-group differences in amygdala activation were found, the typically developing children showed task-related modulation of the amygdala (i.e., increased amygdala activation to emotion matching compared with labeling) while the children with HFA/ASP did not. Similarly, in a study measuring modulation of fear, incremental amygdala activation was observed in healthy adults, findings not shown in the HFA/ASP group (79).

Mirror neuron dysfunction has also been hypothesized as a potential neural mechanism underlying social communication deficit, particularly empathy and "theory of mind" in HFA/ASP. Mirror neurons are unique because they fire both when an individual performs an action and when a person observes someone else performing an action. It has been proposed that the brain translates the observed movements of another person into the patterns of neural activation that mimics their own movements and experiences, thus allowing an observer to "share" the experience of the other person. Abnormalities in the mirror neuron system have been reported in HFA/ASP during observation and imitation of emotional facial expressions (73) and finger movements (81). During both observation and imitation of emotional facial expressions, typically developing children produced greater activation than the HFA/ASP group in pars opercularis—a "mirror area" of the inferior frontal gyrus (73). Further, the pars opercularis activation during the imitation task was correlated to social subscale scores on the autism diagnostic observation schedule (82), and autism diagnostic interview (66), such that more impaired social functioning was associated with reduced activation. In other areas of the brain, a very different pattern of activation was observed between groups. Greater activation was observed in the insular and peri-amygdaloid regions, ventral striatum, and thalamus in the controls, whereas the HFA/ASP children evidenced greater activation in the parietal and right visual association area. In the study investigating motor imitation, reduced activations were demonstrated in the middle occipital, inferior parietal, fusiform, lingual, and the middle temporal gyrus in HFA/ASP. The healthy control group also demonstrated several areas of increased activation, including the left amygdala and bilateral superior temporal gyrus (81). In total, data suggest that mirror neuron regions are altered in HFA/ASP, resulting in vastly different activation patterns in subjects performing tasks in this domain.

Another behavioral challenge in HFA/ASP is reading intentionality from eye gaze. The neural correlates of this behavioral feature in HFA were tested by Pelphrey et al. (83) who examined differences in brain activation to eye gaze shifts toward the direction of a target stimulus (congruent) compared with an eye gaze shift toward empty space (incongruent). In neurologically healthy individuals, eye gaze processing is mediated by the STS. This brain region is also sensitive to social context, via the information conveyed by eye movements and other types of biological motion. In the fMRI experiment by Pelphrey et al., STS activation was modulated by intentionality in the control group but not the HFA/ASP group. That is, the controls exhibited increased activation to trials that violated their expectations (incongruent trials) compared with trials that met their expectations (congruent trials). No difference in STS activation between congruent and incongruent trials was observed in the HFA group, suggesting social context does not modulate STS activation in individuals with HFA/ASP. This failure of task-related modulation in the STS may contribute to the deficits in interpreting and utilizing information from faces present in HFA. In a similar line of inquiry, Baron-Cohen et al. (80) conducted an fMRI study of social intelligence in individuals with HFA/ASP. During the task condition, participants were shown a pair of eyes and asked to decide which of two words best described what the person was thinking. The individuals with HFA/ASP had reduced activation in the left amygdala, right insula, and left inferior frontal gyrus (a mirror area). Increased activation was observed in the bilateral superior temporal gyrus in the HFA/ASP group when compared with the controls.

Although social deficits are the most prominent behavioral feature of individuals with Asperger's syndrome, restricted, repetitive, and stereotyped patterns of behavior are also key features of the disorder and are thought to reflect a failure of inhibition, cognitive rigidity, and a generativity impairment (84). The restricted and repetitive behaviors observed in HFA/ASP include insistence on sameness or highly circumscribed interests (85). Such behaviors may reflect executive dysfunction in individuals with HFA/ASP. fMRI studies of executive functioning in HFA/ASP have included attentional processes (74,86–88), spatial working memory (89,90), inhibition (30), and cognitive switching (30). Increased activation during tasks tapping executive functions has been consistently observed in HFA/ASP. Visual attention tasks have identified increased activation in the frontal lobes (87,88), parietal lobes (86,87), occipital cortex (30,88), and the insula (87) in HFA/ASP. Similarly, increased activation was reported in the left middle, left inferior, and orbital frontal areas during motor inhibition; increased insula activation was observed during cognitive inhibition, and increased parietal lobe activation was reported during cognitive switching (30). In the Schmitz et al. study, increased frontal lobe activation in HFA/ASP was localized to the same area as increased gray matter density (30). For working memory tasks, activations may be decreased in HFA/ASP, with two studies finding decreased activation in prefrontal cortex (89,90), right medial frontal, the anterior cingulate (89), and posterior cingulate (90).

A last area that has been increasingly studied in HFA/ASP is functional connectivity. Functional connectivity is the study of activation patterns between regions, and can be performed in the presence or absence of a task. Although abnormal intra- and intercortical functional connectivity in ASD was first reported in a PET study approximately 20 years ago (91), focus on this phenomenon has resurfaced recently. Studies utilizing functional connectivity MRI (FcMRI) techniques have identified abnormal connectivity between brain regions that mediate complex language, selective attention, visuomotor coordination, emotion perception, and executive functioning tasks (33,74,92–97). Examining such relationships in HFA have revealed reduced connectivity between occipital and frontal regions during a visuomotor sequencing task and a sentence comprehension task (92,94), reduced frontal and parietal connectivity during visually mediated executive functioning tasks (33,93), and an increased connectivity between the amygdala and parahippocampal regions during fearful face processing in HFA/ASP (95). Not all results are consistent. For example, reduced connectivity between the occipital lobes and parietal lobes was reported by one group during a language task requiring visual imagery (96), but not another which required visuomotor sequencing (94). A compelling selective attention study of faces and houses by Bird and colleagues (74) found that connectivity between V1 and the FFA (the brain region that responded the most strongly to faces) was not modulated by attention in HFA/ASP although connectivity between V1 and the parahippocampal place area (the brain region that responded the most strongly to houses) was modulated. It is also possible that weaker connectivity is present in HFA during a resting fixation task, as was recently demonstrated (98). At present, some baseline alterations in connectivity may predispose HFA/ASP subjects to poorer task performance for some domains, with connectivity adding another layer of complexity on top of activation regions and effect direction.

Summary

fMRI studies have made remarkable progress describing how the HFA/ASP brain responds in abnormal ways to language, executive functions, social cues, and face processing. The results can be broadly characterized in three ways, a diminished or absent activation response compared with controls, less connectivity between areas of activations, or a different set of anatomical biases. Notably, it may not be possible to simply conclude that a structure works more poorly across all tasks; whether such a directional dissociation can be demonstrated will be exciting avenue to pursue in future research.

DISCUSSION

Tremendous progress has been made to date toward understanding the volumetric, chemical, and functional regions or networks altered in HFA/ASP. Although the literature is leaner and more variable in some areas than others, important generalities emerge that mark both our current progress, and provide guidance for future work.

First, reduced brain asymmetry and connectivity appears common in HFA/ASP subjects. Such findings may reflect alterations from typical patterns of brain development, which occur during time-points critical to hemispheric specialization, an idea that has been suggested in the neuropsychological literature (99). The corpus callosum is often smaller in area as well, suggesting atypical connectivity between the cerebral hemispheres. In fcMRI studies at rest (fixation crosshair), anterior-posterior connectivity was reduced, perhaps supportive of cortical white matter radiate differences in HFA/ASP (22).

Second, atypical scaling of volume is demonstrated within the HFA/ASP group for many brain tissues/structures. This has been observed in two main domains, comparing total brain volume to volumes of specific nuclei (as for the amygdala), or when examining how the volume of a structure changes across the life span. A liberal reading of the MRS studies to date also support this idea, with decreases in neurochemistry more prevalent in childhood samples, whereas older samples may demonstrate marked regional chemical increases. If correct, the presence of developmental differences across the life span in HFA/ASP versus healthy control subjects would explain some of the literature variability. Further studies examining either longitudinal samples or narrow age ranges, will be instructive to characterize the anatomical backdrop related to the appearance of symptoms particularly, during adolescence and across the adult life span. For example, although both amygdala and hippocampus volume are enlarged in ASD at three to four years of age, only amygdala volume predicted poor social development over the next few years (100).

Having found evidence that many brain structures show altered volumes in individuals with HFA/ASP, we turn to the MRS findings for more specific clues to what may be different about these structures. From MRS data, it appears that the cellular properties of many tissues are abnormal, and they are not necessarily limited to those structures that show volumetric differences. This highlights the challenge faced by the field of integrating the information gained from measurements of brain volume, chemistry, and activation. Simultaneous investigation of these different methods will be invaluable in understanding both how the measures interrelate, and for evaluating which features carry unique information and which are redundant. For example, in a subject where right and left volumetric asymmetry is reversed, are such changes also evident in the brain chemistry? Does low brain chemistry predict poor activation on a task tapping that region? These types of questions along with the integration of other multimodal measures [(e.g., serotonin transporter densities (101)] will be crucial to help clarify these aims.

On a related point, reducing variability in clinical samples in terms of diagnostic criteria will be critical to evaluate how and whether HFA and ASP differ, a distinction that cannot be clearly drawn from the MRI literature to date. This, however, is not a simple task. For example, obtaining a homogeneous subgroup of adults in terms of present verbal IQ may not automatically yield a homogenous group with regard to other potentially important aspects of language functioning (i.e., language acquisition, pragmatics, etc.). At a minimum, obtaining data from well-defined segments of the clinical spectrum may help to clarify some of the heterogeneity present in the available data.

Neuroimaging investigations into HFA/ASP are still quite young. Though much progress has been made describing alterations in morphology, chemistry, and functional activation in signals within ASD, far more work remains ahead, a humbling and exciting reality. As almost all of the literature is based between HFA/ASP and healthy controls, the described findings need to be further replicated, refined, and narrowed toward the individual case. While individual case description may be difficult to achieve because of the many factors that lead to symptom expression, understanding what clusters of genetic, biomarker, and behavioral deficits are present in clinical sample may allow important subgroup segregation. Such an approach may have important utility for understanding developmental course, symptom burden, and evaluating treatment efficacy.

ACKNOWLEDGEMENTS

The authors are tremendously grateful for the collaboration of Drs. Geri Dawson, Stephen Dager, Dennis Shaw, Alan Artru, and the staff of the UW Autism Center. The UW autism study was supported by PO1 HD34565. Dr. Friedman was supported by K01 MH069848. We wish to extend our sincere thanks to the parents and children who participated in the studies described herein.

REFERENCES

1. Lauterbur PC. Image formation by induced local interactions: examples of employing nuclear magnetic resonance. Nature 1973; 242:190–191.
2. Garroway AN, Grannell PK, Mansfield P. Image formation in NMR by a selective irradiative process. J Phys C: Solid State Phys 1974; 7:457–462.

3. Clow H, Young IR. Britian's brains produce first NMR scans. New Sci 1978; 80:588.
4. Ogawa S, Lee TM, Kay AR, et al. Brain magnetic resonance imaging with contrast dependent on blood oxygenation. Proc Natl Acad Sci U S A 1990; 87:9868–9872.
5. Raichle ME. Behind the scenes of functional brain imaging: a historical and physiological perspective. Proc Natl Acad Sci U S A 1998; 95:765–772.
6. Taber KH, Black KJ, Hurley RA. Blood flow imaging of the brain: 50 years experience. J Neuropsychiatry Clin Neurosci 2005; 17:441–446.
7. Kanner L. Autistic disturbances of affective contact. Nerv Child 1943; 2:217–250.
8. Asperger H. Die 'Autistischen Psychopathen' im Kindesalter. Arch Psychiatr Nervenkr 1944; 117:76–136.
9. Palmen SJ, van Engeland H. Review on structural neuroimaging findings in autism. J Neural Transm 2004; 111:903–929.
10. Lainhart JE, Bigler ED, Bocian M, et al. Head circumference and height in autism: a study by the collaborative program of excellence in autism. Am J Med Genet A 2006; 140:2257–2274.
11. Hazlett HC, Poe M, Gerig G, et al. Magnetic resonance imaging and head circumference study of brain size in autism: birth through age 2 years. Arch Gen Psychiatry 2005; 62:1366–1376.
12. Courchesne E, Carper R, Akshoomoff N. Evidence of brain overgrowth in the first year of life in autism. JAMA 2003; 290:337–344.
13. Herbert MR, Ziegler DA, Deutsch CK, et al. Dissociations of cerebral cortex, subcortical and cerebral white matter volumes in autistic boys. Brain 2003; 126:1182–1192.
14. Howard MA, Cowell PE, Boucher J, et al. Convergent neuroanatomical and behavioural evidence of an amygdala hypothesis of autism. Neuroreport 2000; 11:2931–2935.
15. McAlonan GM, Daly E, Kumari V, et al. Brain anatomy and sensorimotor gating in Asperger's syndrome. Brain 2002; 125:1594–1606.
16. Schumann CM, Hamstra J, Goodlin-Jones BL, et al. The amygdala is enlarged in children but not adolescents with autism; the hippocampus is enlarged at all ages. J Neurosci 2004; 24:6392–6401.
17. Hardan AY, Girgis RR, Adams J, et al. Abnormal brain size effect on the thalamus in autism. Psychiatry Res 2006; 147:145–151.
18. Palmen SJ, Durston S, Nederveen H, et al. No evidence for preferential involvement of medial temporal lobe structures in high-functioning autism. Psychol Med 2006; 36:827–834.
19. Dziobek I, Fleck S, Rogers K, et al. The 'amygdala theory of autism' revisited: linking structure to behavior. Neuropsychologia 2006; 44:1891–1899.
20. Palmen SJ, Hulshoff Pol HE, Kemner C, et al. Increased gray-matter volume in medication-naive high-functioning children with autism spectrum disorder. Psychol Med 2005; 35:561–570.
21. Lotspeich LJ, Kwon H, Schumann CM, et al. Investigation of neuroanatomical differences between autism and Asperger syndrome. Arch Gen Psychiatry 2004; 61:291–298.
22. Herbert MR, Ziegler DA, Makris N, et al. Localization of white matter volume increase in autism and developmental language disorder. Ann Neurol 2004; 55: 530–540.

23. McAlonan GM, Cheung V, Cheung C, et al. Mapping the brain in autism. A voxel-based MRI study of volumetric differences and intercorrelations in autism. Brain 2005; 128:268–276.
24. Abell F, Krams M, Ashburner J, et al. The neuroanatomy of autism: a voxel-based whole brain analysis of structural scans. Neuroreport 1999; 10:1647–1651.
25. Chung MK, Robbins SM, Dalton KM, et al. Cortical thickness analysis in autism with heat kernel smoothing. Neuroimage 2005; 25:1256–1265.
26. Haznedar MM, Buchsbaum MS, Wei TC, et al. Limbic circuitry in patients with autism spectrum disorders studied with positron emission tomography and magnetic resonance imaging. Am J Psychiatry 2000; 157:1994–2001.
27. Salmond CH, Ashburner J, Connelly A, et al. The role of the medial temporal lobe in autistic spectrum disorders. Eur J Neurosci 2005; 22:764–772.
28. Hadjikhani N, Joseph RM, Snyder J, et al. Anatomical differences in the mirror neuron system and social cognition network in autism. Cereb Cortex 2006; 16: 1276–1282.
29. Kwon H, Ow AW, Pedatella KE, et al. Voxel-based morphometry elucidates structural neuroanatomy of high-functioning autism and Asperger syndrome. Dev Med Child Neurol 2004; 46:760–764.
30. Schmitz N, Rubia K, Daly E, et al. Neural correlates of executive function in autistic spectrum disorders. Biol Psychiatry 2006; 59:7–16.
31. Chung MK, Dalton KM, Alexander AL, et al. Less white matter concentration in autism: 2D voxel-based morphometry. Neuroimage 2004; 23:242–251.
32. Waiter GD, Williams JH, Murray AD, et al. Structural white matter deficits in high-functioning individuals with autistic spectrum disorder: a voxel-based investigation. Neuroimage 2005; 24:455–461.
33. Just MA, Cherkassky VL, Keller TA, et al. Functional and anatomical cortical underconnectivity in autism: evidence from an fMRI Study of an Executive Function Task and Corpus Callosum Morphometry. Cereb Cortex 2007; 17(4):951–961.
34. Palmen SJ, van Engeland H, Hof PR, et al. Neuropathological findings in autism. Brain 2004; 127:2572–2583.
35. Ciesielski KT, Harris RJ, Hart BL, et al. Cerebellar hypoplasia and frontal lobe cognitive deficits in disorders of early childhood. Neuropsychologia 1997; 35:643–655.
36. Holttum JR, Minshew NJ, Sanders RS, et al. Magnetic resonance imaging of the posterior fossa in autism. Biol Psychiatry 1992; 32:1091–1101.
37. Pierce K, Courchesne E. Evidence for a cerebellar role in reduced exploration and stereotyped behavior in autism. Biol Psychiatry 2001; 49:655–664.
38. Aylward EH, Minshew NJ, Goldstein G, et al. MRI volumes of amygdala and hippocampus in non-mentally retarded autistic adolescents and adults. Neurology 1999; 53:2145–2150.
39. Sparks BF, Friedman SD, Shaw DW, et al. Brain structural abnormalities in young children with autism spectrum disorder. Neurology 2002; 59:184–192.
40. Filipek PA, Richelme C, Kennedy DN, et al. Morphometric analysis of the brain in developmental language disorders and autism. Ann Neurol 1992; 32:475.
41. Saitoh O, Courchesne E, Egaas B, et al. Cross-sectional area of the posterior hippocampus in autistic patients with cerebellar and corpus callosum abnormalities. Neurology 1995; 45:317–324.

42. Haznedar MM, Buchsbaum MS, Hazlett EA, et al. Volumetric analysis and three-dimensional glucose metabolic mapping of the striatum and thalamus in patients with autism spectrum disorders. Am J Psychiatry 2006; 163:1252–1263.

43. Sears LL, Vest C, Mohamed S, et al. An MRI study of the basal ganglia in autism. Prog Neuropsychopharmacol Biol Psychiatry 1999; 23:613–624.

44. Tsatsanis KD, Rourke BP, Klin A, et al. Reduced thalamic volume in high-functioning individuals with autism. Biol Psychiatry 2003; 53:121–129.

45. Casanova MF, Buxhoeveden DP, Switala AE, et al. Asperger's syndrome and cortical neuropathology. J Child Neurol 2002; 17:142–145.

46. Friedman SD, Shaw DW, Artru AA, et al. Gray and white matter brain chemistry in young children with autism. Arch Gen Psychiatry 2006; 63:786–794.

47. Urenjak J, Williams SR, Gadian DG, et al. Proton nuclear magnetic resonance spectroscopy unambiguously identifies different neural cell types. J Neurosci 1993; 13:981–989.

48. Lu ZH, Chakraborty G, Ledeen RW, et al. N-Acetylaspartate synthase is bimodally expressed in microsomes and mitochondria of brain. Brain Res Mol Brain Res 2004; 122:71–78.

49. Bhakoo KK, Craig TJ, Styles P. Developmental and regional distribution of aspartoacylase in rat brain tissue. J Neurochem 2001; 79:211–220.

50. Baslow MH. N-acetylaspartate in the vertebrate brain: metabolism and function. Neurochem Res 2003; 28:941–953.

51. Clark JF, Doepke A, Filosa JA, et al. N-acetylaspartate as a reservoir for glutamate. Med Hypotheses 2006; 67:506–512.

52. Friedman SD, Brooks WM, Jung RE, et al. Quantitative proton MRS predicts outcome after traumatic brain injury. Neurology 1999; 52:1384–1391.

53. Mathiesen HK, Jonsson A, Tscherning T, et al. Correlation of global N-acetylaspartate with cognitive impairment in multiple sclerosis. Arch Neurol 2006; 63:533–536.

54. Brooks WM, Stidley CA, Petropoulos H, et al. Metabolic and cognitive response to human traumatic brain injury: a quantitative proton magnetic resonance study. J Neurotrauma 2000; 17:629–640.

55. Cheng LL, Newell K, Mallory AE, et al. Quantification of neurons in Alzheimer and control brains with ex vivo high resolution magic angle spinning proton magnetic resonance spectroscopy and stereology. Magn Reson Imaging 2002; 20:527–533.

56. Mohanakrishnan P, Fowler AH, Vonsattel JP, et al. An in vitro 1H nuclear magnetic resonance study of the temporoparietal cortex of Alzheimer brains. Exp Brain Res 1995; 102:503–510.

57. Petroff OA, Errante LD, Rothman DL, et al. Neuronal and glial metabolite content of the epileptogenic human hippocampus. Ann Neurol 2002; 52:635–642.

58. Bluml S, Seymour KJ, Ross BD. Developmental changes in choline- and ethanolamine-containing compounds measured with proton-decoupled (31)P MRS in in vivo human brain. Magn Reson Med 1999; 42:643–654.

59. Ross B, Michaelis T. Clinical applications of magnetic resonance spectroscopy. Magn Reson Q 1994; 10:191–247.

60. Pellerin L. How astrocytes feed hungry neurons. Mol Neurobiol 2005; 32:59–72.

61. Chugani DC, Sundram BS, Behen M, et al. Evidence of altered energy metabolism in autistic children. Prog Neuropsychopharmacol Biol Psychiatry 1999; 23:635–641.

62. Friedman SD, Shaw DW, Artru AA, et al. Regional brain chemical alterations in young children with autism spectrum disorder. Neurology 2003; 60:100–107.
63. Minshew NJ, Goldstein G, Dombrowski SM, et al. A preliminary 31P MRS study of autism: evidence for undersynthesis and increased degradation of brain membranes. Biol Psychiatry 1993; 33:762–773.
64. Levitt JG, O'Neill J, Blanton RE, et al. Proton magnetic resonance spectroscopic imaging of the brain in childhood autism. Biol Psychiatry 2003; 54:1355–1366.
65. Murphy DG, Critchley HD, Schmitz N, et al. Asperger syndrome: a proton magnetic resonance spectroscopy study of brain. Arch Gen Psychiatry 2002; 59:885–891.
66. Lord C, Rutter M, Le Couteur A. Autism diagnostic interview-revised: a revised version of a diagnostic interview for caregivers of individuals with possible pervasive developmental disorders. J Autism Dev Disord 1994; 24:659–685.
67. Hadjikhani N, Chabris CF, Joseph RM, et al. Early visual cortex organization in autism: an fMRI study. Neuroreport 2004; 15:267–270.
68. Schultz RT, Gauthier I, Klin A, et al. Abnormal ventral temporal cortical activity during face discrimination among individuals with autism and Asperger syndrome. Arch Gen Psychiatry 2000; 57:331–340.
69. Pierce K, Muller RA, Ambrose J, et al. Face processing occurs outside the fusiform 'face area' in autism: evidence from functional MRI. Brain 2001; 124:2059–2073.
70. Hubl D, Bolte S, Feineis-Matthews S, et al. Functional imbalance of visual pathways indicates alternative face processing strategies in autism. Neurology 2003; 61:1232–1237.
71. Dalton KM, Nacewicz BM, Johnstone T, et al. Gaze fixation and the neural circuitry of face processing in autism. Nat Neurosci 2005; 8:519–526.
72. Hadjikhani N, Joseph RM, Snyder J, et al. Activation of the fusiform gyrus when individuals with autism spectrum disorder view faces. Neuroimage 2004; 22:1141–1150.
73. Dapretto M, Davies MS, Pfeifer JH, et al. Understanding emotions in others: mirror neuron dysfunction in children with autism spectrum disorders. Nat Neurosci 2006; 9:28–30.
74. Bird G, Catmur C, Silani G, et al. Attention does not modulate neural responses to social stimuli in autism spectrum disorders. Neuroimage 2006; 31:1614–1624.
75. Wang AT, Dapretto M, Hariri AR, et al. Neural correlates of facial affect processing in children and adolescents with autism spectrum disorder. J Am Acad Child Adolesc Psychiatry 2004; 43:481–490.
76. Piggot J, Kwon H, Mobbs D, et al. Emotional attribution in high-functioning individuals with autistic spectrum disorder: a functional imaging study. J Am Acad Child Adolesc Psychiatry 2004; 43:473–480.
77. Pierce K, Haist F, Sedaghat F, et al. The brain response to personally familiar faces in autism: findings of fusiform activity and beyond. Brain 2004; 127:2703–2716.
78. Critchley HD, Daly EM, Bullmore ET, et al. The functional neuroanatomy of social behaviour: changes in cerebral blood flow when people with autistic disorder process facial expressions. Brain 2000; 123(pt 11):2203–2212.
79. Ashwin C, Baron-Cohen S, Wheelwright S, et al. Differential activation of the amygdala and the 'social brain' during fearful face-processing in Asperger Syndrome. Neuropsychologia 2007; 45(1):2–14.
80. Baron-Cohen S, Ring HA, Wheelwright S, et al. Social intelligence in the normal and autistic brain: an fMRI study. Eur J Neurosci 1999; 11:1891–1898.

81. Williams JH, Waiter GD, Gilchrist A, et al. Neural mechanisms of imitation and 'mirror neuron' functioning in autistic spectrum disorder. Neuropsychologia 2006; 44:610–621.
82. Lord C, Risi S, Lambrecht L, et al. The autism diagnostic observation schedule-generic: a standard measure of social and communication deficits associated with the spectrum of autism. J Autism Dev Disord 2000; 30:205–223.
83. Pelphrey KA, Morris JP, McCarthy G. Neural basis of eye gaze processing deficits in autism. Brain 2005; 128:1038–1048.
84. Turner MA. Generating novel ideas: fluency performance in high-functioning and learning disabled individuals with autism. J Child Psychol Psychiatry 1999; 40:189–201.
85. Ozonoff S, South M, Miller JN. DSM-IV-defined Asperger syndrome: cognitive, behavioral and early history differentiation from high-functioning autism. Autism 2000; 4:29–46.
86. Belmonte MK, Yurgelun-Todd DA. Functional anatomy of impaired selective attention and compensatory processing in autism. Brain Res Cogn Brain Res 2003; 17:651–664.
87. Haist F, Adamo M, Westerfield M, et al. The functional neuroanatomy of spatial attention in autism spectrum disorder. Dev Neuropsychol 2005; 27:425–458.
88. Ring HA, Baron-Cohen S, Wheelwright S, et al. Cerebral correlates of preserved cognitive skills in autism: a functional MRI study of embedded figures task performance. Brain 1999; 122(pt 7):1305–1315.
89. Silk TJ, Rinehart N, Bradshaw JL, et al. Visuospatial processing and the function of prefrontal-parietal networks in autism spectrum disorders: a functional MRI study. Am J Psychiatry 2006; 163:1440–1443.
90. Luna B, Minshew NJ, Garver KE, et al. Neocortical system abnormalities in autism: an fMRI study of spatial working memory. Neurology 2002; 59:834–840.
91. Horwitz B, Rumsey JM, Grady CL, et al. The cerebral metabolic landscape in autism. Intercorrelations of regional glucose utilization. Arch Neurol 1988; 45:749–755.
92. Just MA, Cherkassky VL, Keller TA, et al. Cortical activation and synchronization during sentence comprehension in high-functioning autism: evidence of under-connectivity. Brain 2004; 127:1811–1821.
93. Koshino H, Carpenter PA, Minshew NJ, et al. Functional connectivity in an fMRI working memory task in high-functioning autism. Neuroimage 2005; 24:810–821.
94. Villalobos ME, Mizuno A, Dahl BC, et al. Reduced functional connectivity between V1 and inferior frontal cortex associated with visuomotor performance in autism. Neuroimage 2005; 25:916–925.
95. Welchew DE, Ashwin C, Berkouk K, et al. Functional disconnectivity of the medial temporal lobe in Asperger's syndrome. Biol Psychiatry 2005; 57:991–998.
96. Kana RK, Keller TA, Cherkassky VL, et al. Sentence comprehension in autism: thinking in pictures with decreased functional connectivity. Brain 2006; 129: 2484–2493.
97. Mizuno A, Villalobos ME, Davies MM, et al. Partially enhanced thalamocortical functional connectivity in autism. Brain Res 2006; 1104:160–174.
98. Cherkassky VL, Kana RK, Keller TA, et al. Functional connectivity in a baseline resting-state network in autism. Neuroreport 2006; 17:1687–1690.
99. Shields J, Varley R, Broks P, et al. Hemispheric function in developmental language disorders and high-level autism. Dev Med Child Neurol 1996; 38:473–486.

100. Munson J, Dawson G, Abbott R, et al. Amygdalar volume and behavioral development in autism. Arch Gen Psychiatry 2006; 63:686–693.
101. Murphy DG, Daly E, Schmitz N, et al. Cortical serotonin 5-HT2A receptor binding and social communication in adults with Asperger's syndrome: an in vivo SPECT study. Am J Psychiatry 2006; 163:934–936.
102. Friedman SD, Jensen JE, Frederick BB, et al. Brain changes to hypocapnia using rapidly interleaved phosphorus-proton magnetic resonance spectroscopy at 4 Tesla. J Cereb Blood Flow Metab 2007; 27(3):646–653.

9

Neuropathological Findings in Asperger Syndrome

Manuel F. Casanova

Department of Psychiatry, University of Louisville, Louisville, Kentucky, U.S.A.

INTRODUCTION

By defining Asperger syndrome as a pervasive developmental disorder (PDD) of childhood in the Diagnostic and Statistical Manual of Mental Disorders-Fourth Edition (DSM-IV-TR), clinicians emphasize its natural history: Asperger syndrome manifests as an amalgamation of continuous, lifelong characteristics affecting function in several broad areas of neurodevelopment.

During development, some autistic patients may overcome the pervasive nature of their language disturbance and "catch-up" with Asperger patients. A clinician taking a cross-sectional view of older patients, unaware of previous behaviors, may consequently be hard pressed to find differences between patients in the autism spectrum. It is common for a child to receive varying diagnoses, depending on the clinician and the diagnostic methods or screening instruments used. This varied diagnosis occurs despite the arbitrary DSM-IV consideration that a child with Asperger may not fulfill criteria for another PDD or schizophrenia.

Owing to the phenotypic overlap and associated difficulties with current diagnostic instruments (1–3), clinicians, unsurprisingly, debate whether conditions within the autism spectrum are separate from each other, whether they represent separate neurobiology, and whether they constitute different expressions of a multideterminant trait. Autistic spectrum disorder encompasses autism, atypical autism (PDD NOS), and Asperger syndrome.

This "broader phenotype" suggests a range of symptom manifestations in different severities from a similar multifactorial diathesis. As discussed elsewhere in this volume, the evidence suggests that common genetic mechanisms may exist for both autism and Asperger disease. According to Szatmari (3), "even if the genes were totally distinct, it is highly likely that the phenotypical effects of those genes would overlap and disrupt the same brain systems."

Unsurprisingly, preliminary data on the neuropathology of Asperger syndrome have revealed similar but less-severe findings as in autism (4). These preliminary findings emphasize changes in the limbic system and cerebellum consisting primarily of small neurons and increase in packing density. Given the considerable overlap in clinical manifestations and family histories, a review on the neurobiology and pathology of Asperger syndrome is by necessity conflated with what is currently known regarding autism.

Limitations of Postmortem Studies

It should be pointed out that almost any research into any PDD of childhood will suffer from severe limitations. Thus, genetic studies are restricted by the lack of further reproduction of affected individuals and a skewed sex ratio. Neuroimaging lacks the resolutions to provide for diagnosis. Structural and physiological deviations in anatomical regions of interest may not necessarily represent pathology. The scarcity of postmortem material has lead to neurochemical assays in peripheral tissues. The results of these studies may not be representative of mechanisms operating at the level of the central nervous system. Given the variability in measurements, small postmortem brain series are biased toward negative findings. It is quite possible that many good leads regarding the neuropathology of PDD have never been published. The following paragraphs relate some limitations of postmortem studies in PDD as related to comorbidities and tissue processing.

The study of postmortem PDD tissue samples entails specific considerations with regard to age of onset (diagnosis) and comorbidities. In the case of autism, a diagnosis is apparent by three years of age but symptoms are most clearly recognizable by four to five years of age (5). A small section of these patients seem to outgrow autism (6). In contrast, because language abilities come at an appropriate age group in Asperger syndrome (e.g., single words are apparent by two years of age and communicative phrases by three years), diagnosis may be delayed. Despite being considered a lifelong disorder with neurodevelopmental underpinnings, the clinical picture of Asperger syndrome often manifests itself differently with aging. Furthermore, comorbidity in Asperger disorder is the rule rather than the exception. Associated disorders include Tourette syndrome, affective disorders, attention deficit hyperactivity disorder, and obsessive-compulsive disorder. Postmortem findings related to older patients may not be representative of the core pathology that causes manifestations at an earlier age. Rather, pathological findings in older age groups are likely the result of "unrelated" comorbid conditions that express themselves with aging.

Studies based on frozen tissue samples may by hampered by thawing artifacts. Since many brain samples are collected at facilities that lack "snap freezing" equipment, tissues are usually slow frozen before being sent to a central tissue repository. Ice crystals formed during slow freezing cause membrane damage. A primary misconception about freezing is that ice crystals cause an increase in cell volume and hence their rupture; instead, it causes cell shrinkage. During slow freezing, extracellular crystallization occurs first, drawing water from within the cell. The use of certain chemicals like isopentane in combination with dry ice accelerates freezing by retarding the Leidenfrost effect that is seen with liquid nitrogen. However, these chemicals (e.g., isopentane) become concentrated in ice crystals creating a potential confound to molecular assays. Furthermore, washing of whole or ground tissue will loosen many intracellular molecules. Leakage of chemicals that cannot be quantified or ascertained makes this type of processed tissue worthless for neurochemical assays.

Sampling frozen tissue for study or distribution offers many limitations. Frozen tissue may shatter when cut, and the resultant fracture may not follow anatomical boundaries. The emphasis on obtaining a homogenous sample can only be achieved by including contaminating tissue, e.g., samples of cortex are usually contaminated with underlying white matter. It is seldom the case that regions of interest are dissected in fresh tissue and then frozen before being sent to a central tissue repository or brain bank.

Limited Interpretations of Select Pathological Parameters (Oxidative Load and Inflammation)

Results of many neuropathological studies on the autism spectrum may reflect the effect of variables such as postmortem intervals, seizures, and medication usage. Certain regions of the brain exhibit a pathoclisis toward hypoxia prompted by seizures and preagonal conditions such as drowning and attempts at resuscitation. These parameters need to be carefully taken into account when interpreting Purkinje cell loss and somatic abnormalities of hippocampal cells within the cornu ammonis. Similarly, parameters of oxidative stress are closely regulated and most likely reflect the preagonal and agonal conditions of the patients rather than the core pathology of the same. Frozen tissue used for postmortem analysis is usually derived from brains that have been sampled many times for the purpose of distribution. Repeated cycles of thawing and freezing serve as an oxidative stressor, which are difficult or impossible to account for when interpreting results of an experiment. Further complications are offered by comorbidities that alter the oxidative load of postmortem tissue from autistic patients, e.g., seizure disorders, metabolic disturbances, low cerebral blood perfusion. Each of these possibilities has to be examined on a case-by-case basis. The fact that some of these variables [e.g., postmortem interval (PMI), cause of death] have not been considered within the statistical analysis of published studies is unsettling.

One of the reasons for studying oxidative loads is the underlying presumption that the same is caused by an inflammatory reaction. Some of the findings suggesting an inflammatory response are derived from peripheral markers. Systemic inflammation may not produce the same effects as inflammatory responses confined to the brain. Rather, subsequent mediators are involved in initiating and sustaining the inflammatory reaction and propitiating brain damage. Chemokines themselves have important roles in brain development. Injection of chemokines into the lateral ventricles of rats during specific postnatal days alters both social and environmental exploratory behavior. Chemokines appear to play an important role during development by mediating the survival of cells and helping orchestrate cellular migration (7). Proinflammatory cytokines increase reactive oxygen species, leading to cell loss. The results are of importance because antioxidants such as N-acetyl-cysteine (NAC) may provide protections against cell damage caused by oxidative injury (8). The findings could be of importance as a disturbance of the blood-brain barrier during specific stages of development by an inflammatory process (e.g., exposure to lipopolysaccharide) leads to local or diffuse white matter damage, with prolonged responses causing decreased white matter volume, astrogliosis, and hypomyelination (9). In this case, microglia and oligodendrocytes participate in a cascade of targeting a late oligodecdrocyte precursor that gives rise to periventricular leukomalacia (10).

It should be stressed that an inflammatory reaction presupposes participation of a vascular component. By definition, inflammation is a local response of tissue to injury that involves small vessels and cells within these vessels. The response is quite stereotyped, manifesting hyperemia, edema, and the adhesion of leukocytes to blood vessels. A vascular response appears not to be present in postmortem studies of PDD. Positive reports appear to be limited to innate cellular components (astrocytes and microglia) and systemic rather than local chemical mediators.

Neuropathology of Autism

Conceptually, autism has been classified as a disorder of the arousal-modulating systems of the brain (11). According to this theory, autistic individuals are in a chronic state of overarousal, and the abnormal behaviors exhibited by the patients are means of diminishing this arousal. Other proposals include the "theory of mind" and "executive dysfunction." The theory of mind explains the autistic inability to interact socially as a difficulty in perceiving the emotions and thoughts of others (12). Many argue that the tasks necessary to guarantee this interactive process are really tests of executive functioning (13,14). Unsurprisingly, autistic patients perform poorly in neuropsychological tests that reflect executive function, e.g., Wisconsin Card Sort test and the Tower of London test. A major problem with these complex theories is the inability to verify them without a known pathophysiological mechanism. Modern days neuropathological studies converge on ideas and findings that may add construct validity to these observations. Whereas previous studies emphasized posterior fossa structures and the limbic system as possible sites of pathology, modern studies suggest a role of the neocortex and attendant white matter connectivity in the pathology of autism.

In recent years, neuropathological studies have revealed abnormalities in various brain regions. Martha Bauman and colleagues (15–17) used whole hemispheres of 19 cases embedded in celloidin to describe the pathology in both Nissl stain and Golgi impregnated sections. Six more cases were added by Bailey et al. (18) and 13 others have appeared as case reports (19–23). These studies (based on 38 patients) reveal increased cell-packing density and reduced cell size in the amygdala, entorhinal cortex, subiculum, mammillary bodies, and septum, with specific dendritic abnormalities of CA1 and CA4 pyramidal cells. In the cerebellum, both Purkinje and granule cells from neocerebellar cortex show reductions in numbers. Cells in the deep cerebellar nuclei (emboliform, globose, and fastigial) are reduced in numbers and those remaining are small and pale staining. Bailey and coworkers (18) have added to the pathology by describing abnormalities in cortical lamination, heterotopias, and increased neurons in all of the six specimens they studied. The data suggest that the neuropathological underpinning of autism affects multiple systems or involves widespread areas of the brain, rather than discrete anatomical structures (24).

Structural abnormalities by brain imaging have included localized hypoplasia of the corpus callosum (25) and variations in cerebral asymmetry (26–29). Findings for the cerebellum have been contradictory with some studies showing reduction in size (30,31) and others unable to find an abnormality (28,32). The imaging literature has been reviewed by Goldberg et al. (33). According to these researchers, most imaging findings lack replication and/or control for confounding variables. They concluded that enlarged brain size (macroencephaly), particularly in the temporoparietal brain region, and decreased size of the posterior corpus callosum are the only independently replicated findings (33).

Clinical studies have made references to enlarged head circumference (macrocephaly) in children with autism (34–38). Although external measures account for, at most, 60% of the variance in cranial capacity (39), both postmortem (22,40) and MRI studies (41) have confirmed the presence of increased brain weight/volume in a subset of autistic individuals (42). This finding appears true after controlling for height, gender, the presence of epilepsy, or other medical disorders (43,44). Enlarged brain regions appear confined to the temporal, parietal, and occipital lobes, but do not affect the frontal lobes (45). The relationship between megalencephaly and performance IQ (high or low IQ autistics) is less clear (43,46,47).

It is noteworthy that mental deficiency and either macro- or megalencephaly has been reported with sex chromosome abnormalities (48–51), some of which present with autistic symptomatology (52) Despite the enlarged brains, no consistent pattern of cerebral dysplasia has been found in these cases. The observation may be of some relevance to autism where affected individuals are primarily males and often exhibit both macroencephaly and mental retardation without evident cortical dysplasia.

The phenomenon of macroencephaly in autism receives further support from functional neuroimaging and neurochemical studies. Concentration of the four major gangliosides has been measured in the cerebrospinal fluid (CSF) of 20 autistic children and 25 controls (53). The level of all gangliosides was significantly higher in the autistic children. Although localized in the outer neuronal membrane, gangliosides are found in highest concentration in the synaptic junction (54,55) and small portions are extruded to the CSF during exocytosis (56). The CSF levels of gangliosides among autistic patients suggest increased synaptic activity and/or an enlarged membrane compartment.

In a pilot study on 31P MRS (magnetic resonance spectroscopy) brain, high-energy phosphate and membrane phospholipid metabolism were investigated in the prefrontal cortex of 11 autistic adolescents and an equal number of age-, gender-, IQ-matched controls (57). The phospholipid data indicated enhanced degradation of brain membranes in autism. The finding is also in agreement with the neuropathological observation of a truncated development of the neuronal dendritic tree (16,58).

Two studies have examined cortical cell density in autism by using the Grey Level Index—the ratio of area covered by Nissl-stained elements to unstained area in postmortem samples (59). These studies have found no significant differences between autistics and controls (60,61). Buxhoeveden et al. (62) reported an increased Grey Level Index in a single autistic patient, although no age-matched control was provided (63). This preliminary study offered little or no information by which to judge the appropriateness of the methodology employed. Some authors relate the lack of Grey Level Index abnormalities to an increased total number of minicolumns as suggestive of diminished cell size. More specifically, the results indicate that pyramidal cells, the backbone of cell arrays in minicolumns, must be reduced in size (Fig. 1) (61). Since pyramidal cell size is related to connectivity, the smaller pyramidal cells in the brains of autistic patients provide a bias, favoring short over longer connections, e.g., u-fibers over commisural projections.

The available literature indicates that autistic individuals have larger brains, increased cell-packing density, and synaptic abnormalities. Several reasons justify the use of minicolumns to elucidate the nature of the reported pathology. First, since minicolumns are a basic functional unit of the brain around which neurons in cortical space congregate (64–67), changes on the basis of circuitry or spatial morphology may be expressed within this fundamental unit of cortical structure. Second, the relative proximity of neurons to one another is reflected in the relative proximity of minicolumns to one another. Therefore, examining the minicolumn is a way of independently confirming the results of cell-counting methods. Lastly, quantifying the density of neurons within cell

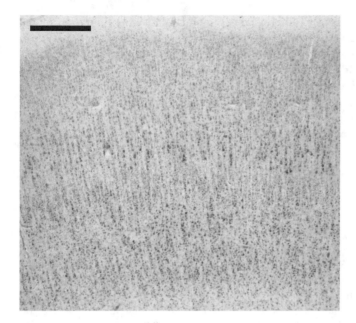

Figure 1 Four different parameters have been used to measure minicolumnar width, these include the spacing between apical dendritic bundles, myelinated bundles, pyramidal cell arrays, and double bouquet cells. The figure illustrates the striking rectilinear arrangement of pyramidal cell arrays. These structural motifs are fragmented by thinner sections (e.g., paraffin embedded) and have traditionally been examined in cellodin 35-μm thick sections (scale bar 500 μm).

columns will enable us to precisely describe the morphology of interneuronal spaces. Reduction in interneuronal space must occur either in the main body of cells that constitutes the visible body of the column in a Nissl stain or in the space that horizontally separates minicolumns, or perhaps both. Determining the location of interneuronal reduction and measuring its extent is vital to any pathological explanations. These compartments differentiate synaptic spaces and areas of unmyelinated interneuronal connections from those providing the major afferent and efferent cortical projections.

Functional activity that occurs in the space surrounding individual minicolumns (the neuropil space) differs from that within the area occupied primarily by the neuronal soma (65,66,68–70). It is known that large diameter axons mingle with the perikarya in a neuronal column (70,71), or are closely adjacent to the pyramidal cells. Moreover, the neuropil space is occupied by dendrites and possibly by small bundles of narrow-diameter axons that originate within the cell columns (68,69,72,73). Therefore, changes in the distributions of transcallosal fibers or thalamic inputs may affect cell soma arrangements, while changes in dendritic processes and intrahemispheric organization may expand or reduce neuropil space. Accurately quantifying the extent of these changes requires analysis of the spatial configuration of the minicolumn in the autistic brain.

The presence of macroencephaly and synaptic abnormalities in autism is suggestive of disturbances in the regulation of germinal cell proliferation. The end result of this abnormality is an increased number of neurons or in the total number of minicolumns. In the following sections, we will elaborate on these possibilities. It is well established that there is an exuberant development of neurons and their connections early in development, which is followed by their partial elimination (cell death). Brain hyperplasia may therefore result from redundant formation of tissue (cell and connections) or from subnormal elimination (74).

After migration, neurons face the issue of survival or death. The young neurons differentiate, i.e., develop processes, organelles, and form synaptic connections. An integral part of the development of the nervous system is the loss of large numbers of differentiated neurons (75,76). It is unclear as to why there is an initial overproduction of cells; and also, the precise reason of their death remains a mystery. Among a variety of ideas put forward to explain the purpose of cell death, the most popular view is that it serves to match the size of the target with its innervation pool. This would imply that the targets are too small to support survival of all associated neurons. The target is believed to provide trophic factors necessary for the survival of neurons. Small targets with lesser amounts of trophic factors will therefore create competitive situation for survival. It is believed that those neurons that were unable to obtain adequate amounts of trophic factors will die. There is experimental evidence in support and against this view (76). A number of trophic factors such as the nerve growth factor, ciliary neurotrophic factor, brain derived neurotrophic factor, and neurotrophins have been shown to rescue neurons from death. Patients with multiple somatic abnormalities may manifest disturbances in programmed cell death (77). These abnormalities may include macrocephaly, dysmorphic features, and syndactyly, all of which have been reported in autism (35).

Minicolumnarity and Asperger Syndrome

It does appear that minicolumnar pathology may provide an overarching explanation to many of the signs and symptoms observed in autism. Supernumerary minicolumns provide for cortical expansions and consequently brain growth. Furthermore, exigencies in terms of connectivity provide for scaled expansion of white matter as the total number of minicolumns increases. A putative minicolumnopathy in autism therefore explains differences in brain size, gray/white matter ratios, and an increase in the outer radiate white matter compartment (78,79). At present, two patients with Asperger have been studied with the same computerized algorithms as those previously used in autism case series (Fig. 2) (80). Three areas (frontal area 9, middle temporal area 21, and superior temporal area 22) were examined in celloidin embedded, 35-μm thick

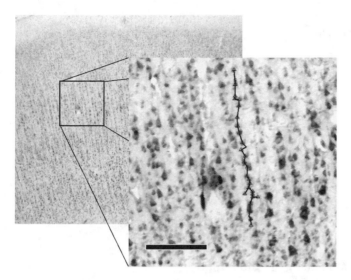

Figure 2 Pyramidal cell arrays can be fragmented by tissue sectioning. Visual methods are inaccurate at quantifying the intricacies of these structures in either two or three dimensions. The figure illustrates an algorithm based on the Euclidean minimum spanning tree that recognizes rectilinear arrangements. The use of this algorithm is based on the supposition that pyramidal cell arrays are remnants of the ontogenetic radial cell column (layer III, scale bar 150 μm).

sections. Neuropathological changes failed to reveal neurodegenerative changes or gliosis. Results indicated that minicolumns were smaller and their components cells more dispersed than normal. Findings were similar with those previously reported in autism except for the magnitude of the changes—patients with Asperger were less affected than those with autism (Fig. 3). This comparison appears proper as both Asperger, autistic, and controls were derived from the same brain collection and were processed in exactly the same manner. Although the total number of specimens (9 autistic and 2 Asperger) is small, there is a trend for the described pathology to improve with aging. The results are in keeping with an autistic spectrum or continuum of symptomatology upon which Frith (81) commented that "Asperger syndrome is the first plausible variant to crystallize from the autism spectrum."

The results of the previously described neuropathological studies are of interests because both autistic and Asperger patients showed diminished mini-columnar width. The compartment most affected in both instances was the peripheral neuropil space as compared to the cell core. In both cases, the percentage amount of diminution was similar. The peripheral neuropil space is the minicolumnar compartment where many interneuronal elements are located. Most strikingly, double bouquet axons provide for a shower curtain of inhibition that wraps around the core of pyramidal cells. A defect in the peripheral neuropil space may provide for signals to suffuse into adjacent minicolumns. The overall

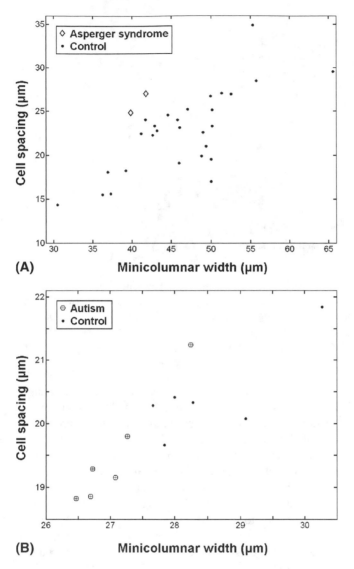

Figure 3 Results of our computerized morphometry plotted as minicolumnar width (CW) versus mean distance between neighboring neurons within a minicolumn (MCS). (**A**) Data are from our Asperger's patients (80) and associated controls in cortical area 22. (**B**) Data from our autism series (61) and associated controls in cortical area 9.

effect is one of amplification and a bias in the signal to noise ratio in favor of signal. The pathological findings in both autistic and Asperger patients provide a cascade of putative abnormalities linking minicolumns to macrocolumns and implicate the inhibitory elements of these cortical modules. The following paragraphs will illustrate the role of inhibition in cortical modularity.

Cortical Modules and Inhibition (Insights Gained from the Barrel Cortex)

The specialized columns in layer IV of rodent somatosensory cortex have been the object of intense study. This is important for understanding how columns process tactile input, which is very significant for the study of PDD of childhood. Stimulation of the thalamus results in activity restricted to a single barrel (82) and demonstrates the input specificity of this module. The spatiotemporal spread of activity in barrel cortex is thought to be based on *N*-methyl-D-aspartate (NMDA) receptor–mediated mechanisms (82). In a study of optical imaging of barrel cortex, it was found that low concentrations of gamma-aminobutyric acid (GABA) A receptor antagonist (bicuculline) increase the amplitude of the optical signals without affecting their spatiotemporal propagation. Enhancement of NMDA receptors dramatically alters the spatiotemporal pattern of excitation, where it spreads to supragranular and infragranular layers and adjacent barrel columns. Similar changes result from short, high frequency pulse stimulation of the thalamus.

Temporal relationships among tactile stimuli are coded by facilitory and inhibitory interactions among neurons located in neighboring barrel columns. That is, the interstimulus intervals are important in determining whether it will facilitate a response. Evidence is that facilitory response is produced by intracortical rather than subcortical mechanisms (83). Inhibition within a barrel serves as a contrast enhancement to differentiate small versus large magnitude responses. Less vigorous responses, such as inputs from nonoptimal deflection angles or noncolumnar whiskers, are strongly depressed (84). In barrel cortex, about 20% of the thalamic afferents terminate on aspinous, presumably GABAergic interneurons (85,86). Layer IV spiny stellates cells are the input neurons that amplify and relay incoming excitation from the periphery. Layer V pyramidal cells integrate signals within and across cortical columns and distribute information to cortical and subcortical regions (87). Layer IV cells act as strong amplifiers of even weak thalamic inputs because they are highly interconnected, whereas layer V pyramidal cells are the major cortical output neurons to subcortical centers.

An in-depth study of feedforward inhibition in the mouse barrel provided findings of importance to a proper understanding of sensory processing in the neocortex and PDD in particular (88). The study found that several distinct classes of interneurons are involved in feedforward inhibition—a diverse population according to electrophysiology, cytochemistry, and morphology. Porter et al (88) also discovered that excitatory neurons were actually less responsive than inhibitory interneurons to thalamic input. Another discovery was that interneurons that discharged in response to thalamocortical input received larger synaptic inputs. The morphology of axonal arbors also varied greatly among types of inhibitory interneurons mediating feedforward inhibition. All of them, except for two cells, had cell bodies located within layer IV or the border of layers IV/V. On the basis of the morphology of the axonal arbors, the authors found five categories regarding lamina distribution and horizontal localization. Two types seemed to have all of their arbors within the minimum minor axis of a barrel (200 μm). However, one type of cell had arbors that extended from 350 μm to 776 μm, which would encompass an additional barrel in the same row on either or both sides. In conclusion, some inhibitory interneurons generate feedforward inhibition within their own barrel; others relay a disynaptic inhibition to upper cortical layers within their own columns as well as to columns outside the barrel of origin. This is a duplication of the finding in monkey cortex, with only the scale changed to match the smaller size of the barrel columns. In both cases, there were a few cells with axons extending to neighboring macrocolumns but seemingly only to an immediate neighbor.

The feedforward inhibitory interneurons also engage in very rapid mutual suppression after the first spike (most feedforward inhibition is based on a single volley). This is thought to allow for faster recovery of the cortex from the initial inhibitory volley. The importance of this is reinforced by recent studies showing that inhibitory interneurons in rat barrel cortex are interconnected by gap junctions. The gap junctions were frequent between inhibitory cells of the same type, while rare for those between differing kinds (89). Another study found a high occurrence of gap junctions between fast-spiking interneurons. None were found for pyramidal cells or between fast-spiking cells and other cortical cells. Electrical coupling is thought to synchronize activity of neurons. Interneurons are thought to generate synchronous inhibitory rhythms in the neocortex (90,91). It is easy to see how a breakdown of this mutual inhibition would result in a distortion of signal processing.

REFERENCES

1. Miller JN, Ozonoff S. Did Asperger's cases have Asperger disorder? J Child Psychol Psychiatry 1997; 38:247–251.
2. Wolff S. Schizoid personality in childhood and Asperger syndrome. In: Klin A, Volkmar FR, Sparrow SS, eds. Asperger Syndrome. New York, NY: Guilford Press, 2000:277–305.
3. Szatmari P. Perspectives on the classification of Asperger syndrome. In: Klin A, Volkmar FR, Sparrow SS, eds. Asperger Syndrome. New York, NY: Guilford Press, 2000:403–417.
4. Bauman ML. Brief report: neuroanatomic observations of the brain in pervasive developmental disorders. J Autism Dev Disord 1996; 26:199–203.
5. Le Couteur A, Rutter M, Lord C, et al. Autism diagnostic interview: a standardized investigator-based instrument. J Autism Dev Disord 1989; 19:363–387.
6. Lord C, Spence S. Autism spectrum disorders: phenotype and diagnosis. In: Moldin SO, Rubenstein JLR, eds. Understanding Autism: From Basic Neuroscience to Treatment. New York, NY: CRC Taylor & Francis, 2006:12–24.
7. Brenneman DE, Hauser J, Spong CY, et al. VIP and D-ala-peptide T-amide release chemokines which prevent HIV-1 GP120-induced neuronal death. Brain Res 1999; 838:27–36.
8. Paintlia MK, Paintlia AS, Barbosa E, et al. N-acetylcysteine prevents endotoxin-induced degeneration of oligodendrocyte progenitors and hypomyelination in developing rat brain. J Neurosci Res 2004; 78:347–361.

9. Stolp HB, Dziegielewska KM, Ek CJ, et al. Long-term changes in blood-brain barrier permeability and white matter following prolonged systemic inflammation in early development in the rat. Eur J Neurosci 2005; 22:2805–2816.

10. Volpe JJ. Neurobiology of periventricular leukomalacia in the premature infant. Pediatr Res 2001; 50:553–562.

11. Hutt C, Hutt SJ, Lee D, et al. Arousal and childhood autism. Nature 1964; 204:908–909.

12. Baron-Cohen S, Leslie AM, Frith U. Does the autistic child have a "theory of mind"? Cognition 1985; 21:37–46.

13. Russell J, Mauthner N, Sharpe S, et al. The "windows task" as a measure of strategic deception in preschoolers and autistic subjects. Br J Dev Psychol 1991; 9:331–349.

14. Hughes C, Russell J. Autistic childrens' difficulty with mental disengagement from an object: its implications for theories of autism. Dev Psychol 1993; 29:498–510.

15. Bauman ML, Kemper TL. Neuroanatomic observations of the brain in autism. In: Bauman ML, Kemper TL, eds. The Neurobiology of Autism. Baltimore, MD: Johns Hopkins University Press, 1994:119–145.

16. Raymond GV, Bauman ML, Kemper TL. Hippocampus in autism: a Golgi analysis. Acta Neuropathol 1995; 91:117–119.

17. Kemper TL, Bauman ML. Neuropathology of infantile autism. J Neuropathol Exp Neurol 1998; 57:645–652.

18. Bailey A, Luthert P, Dean A, et al. A clinicopathological study of autism. Brain 1998; 121:889–905.

19. Williams RS, Hauser SL, Purpura DP, et al. Autism and mental retardation: neuropathological studies performed in four retarded persons with autistic behavior. Arch Neurol 1980; 37:749–753.

20. Coleman PD, Romano J, Lapham LW, et al. Cell counts in cerebral cortex of an autistic patient. J Autism Dev Disord 1985; 15:245–255.

21. Ritvo ER, Freeman BJ, Scheibel AB, et al. Lower Purkinje cell counts in the cerebella of four autistic subjects: initial findings of the UCLA-NSAC Autopsy Research Report. Am J Psychiatry 1986; 143:862–866.

22. Bailey A, Luthert P, Bolton P, et al. Autism and megalencephaly. Lancet 1993; 341:1225–1226.

23. Rodier PM, Ingram JL, Tisdale B, et al. Embryological origin for autism: developmental anomalies of the cranial nerve motor nuclei. J Comp Neurol 1996; 370:247–261.

24. Bailey A, Phillips W, Rutter M. Autism: towards an integration of clinical, genetic, neuropsychological, and neurobiological perspectives. J Child Psychol Psychiatry 1996; 37:39–126.

25. Egaas B, Courchesne E, Saitoh O. Reduced size of corpus callosum in autism. Arch Neurol 1995; 45:317–324.

26. Hauser SL, DeLong GR, Rosman NP. Pneumographic findings in the infantile autism syndrome: a correlation with temporal lobe disease. Brain 1975; 98:667–688.

27. Tsai LY, Jacoby CG, Stewart MA. Morphological cerebral asymmetries in autistic children. Biol Psychiatry 1983; 18:317–327.

28. Rumsey JM, Creasey H, Stepanek JS, et al. Hemispheric asymmetries, fourth ventricular size, and cerebellar morphology in autism. J Autism Dev Disord 1988; 18:127–137.

29. Hendren RL, De Backer I, Pandina GJ. Review of neuroimaging studies of child and adolescent psychiatric disorders from the past 10 years. J Am Acad Child Adolesc Psychiatry 2000; 39:815–828 (review).

30. Courchesne E, Yeung-Courchesne R, Press GA, et al. Hypoplasia of cerebellar vermal lobules VI and VII in autism. N Engl J Med 1988; 318:1349–1354.
31. Murakami JW, Courchesne E, Press GA, et al. Reduced cerebellar hemisphere size and its relationship to vermal hypoplasia in autism. Arch Neurol 1989; 46:689–694.
32. Holttum JR, Minshew NJ, Sanders RS, et al. Magnetic resonance imaging of the posterior fossa in autism. Biol Psychiatry 1992; 32:1091–1101.
33. Goldberg J, Szatmari P, Nahmias C. Imaging of autism: lessons from the past to guide studies in the future. Can J Psychiatry 1999; 44:793–801.
34. Steg JP, Rapoport JL. Minor physical anomalies in normal, neurotic, learning disabled, and severely disturbed children. J Autism Child Schizophr 1975; 5:299–307.
35. Walker HA. Incidence of minor physical anomaly in autism. J Autism Child Schizophr 1977; 7:165–176.
36. Davidovitch M, Patterson BJ, Gartside P. Head circumference measurements in children with autism. J Child Neurol 1996; 11:389–393.
37. Rapin I. Neurological examination. In: Rapin I, ed. Preschool Children with Inadequate Communication: Developmental Language Disorder, Autism, Low IQ. London, UK: Mac Keith Press, 1996:98–122.
38. Woodhouse W, Bailey A, Rutter M, et al. Head circumference in autism and other pervasive developmental disorders. J Child Psychol Psychiatry 1996; 37:665–671.
39. Friedman L, Wiechers IR, Cerny CA, et al. If patients with schizophrenia have small brains, why don't they have small heads? Schizophr Res 2000; 42:1–6.
40. Bauman ML, Kemper TL. Is autism a progressive process? Neurology 1997; 48(suppl 2):A285.
41. Filipek PA, Richelme C, Kennedy DN, et al. Morphometric analysis of the brain in developmental language disorders and autism. Ann Neurol 1992; 32:475.
42. Courchesne E, Müller RA, Saitoh O. Brain weight in autism: normal in the majority of cases, megalencephalic in rare cases. Neurology 1999; 52:1057–1105.
43. Piven J, Arndt S, Bailey J, et al. An MRI study of brain size in autism. Am J Psychiatry 1995; 152:1145–1149.
44. Fombonne E, Rogé B, Claverie J, et al. Microcephaly and macrocephaly in autism. J Autism Dev Disord 1999; 29:113–119.
45. Piven J, Arndt S, Bailey J, et al. Regional brain enlargement in autism: a magnetic resonance imaging study. J Am Acad Child Adolesc Psychiatry 1996; 35:530–536.
46. Lainhart JE, Piven J, Wzorek M, et al. Macrocephaly in children and adults with autism. J Am Acad Child Adolesc Psychiatry 1997; 36:282–290.
47. Stevensen RE, Schroer RJ, Skinner C, et al. Autism and macrocephaly. Lancet 1997; 349:1744–1745.
48. Brun A, Gustavson KH. Cerebral malformations in the XYY syndrome. Acta Pathol Microbiol Scand[A] 1972; 80:627–633.
49. Laxova R. Fragile X syndrome. Adv Pediatr 1994; 41:305–342 (review).
50. Drigo P, Carra S, Laverda AM, et al. Macrocephaly and chromosome disorders: a case report. Brain Dev 1996; 18:312–315.
51. Sabaratnam M. Pathological and neuropathological findings in two males with fragile-X syndrome. J Intellect Disabil Res 2000; 44:81–85.
52. Cohen IL, Sudhalter V, Pfadt A, et al. Why are autism and the fragile-X syndrome associated? Conceptual and methodological issues. Am J Hum Genet 1991; 48:195–202.
53. Lekman A, Skjeldal O, Sponheim E, et al. Gangliosides in children with autism. Acta Paediatr 1995; 84:787–790.

54. Hansson HA, Holmgren J, Svennerholm L. Ultrastructural localization of cell membrane GM1 ganglioside by cholera toxin. Proc Natl Acad Sci U S A 1977; 74:3782–786.
55. Svennerholm L, Boström K, Fredman P, et al. Human brain gangliosides: developmental changes from early fetal stage to advance age. Biochim Biophys Acta 1989; 1005:109–117.
56. Svennerholm L. Gangliosides in synaptic transmission. In: Svennerholm L, Mandel P, Dreyfus H, et al., eds. Structure and Function of Gangliosides. New York, NY: Plenum Press, 1980:533–544.
57. Minshew NJ, Goldstein G, Dombrowski SM, et al. A preliminary 31P MRS study of autism: evidence for undersynthesis and increased degradation of brain membranes. Biol Psychiatry 1993; 33:762–773.
58. Bauman ML, Kemper TL. Histoanatomic observations of the brain in early infantile autism. Neurology 1985; 35:866–874.
59. Schlaug G, Schleicher A, Zilles K. Quantitative analysis of the columnar arrangement of neurons in the human cingulate cortex. J Comp Neurol 1995; 351:441–452.
60. Casanova MF, Buxhoeveden DP, Switala AE, et al. Neuronal density and architecture (gray level index) in the brains of autistic patients. J Child Neurol 2002; 17:515–521.
61. Casanova MF, van Kooten IAJ, Switala AE, et al. Minicolumnar abnormalities in autism. Acta Neuropathol 2006; 112:287–303.
62. Buxhoeveden DP, Semendeferi K, Schenker N, et al. Decreased cell column spacing in autism. Abstr Soc Neurosci 2004; 30:582.6.
63. Courchesne E, Pierce K. Why the frontal cortex in autism might be talking only to itself: local over-connectivity but long-distance disconnection. Curr Opin Neurobiol 2005; 15:225–230.
64. Tommerdahl MA, Favorov OV, Whitsel BL, et al. Minicolumnar activation patterns in cat and monkey S1 cortex. Cereb Cortex 1993; 3:399–411.
65. Favorov OV, Kelly DG. Minicolumnar organization within somatosensory cortical segregates, I: development of afferent connections. Cereb Cortex 1994; 4:408–427.
66. Favorov OV, Kelly DG. Minicolumnar organization within somatosensory cortical segregates, II: emergent functional properties. Cereb Cortex 1994; 4:428–442.
67. Mountcastle VB. The columnar organization of the neocortex. Brain 1997; 120: 701–722.
68. Seldon HL. Structure of human auditory cortex, I: cytoarchitectonics and dendritic distributions. Brain Res 1981; 229:277–294.
69. Seldon HL. Structure of human auditory cortex, II. Axon distributions and morphological correlates of speech perception. Brain Res 1981; 229:295–310.
70. Ong WY, Garey LJ. Neuronal architecture of the human temporal cortex. Anat Embryol (Berl) 1990; 181:351–364.
71. Seldon HL. The anatomy of speech perception: human auditory cortex. In: Jones EG, Peters A, eds. Association and Auditory Cortices. New York, NY: Plenum Press, 1985:273–327.
72. Jones EG, Burton H. Cytoarchitecture and somatic sensory connectivity of thalamic nuclei other than the ventrobasal complex in the cat. J Comp Neurol 1974; 154:395–432.
73. Szentágothai J. The modular architectonic principle of neural centers. Rev Physiol Biochem Pharmacol 1983; 98:11–61.
74. Friede RL. Developmental Neuropathology. 2nd ed. Berlin, Germany: Springer-Verlag, 1989.

75. Oppenheim RW. Cell death during development of the nervous system. Annu Rev Neurosci 1991; 14:453–501.
76. Sohal GS. The role of target size in neuronal survival. J Neurobiol 1992; 23: 1124–1130.
77. Hennekam RC, Cohen MM Jr. Hypothesis: patient with possible disturbance in programmed cell death. Eur J Hum Genet 1995; 3:374–377.
78. Casanova MF, Buxhoeveden D, Switala A, et al. Minicolumnar pathology in autism. Neurology 2002; 58:428–432.
79. Casanova MF, Buxhoeveden DP, Brown C. Clinical and macroscopic correlates of minicolumnar pathology in autism. J Child Neurol 2002; 17:692–695.
80. Casanova MF, Buxhoeveden D, Switala A, et al. Asperger's syndrome and cortical neuropathology. J Child Neurol 2002; 17:142–145.
81. Frith U. Autism and Asperger Syndrome. Cambridge, UK: Cambridge University Press, 1991.
82. Laaris N, Carlson GC, Keller A. Thalamic-evoked synaptic interactions in barrel cortex revealed by optical imaging. J Neurosci 2000; 20:1529–1537.
83. Shimegi S, Ichikawa T, Akasaki T, et al. Temporal characteristics of response integration evoked by multiple whisker stimulations in the barrel cortex of rats. J Neurosci 1999; 19:10164–10175.
84. Brumberg JC, Pinto DJ, Simons DJ. Spatial gradients and inhibitory summation in the rat whisker barrel system. J Neurophysiol 1996; 76:130–140.
85. Benshalom G, White EL. Quantification of thalamocortical synapses with spiny stellate neurons in layer IV of mouse somatosensory cortex. J Comp Neurol 1986; 253:303–314.
86. White EL, Rock MP. A comparison of thalamocortical and other synaptic inputs to dendrites of two non-spiny neurons in a single barrel of mouse SmI cortex. J Comp Neurol 1981; 195:265–277.
87. Feldmeyer D, Sakmann B. Synaptic efficacy and reliability of excitatory connections between the principal neurones of the input (layer 4) and output layer (layer 5) of the neocortex. J Physiol 2000; 525:31–39.
88. Porter JT, Johnson CK, Agmon A. Diverse types of interneurons generate thalamus-evoked feedforward inhibition in the mouse barrel cortex. J Neurosci 2001; 21: 2699–2710.
89. Gibson JR, Beierlein M, Connors BW. Two networks of electrically coupled inhibitory neurons in neocortex. Nature 1999; 402:75–79.
90. Benardo LS. Recruitment of GABAergic inhibition and synchronization of inhibitory interneurons in rat neocortex. J. Neurophysiol 1997; 77:3134–3144.
91. Jefferys JGR, Traub RD, Whittington MA. Neuronal networks for induced "40 Hz" rhythms. Trends Neurosci 1996; 19:202–208.

10

The Genetics, Epigenetics and Proteomics of Asperger's Disorder

Maria E. Johnson

BrainScience Augusta and Developmental Disability Psychiatric Consultation-Liaison, Gracewood Hospital, Augusta, Georgia, U.S.A.

Jeffrey L. Rausch

BrainScience Augusta and Department of Psychiatry and Health Behavior, Medical College of Georgia, Augusta, Georgia, U.S.A.

INTRODUCTION

Hans Asperger, in his original work, wrote that

"The idea that psychopathic states are constitutional and, hence, inheritable has long been confirmed....

"We have been able to discern related incipient traits in parents or relatives in every single case where it was possible for us to make a closer acquaintance. Usually certain autistic peculiarities were present, but often we also found the fully fledged autistic picture starting with abnormalities of expressive functions and gaucheness up to the higher level of 'integration difficulties.'

However, it is a vain hope to think there may be a clear and simple mode of inheritance. These states are undoubtedly polygenetic, but it is as yet impossible to know whether such a trait is dominant or recessive.....

It is fascinating to note that the autistic children we have seen here are almost exclusively boys. .... There is certainly a strong hint at a sex-linked or at least sex-limited mode of inheritance. " (1)

From the above, is apparent that Hans Asperger made four broad hypotheses regarding the biological etiology of his disorder: (*i*) it was inheritable, (*ii*) the traits were expressed as a spectrum in family members from less to more affected, (*iii*) the condition was undoubtedly polygenetic, and (*iv*) the inheritance was "sex-linked or at least sex-limited."

His predictions have been validated by subsequent research. The following chapter explores that research. Differences in terminology, diagnostic criteria, and categorization complicate the study of Asperger's disorder. This chapter uses the term Asperger's to designate DSM-IV (*Diagnostic and Statistical Manual of Mental Disorders, Fourth Edition*) Asperger's disorder, ICD-10 (International Statistical Classification of Diseases) Asperger syndrome as well as the criteria proposed by Prof. Gillberg.

HERITABILITY OF ASPERGER'S DISORDER

Published clinical observations (2), pedigree family studies (3), and case-controlled family history studies (4,5) support Asperger's first hypothesis that the condition is an inheritable phenotype.

Autism and Asperger's disorder are inherited in the same families (2,6–15). Historically, in one of the earliest reports on Asperger's disorder, van Krevelen described a family where "one of the three children had the typical features of an autistic psychopath (Asperger's definition) and another (the youngest) could be unmistakably diagnosed as suffering from infantile autism (Kanner's definition) (9). Molecular studies of both Asperger's (13) and autism confirm the genetic basis implicated by family studies (6,11,14,16). Including less or more affected autism phenotypes in genetic studies gains statistical power to detect loci, lending evidence to a common inheritance (13,17–21).

Studies of autism spectrum disorders (ASDs) have shown a 45 times greater autism risk in siblings than in the general population. Twin studies in ASDs have documented a higher concordance rate in monozygotic (60–91%) than in dizygotic twins (0–6%) (11,14). Familial inheritance may be as large as 71% (22) when one considers autism, Asperger's, and suspicion of Asperger's in the analysis.

Some have proposed a higher frequency of transmission in families of Asperger's disorder than autism (4,5). This may indicate a greater genetic basis for Asperger's disorder and perhaps leave more room for an environmental contribution to autism. The decrease in obstetric risk factors, the lack of identified environmental contributions compared with autism, and the normal IQ in Asperger's may imply inheritance of multiple autistic trait distribution otherwise diluted in the normal population.

HERITABILITY OF AUTISTIC TRAITS

Autistic Social Traits in the General Population

Autistic social traits unrelated to IQ have been shown to be common in the general population (10,23–26), and are increased in families with pervasive developmental disorder (27). These traits appear to be highly heritable (23,28). A study of school-age twin boys in the general population examined autistic traits and found 0.73 concordance for monozygotic twins ($N = 98$ pairs) and 0.37 concordance for dizygotic twins ($N = 143$ pairs) (23). However, the heritability of the triad of social impairments, communication impairments, and restricted repetitive behaviors and interests required for a diagnosis of Asperger's may only modestly overlap when combined (28). With this information, a dimensional endophenotype approach to genetic study of autistic social traits may be useful.

Broader Autism Phenotype

Hans Asperger originally and most emphasized his observations of unusual social traits in family members of 200 cases (1), and evidence accrued since validates his contention (hypothesis 2). Family members show a spectrum of expressivity of the phenotype, now termed the broader autism phenotype. In case studies (2,4,22,29–31), and family history studies (5,6,32), family members of individuals with Asperger's have unusual traits that have been noted in the diagnostic phenotype of Asperger's.

　　　Preferences for solitary activities, having few friends, rigidity, a preference for sameness, and resistance to change, and abnormalities of social and narrative language (31,32) have been described. In one family study, the traits of social motivation and range of interest or flexibility were the most highly heritable (33).

"Ways of Thinking" in the General Population

Increased levels of systemizing are part of the broader autism phenotype (34,35). The hyper-systemizing, assortive mating theory of autism proposes that mating between two individuals with an increased systemizing way of thinking will result in an increased likelihood for the development of Asperger's and autism (36,37). Dr. Baron-Cohen has shown evidence that humans' ways of thinking or "mentalizing" are sexually dimorphic in the population (38,39) across a spectrum of "empathizing" to "systemizing" (37–40). Both ways of thinking have been shown to be heritable (40–42).

　　　Empathizing is an instinctual way of thinking that is inherited as neurobiological "hardware" to make sense of the social world (41,42). Empathizing components are evident in early life in human children (3 months to 4 years of age). The components include the automatic detection of eye direction, automatic detection of emotions, and an ability to infer another's mental state (38,43,44). Developmental experience then helps teach the subtleties of empathy (38,41,42).

Systemizing is a way of thinking, to predict laws governing change and reveal the structure or laws of nature, a key feature being that single observations are recorded in a standardized manner (38). This way of thinking can be inadequate to manage the high variance and change in human social behavioral interaction.

MATERNAL VS. PATERNAL INHERITANCE OF AUTISTIC TRAITS

While maternal inheritance of autistic traits has been noted (2,45), paternal inheritance is better documented in Asperger's disorder. van Krevelen proposed the child's "autistic psychopathy is transmitted genetically via the father" (9). Volkmar reported a case where a father and son both had the condition. Others also have noted paternal inheritance.(7,46,47). Gillberg found that about 50% of all boys with Asperger's had a paternal family history of autism spectrum disorder (22). Increased maternal and paternal age have also been identified and are discussed below (48–52).

LINKAGE AND ASSOCIATION STUDIES

Linkage studies reveal chromosomal regions that may be associated with a phenotype in pedigree or population analysis. Linkage studies test gene markers through genome scans and measure the likelihood that the region near the markers cosegregates with a trait or disease gene but do not necessarily identify the susceptibility allele.

In a strictly defined study of Asperger's disorder, the authors chose to study only families that had a unilineal dominant mode of inheritance (i.e., only families in which both the patient and one of their parents was affected.) The highest two-point LOD (logarithm of the odds) (the logarithm of: probability genes linked/probability genes not linked) scores were observed on chromosomes 1q-21-22, 3p14-24, and 13q31-33 (17). A replication of the finding on 3p21-24 has been published (53,54). While it is unclear what gene is implicated on 3p21-24 in Asperger's disorder, 3p24-26 was implicated in a larger screen of both the Finnish sample and Autism Genetic Resource Exchange (AGRE) (54) and is the region where the oxytocin receptor is localized.

Association studies measure linkage disequilibrium for alleles through genome scans and can be family or population, case-control based. Linkage disequilibrium is the likelihood that alleles or genetic markers occur more or less frequently than would be expected by chance in the study population. Association studies may reveal different findings in different ethnic populations. For the purpose of studying Asperger's disorder the results of more strict scans of the phenotype are tabulated and illustrated in Table 1 and Figure 1.

Table 1 Chromosomal Regions Identified in Linkage and Association Studies Asperger's

Region	Marker	Population	Sample size $N =$	Refs.
1q21-22	D1S1675	ASD	72	(18)
1q21-22	D1S484	Asperger's	72	(17)
1q21-23	D1S1484	Asperger's	114	(53)
3p14-24	D3S2432	Asperger's	72	(17)
3p21-24	D3S2432	Asperger's	114	(53)
	D3S1619	Asperger's	114	(53)
	D3S1298	Asperger's	114	(53)
	D3S3678	Asperger's	114	(53)
	D3S1767	Asperger's	114	(53)
	D3S2456	Asperger's	114	(53)
	D3S1768	Asperger's	42	(53)
	D3S3547	Asperger's	42	(53)
3p24-26	unk	ASD	unk	(54)
3q25-27	D3S3037	ASD	72	(18)
	D3S3699			(17)
4p15	D4S3001	Asperger's	42	(53,215)
5	D5S2494	ASD	118	(19,215)
7q	D7S483	ASD	118	(19)
7q22-32	D7S1824	ASD	634	(18) (21)
10p12-q11.1	unk	ASD	634	(21) (215)
11p12-p13	unk	ASD	unk	(146)
13q31-33	D13S793	Asperger's	72	(17)
17p12-q22		ASD	634	(21)
17q11	D17S1294	ASD	Male specific; 314	(215,216)
X	DXS7132	ASD	40	(18)
X	DXS1047-maternal allele	ASD	118	(19)

Abbreviations: ASD, autism spectrum disorder; unk, unknown.

Asperger's Disorder

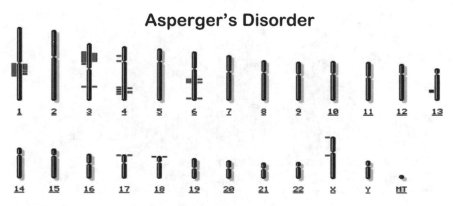

Figure 1 Chromosome regions of interest in Asperger's. Chromosome regions in linkage disequilibrium with Asperger's disorder from population studies. *Source*: From Ref. 70.

MENDELIAN GENETIC PERSPECTIVE

Hans Asperger noted the particular interest for the sex-linked or limited modes of inheritance hold (1) (hypothesis 4). The male-to-female prevalence ratio is 4:1 in autism and 8:1 in Asperger syndrome (11,30,55).

The most straightforward approach to the male predominance in Asperger's disorders would be a Mendelian model for sex-linked genetics. Humans have 46 chromosomes with potential Mendelian interactions (Figs. 2, 3, and 4). Since only males inherit a Y chromosome, a genetic disorder more prominent in males could be explained by Y chromosome transmission of a causative gene.

Y-Linked Inheritance

The increased (8:1) expression and prevalence in males as well as the documentation of paternal inheritance would imply Y-linked inheritance. The pseudoautosomal regions of the X and Y chromosomes could hold a Y dominant

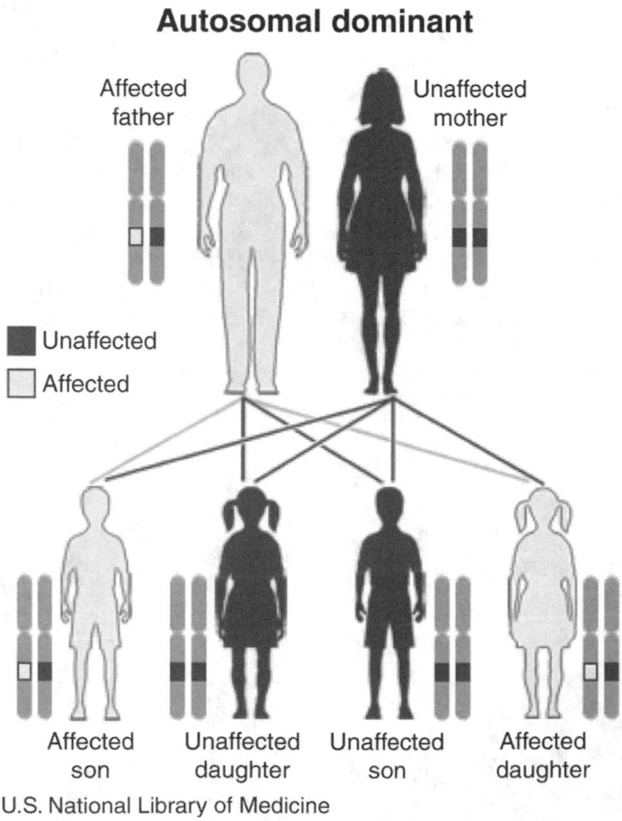

Figure 2   Mendelian autosomal dominant inheritance. With autosomal dominant inheritance, laws of independent assortment predict that 50% of progeny will have the dominant trait. *Source:* Public Domain. U.S. National Library of Medicine, 8600 Rockville Pike, Bethesda, Maryland   20894.

Autosomal Recessive

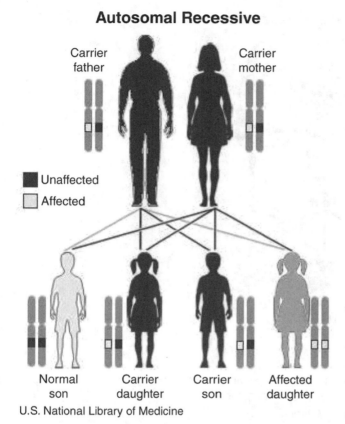

U.S. National Library of Medicine

Figure 3 Autosomal recessive inheritance. With a carrier mother and carrier father, laws of independent assortment will predict expression of the trait in 25% of progeny and carrier status in 50% of progeny. With one carrier parent, independent assortment would predict carrier status in 50% of the progeny with no expression of the trait in the progeny.

gene. In this case, the inheritance would show an autosomal dominant pattern but only males would be affected (Fig. 2). However, while there are reports of Y anomalies (56–58), Y chromosome genes are unlikely to be frequent contributors to Asperger's disorder.

Studies have not revealed linkage disequilibrium on the Y chromosome (59) in Asperger's cohorts and have not supported the Y chromosome in susceptibility to Asperger's disorder (60). The Y chromosome contains few genes compared with the X chromosome (61,62). Mosaicism (some cells XO other XY) of a missing Y chromosome has been reported in one male case with Asperger's (63).

X-Linked Recessive Inheritance

In Mendelian genetics, males would have greater vulnerability to X-linked recessive mutations since there is no second X chromosome available to provide

X-linked recessive, carrier mother

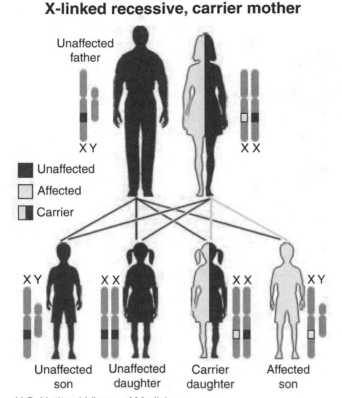

Unaffected
father

■ Unaffected
□ Affected
▨ Carrier

X Y   X X

X Y   X X   X X   X Y

Unaffected   Unaffected   Carrier   Affected
son   daughter   daughter   son

U.S. National Library of Medicine

Figure 4 Mendelian sex-linked inheritance. The law of independent assortment of an X-linked recessive allele predicts that 50% of sons will express the trait and 50% of daughters will be carriers of the trait.

a "normal" gene (Fig. 4), (except in the rare case of a homologous gene on the Y chromosome; homologous X-Y genes are apparent in the pseudoautosomal region). Unaffected mothers and daughters would retain protein function as a result of the presence of one copy of the nonmutated gene. With this understanding, one would expect males with the phenotype associated with the X-linked mutation to inherit the mutation from their mother, as seen in other X-linked conditions (e.g., color blindness, hemophilia, muscular dystrophy) (64).

The X chromosome has been implicated in genome-wide scans of ASDs (19,65), and X genes are important in mental functioning, thus the X chromosome is a region of interest (66). Prosocial behavior, peer problems, and verbal ability may be influenced by X chromosome genes (67).

Three females with autistic features and a distal Xp deletion have been reported. One of these appears relevant to Asperger's—she showed a precocious use of language and was considered to have high-functioning autism (68). Maternally inherited point mutations of the X chromosome (X-linked recessive) have been found in two males with Asperger's disorder (69–71) in one report.

While examples of Mendelian genetics are frequent in medicine, no such pattern has emerged in Asperger's disorder. The mechanisms of inheritance, penetrance, and expressivity of most human traits are more complicated (72–74), and different mutations in the same allele or mutations in different genes can cause the same trait (genetic heterogeneity).

So, sex-linked and autosomal inheritance and penetrance in Asperger's disorder may not show classical Mendelian inheritance.

NO CLEAR AND SIMPLE GENETIC MECHANISM

Fifty years later, it remains, as predicted by Hans Asperger, "a vain hope to think there may be a clear and simple genetic mechanism" (1) (hypothesis 3) behind the Aspergian phenotype. Unlike Rett's disorder, where a single gene is clearly implicated, no single gene or chromosomal region has been determined to "cause" Asperger's disorder, despite much work towards such a goal.

Genetic heterogeneity in the ASDs (15) may obscure genetic associations to the autism spectrum group, so that no simple genetic mechanism is likely for the group. While single gene polymorphisms have been associated with unique cases of Asperger's disorder in certain pedigrees (69), current evidence indicates that genetic transmission of autism and Asperger's disorder is the result of multiple interacting genes (31,75) with likely contribution of epigenetic and/or environmental factors. It has been predicted that ASDs are likely the result of at least 15 different genes (75).

Putative genetic mechanisms being explored (not exclusive of each other) in the development of Asperger's disorder include (*i*) sex chromosome-linked inheritance, (*ii*) multilocus, epistatic inheritance, (*iii*) epigenetic effects (parent-of-origin, gender-related gene expression), and (*iv*) gene or environment interactions.

Epistasis, the interaction of genes where the phenotypic expression of one gene depends upon the genotype of another, likely contributes to inheritance of Asperger's. An epistatic interaction can increase or decrease the risk of disease (76,77). Epistatic interactions have been noted in ASDs (78,79).

A quantitative trait is one where cumulative effects of normal variation result in the phenotype. Unlike Mendelian traits, quantitative traits show a gradient of gene expression over a continuum. These traits are attributable to two or more genes and their interaction with each other and the environment. Evidence implicates polymorphisms in loci contributing to quantitative traits in ASDs (80–83). Markers that contribute to complex traits are termed quantitative trait loci (QTL). QTLs can by analyzed to identify the effects of pairwise sets of

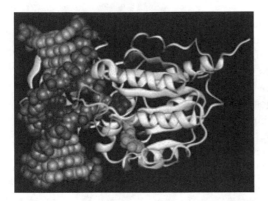

Figure 5 DNA methylation. The white methylating enzyme binds to the DNA. *Source*: From Ref. 110.

markers (84,85), and the magnitude or number of these effects may be more important than additive effects (84). Autism and Asperger's may share susceptibility QTLs.

EPIGENETIC FACTORS

The Epigenome

The epigenome mediates the expression of the genome. At this time, the best understood aspects of the epigenome are the chromatin/histone formation and DNA methylation (86–89). The processes of chromatin remodeling and DNA methylation are genetically programmed, but also susceptible to environmental influence (90,91). Chromatin remodeling mediates transcription and results when the protruding histone tails of the chromatin are chemically modified. DNA methylation is a process where enzymes donate methyl groups—the methylation usually silences gene expression (92) (Fig. 5).

These two epigenetic processes among others can be programmed and can also allow an organism to respond to the environment through changes in gene expression (93). Epigenetic changes in gene expression may be heritable through generations (90,94,95) and programmed in the germ line (88,89,96). Changes in the epigenome are notable in development and continue throughout life and can result in disease (97). The epigenome is particularly susceptible to dysregulation in early development (98). Environmental pressure may affect the expression of the genes leading to a different phenotype or diagnosis (Chap. 11).

Germ Line Mutation

Epigenetic effects are implicated in the increased de novo germ line mutation seen with increasing parental age. Advanced maternal (48) and paternal (50) age have been shown to be independently associated with ASDs (99). Later, paternal age may lower nonverbal IQ scores more than verbal IQ scores (100). The tendency for better verbal IQ is seen frequently in Asperger's.

Germ line mutations (101) including de novo copy number variations (102) have been associated with ASDs. A mutation of mitochondrial DNA [mt DNA (always inherited from the mother)] has been associated with Asperger's disorder (103) and autistic features (104).

Epigenetics—X-Inactivation

X-inactivation has traditionally been understood as a process in females where one of the X chromosomes is randomly and completely inactivated to avoid what would otherwise be an over dosage of the X genes (105). Some X-linked genes in females and some X-linked genes outside the pseudoautosomal regions of the X and Y chromosomes escape X-inactivation in males and females (105–107), implying an improved fitness effect for certain X genes. X-inactivation is hypothesized to contribute to a dampening of autistic traits. Also, X chromosome inactivation divergent from the normal, random pattern has been noted in autistic females (108).

One example of these effects is noted in Rett's disorder, where there are mutations in the gene MECP2 (Xq28) (109). The protein coded by MECP2, X-linked methyl-CpG-binding protein (MeCP2), mediates transcriptional repression through histone modification (110), among other functions (111,112). Affected individuals develop normally until 6 to 18 months of age; they then regress, losing speech, developing autism, and stereotypies among other problems (113,114).

Mutations of the MECP2 gene have been identified only rarely in autism (113), although the protein product has been shown to be differentially expressed in the brains of people with autism (115). Importantly, for the study of inheritance, MeCP2 has been implicated in the regulation of specific imprinted autism candidate genes and loci (112,116).

Epigenetics—Imprinting

Imprinting is the expression or nonexpression of a gene based on whether it is inherited from the mother or father (117). Imprinted genes express in the brain, are important in neurodevelopment (117), growth, and mother-offspring interactions (118). It has been shown that the gametes' development in the germ cells affects the chromatin modeling and methylation (50,119–121) of imprinted genes. Both sex chromosome and autosome genes are subject to imprinting (122,123) (Fig. 6).

Imprinting is implicated in social function, neuroanatomy (64), and language development. A classic example is the finding of imprinting and social function Turner's syndrome (XO). If the father donates the X chromosome, the

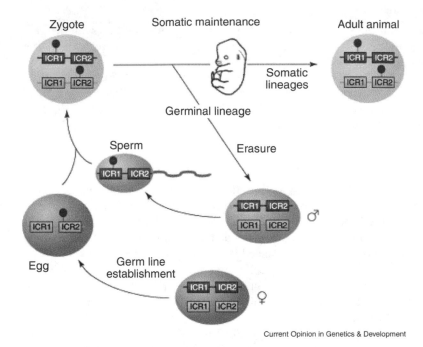

Figure 6 Imprinting. Imprinted genes are expressed from only one allele. Imprinted alleles are established in spermatogenesis or oogenesis at "imprinting control regions (ICRs)." Lollipops in the figure indicate DNA methylation, a marker of imprinted genes. The imprinted status is maintained throughout the cell line lineage of the organism. The imprinting is erased in the germ line. The erasure continues the inheritance process where imprinting status is determined by the gender of the parent. *Source*: From Ref. 119.

daughter will have better social function compared with daughters who inherited the X chromosome maternally (124–126).

It has been suggested that females may experience a phenotypic dampening of autistic traits through "an imprinted X liability threshold mechanism" or X-inactivation (10) with interaction with genetic and environmental influences.

Epigenetics in Development in Asperger's

While epigenetic effects are not clearly understood in the etiology of Asperger's disorder, transcriptional changes must underlie subsequent development and impairment. In a case of twins with Asperger's disorder with confirmed monozygocity of 99.999999%, the twins developed a disparity in their future functioning: The older developed depression and scored lower on IQ testing, while the younger developed seizures and was treated with valproate (13). Interestingly, valproate has been reported to cause demethylation of certain genes.

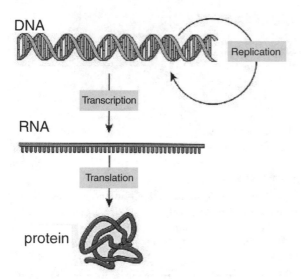

Figure 7   Transcription and translation. The protein is the end result of the genomic processes.

Considering the likely continuous distribution of autistic traits in the general population (10), epigenetic factors may be important in developing Asperger's disorder in comparison with a lesser expression in manifestation of the broader autism phenotype. Epigenetic factors in the regulation of the expression of genes are important to the protein synthesis necessary for of synaptic plasticity.

Further support for activity-dependent and epigenetic effects comes from observations of decreased methylation capacity in autistic children relative to age-matched controls (127), and alterations in gliogenesis and glial plasticity in ASDs (128).

It is important to note that sex-linked genes may express differently depending on gender in different regions of the brain (129), emphasizing the importance of studies of protein expression. For example, asymmetric distribution of messenger ribonucleic acid (mRNAs) can be observed with temporal and regional neural patterns of protein change (130).

Thus, while a human being may have a certain genome, protein expression is the point where the potential of the genetic code becomes apparent (Fig. 7). The neuronal synapse is the most widely studied area of protein expression in Asperger's.

SYNAPTIC PLASTICITY

Neuronal synapses are able to modify their strength in response to external and internal stimuli (131). When a neuron is activated, it elicits a change in the structure. This activity-dependent change is termed synaptic plasticity (132). Synaptic plasticity is fundamental to the nervous system and is a key process in learning and memory (133). Components of synaptic plasticity identified in Asperger's disorder involve neuroligins, neurexins, glutamate, and serotonin (5-HT).

Neuroligins

The two X-linked recessive alleles identified in Asperger's occur on the neuroligin N3 (NLGN3) (Xq13.1) and N4 gene (NLGN4) (Xp22.33) (69,71,134). A NLGN4 mutation has also been identified in a French sample with autism and X-linked MR (71). Interestingly, normal cognitive development may be achieved despite the deletion of NLGN4 (135).

Neuroligin genes code for postsynaptic cell-adhesion molecules and for structure and binding properties of the dendrite (69,70,136). Five genes encoding neuroligins have been identified in the human genome: NLGN3 (Xq13.1), NLGN4 (Xp22.3), NLGN1 (3q26.31), NLGN2 (17p13.1), and NLGN4Y (Yq11.2).

A gene screen of a wider spectrum of Asperger's disorder has identified significant linkage on 3q25-27 (18,137). As above, the NLGN1 gene is located at 3q26. However, Ylisaukko-oja and colleagues, as above, further analyzed their sample for NLGN1, 3, 4, and 4Y polymorphisms, and none of those identified seemed to be polymorphisms with functional consequences (138). 17p13, a region containing the gene NLGN2, has been implicated in chromosomal studies (139,140).

Not identified in other samples (11,138,141–143), it may be that mutations of neuroligins rarely contribute to the etiology of Asperger's disorder and autism (138). However, the function, location, and classification of the neuroligin protein may explain possible causes of Asperger's disorder at the neuronal synapse.

The X-linked recessive mutation of NLGN3 is a C-to-T transition in the gene. The transition changes arginine to cysteine in a domain conserved in all known neuroligins (69). Per Jamain et al., the transition is in a domain "known to confer structural integrity and Ca^{++} dependent functional properties...since binding is only observed in the presence of Ca^{++}, the mutation may modify binding of neuroligins to their pre-synaptic binding partners, neurexins..." (69).

This hypothesis has been validated; the NLGN3 mutation has been shown to result in diminished beta-neurexin-1 (NX1beta) binding (144,145).

Neurexins

The binding of neuroligins to their presynaptic partners, the neurexins is core to the development of glutamatergic (146) and GABAergic synapses (147). A scan of 1,168 autism spectrum disorder families implicated neurexins as candidate genes (146). Neurexins, like neuroligins, are coded by multiple genes (148). Each can trigger formation of a hemisynapse: Neuroligins can trigger

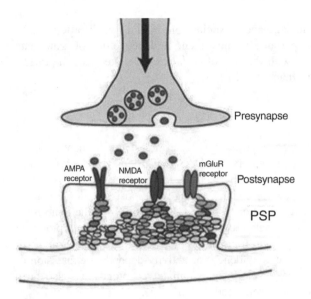

Figure 8 Postsynaptic proteome. Illustration of the postsynaptic proteome of a glutamatergic excitatory synapse. The NMDA, AMPA, and mGLuR subtypes of glutamate receptors connect to the complexes of proteins that process the signals of neuronal communication and plasticity. *Source*: From Ref. 70.

presynaptic differentiation, and neurexins (146) can trigger postsynaptic differentiation (147,149).

The formation and function of a synaptic connection and a neuronal circuit in the developing brain and subsequent plasticity is dependent upon alignment of postsynaptic dendritic neurotransmitter receptors with presynaptic axonal neurotransmitter release sites (136,147,150)(Fig. 8). NLGN1, NLGN3, and NLGN4 localize to glutamate postsynaptic sites, and NLGN2 localizes to GABA postsynaptic sites (147).

Postsynaptic Density

Neuroligins are part of the postsynaptic density (PSD) (70). The PSD is visible by electron microscopy as a large electron-dense complex of proteins below the postsynaptic membrane (151). PSD proteins organize signaling to coordinate functional changes in synapses (152) and are the molecular basis for rapid structural changes of cytoskeletal components (131) (Fig. 8). Mutations in different genes coding for postsynaptic density proteins are significant in that PSD function together in complexes.

X-linked mutations of PSD proteins have been noted to be highly expressed in psychiatric disorders with mental retardation (70). A postsynaptic density protein, the scaffolding protein SHANK3 (22q13.3) is a binding partner of neuroligins and regulates the organization of dendritic spines (153). If mutated,

SHANK3 can result in language and/or social communication disorders (153). The PSD proteins are important in movement and recycling of glutamate receptors (152) and interact with the neuroligin/neurexin system for the differentiation of glutamatergic synapses (146,147).

Glutamate

The presence of a PSD (131) characterizes glutamatergic synapses. There are three classes of ionotropic glutamate receptors, NMDA, AMPA, and kainate, as well as metabotropic receptors (133). Glutamate receptors mediate the majority of excitatory neurotransmission in the brain and changes in postsynaptic glutamate receptors change with synaptic plasticity (132). GRIK2 (6q21) is the gene for a kainate glutamate receptor, glutamate receptor 6. Glutamate-kainate receptors can cause long-term changes in synaptic transmission (133) and are likely important for learning and memory. There is evidence for activity-dependent expression of kainate receptors (154) during development. Kainate receptors have also been demonstrated to be a target for steroid modulation (155).

GRIK 2 has been implicated in ASDs (156–158). Maternal transmission disequilibrium of the allele has been noted (159) as well as evidence of the epigenetic marker histone methylation (160). GRIK2 may be subject to RNA editing (161).

It has been hypothesized that autism is a hypoglutamatergic disorder through interaction with 5-HT1a receptor (162,163). The glutamate system has much cross-talk with the 5-HT system (164,165) and both systems are implicated in Asperger's, neuronal growth, and neuronal plasticity (166).

Reelin

The reelin protein is important in early development and has been located in the PSD in human brain (167,168). The protein plays a role in migration of neurons (169) and development of neural connections and cell-positioning in the brain. The long arm of chromosome 7 (7q) contains the reelin gene (RELN) and, interestingly, the region is subject to imprinting (170). Hypermethylation of the promoter is associated with decreased RELN gene expression. Mutation or hypermethylation of RELN promoters may lead to cognitive deficits (168). Reelin protein and 7q are implicated in autism (14,171–174). The finding of Zhang et al. (175) is interesting for Asperger's disorder, where per DSM-IV diagnostic criteria, speech is not delayed. The authors found that larger repeats of CGG alleles of the long arm of chromosome 7 were transmitted more often than expected to affected autism spectrum children, and noted a trend for children without delayed phrase speech (first phrase $\leq$36 months) to have a least one long ($>$11) CGG repeat allele (175).

SEROTONIN SYSTEM

Hyperserotonemia

It may be that 5-HT is the neurotransmitter most supported to have a role in autism (176). Hyperserotonemia is a well-replicated finding in autism, although no data have yet implicated hyperserotonemia in Asperger's (177,178). Hyperserotonemia in autism is correlated with decreased speech development (179), and thus may possibly define an endophenotype that excludes Asperger's. Serotonin is known to enhance synapse refinement (180).

SERT

The serotonin transporter (5-HTT) gene (SLC6A4 or SERT) has been localized to17q11 (181). A major male-specific linkage peak at chromosome 17q11 has been identified in ASDs (182,183). This 17q11 locus may be subject to imprinting (184).

While multiple autism studies have not supported a role 5-HTT gene alleles to be associated with autism (185–189), the importance of SERT is supported by the observations that the selective serotonin reuptake inhibitors (SSRIs) are known to be efficacious for depression, anxiety, and reduction of obsessive and ritualistic behavior in ASDs (190–193).

5HTTLPR

A number of polymorphisms have been identified in the SLC 6A4 or SERT, but the best understood is the 5-HT long promotor region variant (5HTTLPR). The presence or absence of a promoter region deletion determines the level of SERT translated as mRNA, in turn determining the expression of the 5-HT transporter protein (5-HTT). The same gene encodes for 5-HTT in both platelet and brain. In so far as platelets regulate serotonemia, a potential relationship between 5-HT in the blood and brain could be manifest through a SERT mechanism, i.e., a 5-HTT mechanism. The 5-HTT functions to partition 5-HT across the cell membrane in both platelet and brain. The two tissues correlate in aspects of their 5-HTT protein kinetics (194).

Through genetic analysis of the SERT gene 5HTTLPR, individuals can be most simply classified as SS, SL, or LL 5HTTLPR allele. Individuals with Asperger's Disorder have been shown to have more relatives with depression than subjects with high functioning autism (5). The emotional responsiveness of the amygdala to social cues has been shown to be influenced by functional polymorphisms in the promoter of the 5-HTT gene (66).

A study in Korean trials identified an overtransmission of the L allele in ASD subjects (195) and LL was identified in two severely affected brothers (multiple comorbidities) with Asperger's disorder who also had an unusual Ile425Val mutation of the transporter (196).

This latter mutation, Ile425Val, holds particular interest as a potential etiology of Asperger's disorder. This polymorphism in the coding region constitutes a gain of function mutation associated with cognitive and behavioral stereotypies noted in clinical samples. Unlike the 5HTTLPR polymorphism, which is ubiquitous throughout the population, the Ile425Val mutation is rare, although more recent estimates suggest its prevalence at 1.5% (197). The Ile425Val mutation is in the coding region. It has pronounced effects on behavior and is infrequent. Conversely, the 5HTTLPR is in the noncoding region; it is in the promoter region. The 5HTTLPLPR has behavioral activity of a much more subtle extent and is frequent. To date, most genetic samples have not reported genotyping for the Ile425Val amino acid substitution. Given the fact that Asperger's disorder is not a common condition, it is unlikely that the prevalent 5HTTLPR would directly cause Asperger's disorder, although it may constitute a modifying factor.

Other 5HTTLPR associations have been suggested for the SS genotype as well as the LL genotype. It has been hypothesized that the SS allele may be "a sufficient serotonin dose" for autism and homozygosity for the long allele may be a protective factor in autism. Also, the ITGB3 gene, the beta subunit of the platelet membrane adhesive protein receptor complex GP IIb/IIIa (17q21.32), can influence the effect of the 5HTTLPR and SERT (55,78,198).

Clinical heterogeneity (199) and other 5-HTT polymorphisms (200) may affect the interpretation of the data. Mutations of the 5-HTT gene have been associated with increased rigid-compulsive behaviors (183,199). Some evidence suggests that 5HTTLPR may mediate endophenotypic manifestations in ASD. It has been noted that presence of the short allele (SS or SL) in an autistic sample correlated with "failure to use nonverbal communication to regulate social interaction," while the homozygous LL subjects were more severe on "stereotyped and repetitive motor mannerisms" and aggression (201).

HTR2A

The 5-HT2a receptor gene (HTR2A 13q14-21) is implicated in ASDs (195). The gene is subject to imprinting and, interestingly, has been shown to express only from the maternal allele (202), though the imprinting may be polymorphic in the population (i.e., imprinted in some but not other individuals) (203). Regional reductions in cortical 5-HT2a binding in have been identified in Asperger's disorder. The reduced 5-HT2a receptor binding was significantly related to abnormal social communication (204). Further evidence for a 5-HT2a contribution is the relationship with the oxytocin system discussed in chapter 12.

HTR1D

The 5-HT1d receptor is a 5-HT terminal inhibitory autoreceptor. The 5-HT1d receptor stimulates release of growth hormone. Compared with controls, growth hormone response to sumatriptan has been found to be increased in Asperger's disorder (205), and severity of repetitive compulsive behaviors in Asperger's has been correlated with the hypersensitivity of the 5-HT1d receptor (206).

ASMT

During the light hours of the day, tryptophan is converted to 5-HT. In darkness, 5-HT is converted to melatonin (207). A polymorphism in the acetylserotoninmethyltransferase (ASMT) gene on the pseudo autosomal regions of the sex chromosomes (Xpter- p22.32 and Ypter-p11.2) (208) has been identified in ASDs. As alluded to above, pseudoautosomal genes are sex chromosome genes located at the telomeres of the X and Y genes. They are inherited just as other autosomal genes (Figs. 1 and 2).

Children with Asperger's disorder have difficulty maintaining and initiating sleep (209–211); treatment with metalonin may improve their sleep disorder (212). Decreased nocturnal melatonin excretion has been noted in autism (213).

The 5-HT system is notable for its sexual dimorphism, an important finding to interpret the male-female bias in prevalence in Asperger's disorder. Other gene polymorphisms in sexually dimorphic systems have been identified (Table 2) and are discussed in chapter 12.

CONCLUSIONS

Genetic modes of inheritance implicated in Asperger's disorder include sex-linked genes, epistatic interactions, and heritable or environmentally modified epigenetic mechanisms such as imprinting or germ line mutation. While there is no clear sex-linked gene identified, there is likely a genetic contribution from X chromosome genes. The susceptibility genes may likely be distributed largely in QTLs throughout the genome given the evidence for autistic traits in the general population. Sex-limitation of gene expression and sex-dependent gene findings are discussed in chapter 8. Polymorphisms identified thus far in the neuroligin/neurexin, glutamate, and 5-HT systems highlight the importance of synapse formation and plasticity, implicating mechanisms of learning and association in Asperger's disorder.

Synaptic plasticity and learning are integral to overcoming environmental challenges and reaching homeostasis of mood, relationships, and functioning. Enhancing synaptic plasticity through psychosocial or pharmacological methods is important in the treatment of all psychiatric disorders, particularly those implicated in development.

Humans are a nondeterministic system. "Predisposition is not fate but a possible fate"(214). Humans may choose to overcome disabilities if the techniques are made available through science and medicine. With human genome mapping, the "vain hope" for an inheritance mechanism will likely yield helpful treatments through analysis of candidate gene and protein function.

21. Trikalinos TA, Karvouni A, Zintzaras E, et al. A heterogeneity-based genome search meta-analysis for autism-spectrum disorders. Mol Psychiatry 2006; 11(1): 29–36.

22. Gillberg C, Cederlund M. Asperger syndrome: familial and pre- and perinatal factors. J Autism Dev Disord 2005; 35(2):159–166.

23. Constantino JN, Todd RD. Genetic structure of reciprocal social behavior. Am J Psychiatry 2000; 157(12):2043–2045.

24. Constantino JN, Todd RD. Intergenerational transmission of subthreshold autistic traits in the general population. Biol Psychiatry 2005; 57(6):655–660.

25. Hoekstra RA, Bartels M, Verweij CJ, et al. Heritability of autistic traits in the general population. Arch Pediatr Adolesc Med 2007; 161(4):372–377.

26. Skuse DH, Mandy WP, Scourfield J. Measuring autistic traits: heritability, reliability and validity of the Social and Communication Disorders Checklist. Br J Psychiatry 2005; 187:568–572.

27. Constantino JN, Lajonchere C, Lutz M, et al. Autistic social impairment in the siblings of children with pervasive developmental disorders. Am J Psychiatry 2006; 163(2):294–296.

28. Ronald A, Happe F, Price TS, et al. Phenotypic and genetic overlap between autistic traits at the extremes of the general population. J Am Acad Child Adolesc Psychiatry 2006; 45(10):1206–1214.

29. Kracke I. Developmental prosopagnosia in Asperger syndrome: presentation and discussion of an individual case. Dev Med Child Neurol 1994; 36(10):873–886.

30. Gillberg C. Asperger syndrome in 23 Swedish children. Dev Med Child Neurol 1989; 31(4):520–531.

31. Folstein S, Santangelo S. Does Asperger syndrome aggregate in families? In: Klin A, Volkmar Fred R, Sparrow Sara S, eds. Asperger Syndrome. New York: The Guilford Press, 2000:161–168.

32. Piven J, Palmer P, Jacobi D, et al. Broader autism phenotype: evidence from a family history study of multiple-incidence autism families. Am J Psychiatry 1997; 154(2): 185–190.

33. Sung YJ, Dawson G, Munson J, et al. Genetic investigation of quantitative traits related to autism: use of multivariate polygenic models with ascertainment adjustment. Am J Hum Genet 2005; 76(1):68–81.

34. Baron-Cohen S, hammer J. Parents of children with Asperger syndrome: what is the cognitive phenotype? J Cogn Neurosci 1997; 9(4):548–554 (abstr).

35. Wheelwright S, Baron-Cohen S. The link between autism and skills such as engineering, maths, physics and computing: a reply to Jarrold and Routh. Autism 2001; 5(2):223–227.

36. Baron-Cohen S, Richler J, Bisarya D, et al. The systemizing quotient: an investigation of adults with Asperger syndrome or high-functioning autism, and normal sex differences. Philos Trans R Soc Lond B Biol Sci 2003; 358(1430):361–374.

37. Baron-Cohen S, Wheelwright S. The empathy quotient: an investigation of adults with Asperger syndrome or high functioning autism, and normal sex differences. J Autism Dev Disord 2004; 34(2):163–175.

38. Baron-Cohen S. The hyper-systemizing, assortative mating theory of autism. Prog Neuropsychopharmacol Biol Psychiatry 2006; 30(5):865–872.

39. Wakabayashi A, Baron-Cohen S, Wheelwright S. [Individual and gender differences in Empathizing and Systemizing: measurement of individual differences by

the Empathy Quotient (EQ) and the Systemizing Quotient (SQ)]. Shinrigaku Kenkyu 2006; 77(3):271–277.

40. Baron-Cohen S. Autism: research into causes and intervention. Pediatr Rehabil 2004; 7(2):73–78.
41. Chakrabarti B, Baron-Cohen S. Empathizing: neurocognitive developmental mechanisms and individual differences. Prog Brain Res 2006; 156:403–417.
42. Leiberg S, Anders S. The multiple facets of empathy: a survey of theory and evidence. Prog Brain Res 2006; 156:419–440.
43. Premack D. The infant's theory of self-propelled objects. Cognition 1990; 36(1):1–16.
44. Giannoni M, Corradi M. How the mind understands other minds: cognitive psychology, attachment and reflective function. J Anal Psychol 2006; 51(2):271–284.
45. Asperger H. Die 'Autisitic Psychopathen' im kindesalter. Arch Psychiatr Nervenkr 1944; 117:76–136.
46. Bowman EP. Asperger's syndrome and autism: the case for a connection. Br J Psychiatry 1988; 152:377–382.
47. Gillberg C, Gillberg IC, Steffenburg S. Siblings and parents of children with autism: a controlled population-based study. Dev Med Child Neurol 1992; 34(5):389–398.
48. Gillberg C. Maternal age and infantile autism. J Autism Dev Disord 1980; 10(3): 293–297.
49. Miller MC. Older father, autistic child. Harv Ment Health Lett 2006; 23(6):8.
50. Reichenberg A, Gross R, Weiser M, et al. Advancing paternal age and autism. Arch Gen Psychiatry 2006; 63(9):1026–1032.
51. Mouridsen SE, Rich B, Isager T. Brief report: parental age in infantile autism, autistic-like conditions, and borderline childhood psychosis. J Autism Dev Disord 1993; 23(2):387–396.
52. Is a child's autism related to his father's age? Child Health Alert 2006; 24:1–2.
53. Rehnstrom K, Ylisaukko-oja T, Nieminen-von WT, et al. Independent replication and initial fine mapping of 3p21-24 in Asperger syndrome. Hum Genet 2002; 111(4–5):305–309.
54. Ylisaukko-oja T, Alarcon M, Cantor RM, et al. Search for autism loci by combined analysis of Autism Genetic Resource Exchange and Finnish families. Ann Neurol 2006; 59(1):145–155.
55. Weiss LA, Abney M, Parry R, et al. Variation in ITGB3 has sex-specific associations with plasma lipoprotein(a) and whole blood serotonin levels in a population-based sample. Hum Genet 2005; 117(1):81–87.
56. Blackman JA, Selzer SC, Patil S, et al. Autistic disorder associated with an iso-dicentric Y chromosome. Dev Med Child Neurol 1991; 33(2):162–166.
57. Gillberg C, Wahlstrom J. Chromosome abnormalities in infantile autism and other childhood psychoses: a population study of 66 cases. Dev Med Child Neurol 1985; 27(3):293–304.
58. Nicolson R, Bhalerao S, Sloman L. 47,XYY karyotypes and pervasive developmental disorders. Can J Psychiatry 1998; 43(6):619–622.
59. Jamain S, Quach H, Quintana-Murci L, et al. Y chromosome haplogroups in autistic subjects. Mol Psychiatry 2002; 7(2):217–219.
60. Durand CM, Kappeler C, Betancur C, et al. Expression and genetic variability of PCDH11Y, a gene specific to Homo sapiens and candidate for susceptibility to psychiatric disorders. Am J Med Genet B Neuropsychiatr Genet 2006; 141(1): 67–70.

61. Waters PD, Wallis MC, Marshall Graves JA. Mammalian sex–Origin and evolution of the Y chromosome and SRY. Semin Cell Dev Biol 2007; 18(3):389–400.
62. Ross MT, Grafham DV, Coffey AJ, et al. The DNA sequence of the human X chromosome. Nature 2005; 434(7031):325–337.
63. Fontenelle LF, Mendlowicz MV, Bezerra de MG, et al. Asperger Syndrome, obsessive-compulsive disorder, and major depression in a patient with 45,X/46,XY mosaicism. Psychopathology 2004; 37(3):105–109.
64. Good CD, Lawrence K, Thomas NS, et al. Dosage-sensitive X-linked locus influences the development of amygdala and orbitofrontal cortex, and fear recognition in humans. Brain 2003; 126(pt 11):2431–2446.
65. Gauthier J, Joober R, Dube MP, et al. Autism spectrum disorders associated with X chromosome markers in French-Canadian males. Mol Psychiatry 2006; 11(2): 206–213.
66. Skuse D. Genetic influences on the neural basis of social cognition. Philos Trans R Soc Lond B Biol Sci 2006; 361(1476):2129–2141.
67. Loat CS, Asbury K, Galsworthy MJ, et al. X inactivation as a source of behavioural differences in monozygotic female twins. Twin Res 2004; 7(1):54–61.
68. Thomas NS, Sharp AJ, Browne CE, Skuse D, Hardie C, Dennis NR. Xp deletions associated with autism in three females. Hum Genet 1999; 104(1):43–48.
69. Jamain S, Quach H, Betancur C, et al. Mutations of the X-linked genes encoding neuroligins NLGN3 and NLGN4 are associated with autism. Nat Genet 2003; 34(1): 27–29.
70. Laumonnier F, Cuthbert PC, Grant SG. The role of neuronal complexes in human X-linked brain diseases. Am J Hum Genet 2007; 80(2):205–220.
71. Laumonnier F, Bonnet-Brilhault F, Gomot M, et al. X-linked mental retardation and autism are associated with a mutation in the NLGN4 gene, a member of the neuroligin family. Am J Hum Genet 2004; 74(3):552–557.
72. Skuse D. X-linked genes and the neural basis of social cognition. Novartis Found Symp 2003; 251:84–98.
73. Arnold AP, Burgoyne PS. Are XX and XY brain cells intrinsically different? Trends Endocrinol Metab 2004; 15(1):6–11.
74. Bocklandt S, Vilain E. Sex differences in brain and behavior: hormones versus genes. Adv Genet 2007; 59:245–266.
75. Risch N, Spiker D, Lotspeich L, et al. A genomic screen of autism: evidence for a multilocus etiology. Am J Hum Genet 1999; 65(2):493–507.
76. Keller F, Persico AM. The neurobiological context of autism. Mol Neurobiol 2003; 28(1):1–22.
77. Nagel RL. Epistasis and the genetics of human diseases. C R Biol 2005; 328(7): 606–615.
78. Weiss LA, Ober C, Cook EH Jr. ITGB3 shows genetic and expression interaction with SLC6A4. Hum Genet 2006; 120(1):93–100.
79. Weiss LA, Kosova G, Delahanty RJ, et al. Variation in ITGB3 is associated with whole-blood serotonin level and autism susceptibility. Eur J Hum Genet 2006; 14(8): 923–931.
80. Alarcon M, Yonan AL, Gilliam TC, et al. Quantitative genome scan and Ordered-Subsets Analysis of autism endophenotypes support language QTLs. Mol Psychiatry 2005; 10(8):747–757.

81. Chen GK, Kono N, Geschwind DH, et al. Quantitative trait locus analysis of nonverbal communication in autism spectrum disorder. Mol Psychiatry 2006; 11(2): 214–220.
82. Weiss LA, Purcell S, Waggoner S, et al. Identification of EFHC2 as a quantitative trait locus for fear recognition in Turner syndrome. Hum Mol Genet 2007; 16(1):107–113.
83. Duvall JA, Lu A, Cantor RM, et al. A quantitative trait locus analysis of social responsiveness in multiplex autism families. Am J Psychiatry 2007; 164(4):656–662.
84. Malmberg RL, Mauricio R. QTL-based evidence for the role of epistasis in evolution. Genet Res 2005; 86(2):89–95.
85. Reif A, Lesch KP. Toward a molecular architecture of personality. Behav Brain Res 2003; 139(1–2):1–20.
86. Szyf M, Weaver I, Meaney M. Maternal care, the epigenome and phenotypic differences in behavior. Reprod Toxicol 2007; 24(1):9–19.
87. Weaver IC, Champagne FA, Brown SE, et al. Reversal of maternal programming of stress responses in adult offspring through methyl supplementation: altering epigenetic marking later in life. J Neurosci 2005; 25(47):11045–11054.
88. Morgan HD, Sutherland HG, Martin DI, et al. Epigenetic inheritance at the agouti locus in the mouse. Nat Genet 1999; 23(3):314–318.
89. Kaati G, Bygren LO, Pembrey M, et al. Transgenerational response to nutrition, early life circumstances and longevity. Eur J Hum Genet 2007; 15(7):784–790.
90. Hatchwell E, Greally JM. The potential role of epigenomic dysregulation in complex human disease. Trends Genet 2007; 23(11):588–595.
91. Abdolmaleky HM, Smith CL, Faraone SV, et al. Methylomics in psychiatry: Modulation of gene-environment interactions may be through DNA methylation. Am J Med Genet B Neuropsychiatr Genet 2004; 127(1):51–59.
92. D'Alessio AC, Szyf M. Epigenetic tete-a-tete: the bilateral relationship between chromatin modifications and DNA methylation. Biochem Cell Biol 2006; 84(4): 463–476.
93. Jaenisch R, Bird A. Epigenetic regulation of gene expression: how the genome integrates intrinsic and environmental signals. Nat Genet 2003; 33 Suppl:245–254.
94. Gluckman PD, Hanson MA, Beedle AS. Non-genomic transgenerational inheritance of disease risk. Bioessays 2007; 29(2):145–154.
95. Pembrey ME, Bygren LO, Kaati G, et al. Sex-specific, male-line transgenerational responses in humans. Eur J Hum Genet 2006; 14(2):159–166.
96. Whitelaw NC, Whitelaw E. How lifetimes shape epigenotype within and across generations. Hum Mol Genet 2006; 15 Spec No 2:R131–R137.
97. Feinberg AP. Phenotypic plasticity and the epigenetics of human disease. Nature 2007; 447(7143):433–440.
98. Dolinoy DC, Das R, Weidman JR, et al. Metastable epialleles, imprinting, and the fetal origins of adult diseases. Pediatr Res 2007; 61(5 pt 2):30R–37R.
99. Croen LA, Najjar DV, Fireman B, et al. Maternal and paternal age and risk of autism spectrum disorders. Arch Pediatr Adolesc Med 2007; 161(4):334–340.
100. Malaspina D, Reichenberg A, Weiser M, et al. Paternal age and intelligence: implications for age-related genomic changes in male germ cells. Psychiatr Genet 2005; 15(2):117–125.
101. Butler MG, Dasouki MJ, Zhou XP, et al. Subset of individuals with autism spectrum disorders and extreme macrocephaly associated with germline PTEN tumour suppressor gene mutations. J Med Genet 2005; 42(4):318–321.

102. Sebat J, Lakshmi B, Malhotra D, et al. Strong Association of De Novo Copy Number Mutations with Autism. Science 2007; 316:445–449.

103. Kent L, Lambert C, Pyle A, et al. The mitochondrial DNA A3243A>G mutation must be an infrequent cause of Asperger syndrome. J Pediatr 2006; 149(2):280–281.

104. Pons R, Andreu AL, Checcarelli N, et al. Mitochondrial DNA abnormalities and autistic spectrum disorders. J Pediatr 2004; 144(1):81–85.

105. Salstrom JL. X-inactivation and the dynamic maintenance of gene silencing. Mol Genet Metab 2007; 92(1–2):56–62.

106. Hoffbuhr KC, Moses LM, Jerdonek MA, et al. Associations between MeCP2 mutations, X-chromosome inactivation, and phenotype. Ment Retard Dev Disabil Res Rev 2002; 8(2):99–105.

107. Skuse DH. X-linked genes and mental functioning. Hum Mol Genet 2005; 14 Spec No 1:R27–R32.

108. Talebizadeh Z, Bittel DC, Veatch OJ, et al. Brief report: non-random X chromosome inactivation in females with autism. J Autism Dev Disord 2005; 35(5):675–681.

109. Amir RE, Van dV, I, Wan M, et al. Rett syndrome is caused by mutations in X-linked MECP2, encoding methyl-CpG-binding protein 2. Nat Genet 1999; 23(2):185–188.

110. Dennis C. Epigenetics and disease: Altered states. Nature 2003; 421(6924):686–688.

111. Yasui DH, Peddada S, Bieda MC, et al. Integrated epigenomic analyses of neuronal MeCP2 reveal a role for long-range interaction with active genes. Proc Natl Acad Sci U S A 2007; 104(49):19416–19421.

112. Samaco RC, Hogart A, LaSalle JM. Epigenetic overlap in autism-spectrum neurodevelopmental disorders: MECP2 deficiency causes reduced expression of UBE3A and GABRB3. Hum Mol Genet 2005; 14(4):483–492.

113. Carney RM, Wolpert CM, Ravan SA, et al. Identification of MeCP2 mutations in a series of females with autistic disorder. Pediatr Neurol 2003; 28(3):205–211.

114. Beyer KS, Blasi F, Bacchelli E, et al. Mutation analysis of the coding sequence of the MECP2 gene in infantile autism. Hum Genet 2002; 111(4–5):305–309.

115. Nagarajan RP, Hogart AR, Gwye Y, et al. Reduced MeCP2 expression is frequent in autism frontal cortex and correlates with aberrant MECP2 promoter methylation. Epigenetics 2006; 1(4):e1–e11.

116. LaSalle JM. The Odyssey of MeCP2 and parental imprinting. Epigenetics 2007; 2(1): 5–10.

117. Wilkinson LS, Davies W, Isles AR. Genomic imprinting effects on brain development and function. Nat Rev Neurosci 2007; 8(11):832–843.

118. Isles AR, Holland AJ. Imprinted genes and mother-offspring interactions. Early Hum Dev 2005; 81(1):73–77.

119. Delaval K, Feil R. Epigenetic regulation of mammalian genomic imprinting. Curr Opin Genet Dev 2004; 14(2):188–195.

120. Rousseaux S, Caron C, Govin J, et al. Establishment of male-specific epigenetic information. Gene 2005; 345(2):139–153.

121. Stemkens D, Roza T, Verrij L, et al. Is there an influence of X-chromosomal imprinting on the phenotype in Klinefelter syndrome? A clinical and molecular genetic study of 61 cases. Clin Genet 2006; 70(1):43–48.

122. Cassidy SB, Schwartz S. Prader-Willi and Angelman syndromes. Disorders of genomic imprinting. Medicine (Baltimore) 1998; 77(2):140–151.

123. Veltman MW, Craig EE, Bolton PF. Autism spectrum disorders in Prader-Willi and Angelman syndromes: a systematic review. Psychiatr Genet 2005; 15(4):243–254.

124. Skuse DH, James RS, Bishop DV, et al. Evidence from Turner's syndrome of an imprinted X-linked locus affecting cognitive function. Nature 1997; 387(6634): 705–708.
125. Skuse DH. Imprinting, the X-chromosome, and the male brain: explaining sex differences in the liability to autism. Pediatr Res 2000; 47(1):9–16.
126. Strous RD, Maayan R, Weizman A. The relevance of neurosteroids to clinical psychiatry: from the laboratory to the bedside. Eur Neuropsychopharmacol 2006; 16(3): 155–169.
127. James SJ, Melnyk S, Jernigan S, et al. Metabolic endophenotype and related genotypes are associated with oxidative stress in children with autism. Am J Med Genet B Neuropsychiatr Genet 2006; 141(8):947–956.
128. Dong WK, Greenough WT. Plasticity of nonneuronal brain tissue: roles in developmental disorders. Ment Retard Dev Disabil Res Rev 2004; 10(2):85–90.
129. Vawter MP, Evans S, Choudary P, et al. Gender-specific gene expression in postmortem human brain: localization to sex chromosomes. Neuropsychopharmacology 2004; 29(2):373–384.
130. Bramham CR, Wells DG. Dendritic mRNA: transport, translation and function. Nat Rev Neurosci 2007; 8(10):776–789.
131. Boeckers TM. The postsynaptic density. Cell Tissue Res 2006; 326(2):409–422.
132. Genoux D, Montgomery JM. Glutamate receptor plasticity at excitatory synapses in the brain. Clin Exp Pharmacol Physiol 2007; 34(10):1058–1063.
133. Bortolotto ZA, Clarke VR, Delany CM, et al. Kainate receptors are involved in synaptic plasticity. Nature 1999; 402(6759):297–301.
134. Talebizadeh Z, Lam DY, Theodoro MF, et al. Novel splice isoforms for NLGN3 and NLGN4 with possible implications in autism. J Med Genet 2006; 43(5):e21.
135. Macarov M, Zeigler M, Newman JP, et al. Deletions of VCX-A and NLGN4: a variable phenotype including normal intellect. J Intellect Disabil Res 2007; 51(pt 5): 329–333.
136. Lise MF, El-Husseini A. The neuroligin and neurexin families: from structure to function at the synapse. Cell Mol Life Sci 2006; 63(16):1833–1849.
137. Auranen M, Varilo T, Alen R, et al. Evidence for allelic association on chromosome 3q25-27 in families with autism spectrum disorders originating from a subisolate of Finland. Mol Psychiatry 2003; 8(10):879–884.
138. Ylisaukko-oja T, Rehnstrom K, Auranen M, et al. Analysis of four neuroligin genes as candidates for autism. Eur J Hum Genet 2005; 13(12):1285–1292.
139. Tentler D, Johannesson T, Johansson M, et al. A candidate region for Asperger syndrome defined by two 17p breakpoints. Eur J Hum Genet 2003; 11(2):189–195.
140. Anneren G, Dahl N, Uddenfeldt U, et al. Asperger syndrome in a boy with a balanced de novo translocation: t(17;19)(p13.3;p11). Am J Med Genet 1995; 56(3): 330–331.
141. Blasi F, Bacchelli E, Pesaresi G, et al. Absence of coding mutations in the X-linked genes neuroligin 3 and neuroligin 4 in individuals with autism from the IMGSAC collection. Am J Med Genet B Neuropsychiatr Genet 2006; 141(3):220–221.
142. Chaste P, Nygren G, Anckarsater H, et al. Mutation screening of the ARX gene in patients with autism. Am J Med Genet B Neuropsychiatr Genet 2007; 144(2):228–230.
143. Vincent JB, Kolozsvari D, Roberts WS, et al. Mutation screening of X-chromosomal neuroligin genes: no mutations in 196 autism probands. Am J Med Genet B Neuropsychiatr Genet 2004; 129(1):82–84.

144. Comoletti D, De JA, Jennings LL, et al. The Arg451Cys-neuroligin-3 mutation associated with autism reveals a defect in protein processing. J Neurosci 2004; 24(20):4889–4893.

145. Chubykin AA, Liu X, Comoletti D, et al. Dissection of synapse induction by neuroligins: effect of a neuroligin mutation associated with autism. J Biol Chem 2005; 280(23):22365–22374.

146. Szatmari P, Paterson AD, Zwaigenbaum L, et al. Mapping autism risk loci using genetic linkage and chromosomal rearrangements. Nat Genet 2007; 39(3):319–328.

147. Graf ER, Zhang X, Jin SX, et al. Neurexins induce differentiation of GABA and glutamate postsynaptic specializations via neuroligins. Cell 2004; 119(7): 1013–1026.

148. Chih B, Gollan L, Scheiffele P. Alternative splicing controls selective trans-synaptic interactions of the neuroligin-neurexin complex. Neuron 2006; 51(2):171–178.

149. Craig AM, Kang Y. Neurexin-neuroligin signaling in synapse development. Curr Opin Neurobiol 2007; 17(1):43–52.

150. Lardi-Studler B, Fritschy JM. Matching of pre- and postsynaptic specializations during synaptogenesis. Neuroscientist 2007; 13(2):115–126.

151. de BA, Fiore G. Postsynaptic density scaffolding proteins at excitatory synapse and disorders of synaptic plasticity: implications for human behavior pathologies. Int Rev Neurobiol 2004; 59:221–254.

152. Kim E, Ko J. Molecular organization and assembly of the postsynaptic density of excitatory brain synapses. Results Probl Cell Differ 2006; 43:1–23.

153. Durand CM, Betancur C, Boeckers TM, et al. Mutations in the gene encoding the synaptic scaffolding protein SHANK3 are associated with autism spectrum disorders. Nat Genet 2007; 39(1):25–7. Epub 2006 Dec 17.

154. Kidd FL, Isaac JT. Developmental and activity-dependent regulation of kainate receptors at thalamocortical synapses. Nature 1999; 400(6744):569–573.

155. Dubrovsky BO. Steroids, neuroactive steroids and neurosteroids in psychopathology. Prog Neuropsychopharmacol Biol Psychiatry 2005; 29(2):169–192.

156. Jamain S, Betancur C, Quach H, et al. Linkage and association of the glutamate receptor 6 gene with autism. Mol Psychiatry 2002; 7(3):302–310.

157. Kim SA, Kim JH, Park M, et al. Family-based association study between GRIK2 polymorphisms and autism spectrum disorders in the Korean trios. Neurosci Res 2007; 58(3):332–335.

158. Shuang M, Liu J, Jia MX, et al. Family-based association study between autism and glutamate receptor 6 gene in Chinese Han trios. Am J Med Genet B Neuropsychiatr Genet 2004; 131(1):48–50.

159. Bah J, Quach H, Ebstein RP, et al. Maternal transmission disequilibrium of the glutamate receptor GRIK2 in schizophrenia. Neuroreport 2004; 15(12):1987–1991.

160. Stadler F, Kolb G, Rubusch L, et al. Histone methylation at gene promoters is associated with developmental regulation and region-specific expression of ionotropic and metabotropic glutamate receptors in human brain. J Neurochem 2005; 94(2):324–336.

161. Paschen W, Hedreen JC, Ross CA. RNA editing of the glutamate receptor subunits GluR2 and GluR6 in human brain tissue. J Neurochem 1994; 63(5):1596–1602.

162. Calcagno E, Carli M, Invernizzi RW. The 5-HT(1A) receptor agonist 8-OH-DPAT prevents prefrontocortical glutamate and serotonin release in response to blockade of cortical NMDA receptors. J Neurochem 2006; 96(3):853–860.

163. Carlsson ML. Hypothesis: is infantile autism a hypoglutamatergic disorder? Relevance of glutamate - serotonin interactions for pharmacotherapy. J Neural Transm 1998; 105(4–5):525–535.

164. Sodhi MS, Sanders-Bush E. Serotonin and brain development. Int Rev Neurobiol 2004; 59:111–174.

165. de AJ, Mengod G. Quantitative analysis of glutamatergic and GABAergic neurons expressing 5-HT(2A) receptors in human and monkey prefrontal cortex. J Neurochem 2007; 103(2):475–486.

166. Boylan CB, Blue ME, Hohmann CF. Modeling early cortical serotonergic deficits in autism. Behav Brain Res 2007; 176(1):94–108.

167. Roberts RC, Xu L, Roche JK, et al. Ultrastructural localization of reelin in the cortex in post-mortem human brain. J Comp Neurol 2005; 482(3):294–308.

168. Fatemi SH. Reelin glycoprotein: structure, biology and roles in health and disease. Mol Psychiatry 2005; 10(3):251–257.

169. Roman GC. Autism: transient in utero hypothyroxinemia related to maternal flavonoid ingestion during pregnancy and to other environmental antithyroid agents. J Neurol Sci 2007; 262(1–2):15–26.

170. Schanen NC. Epigenetics of autism spectrum disorders. Hum Mol Genet 2006; 15 Spec No 2:R138–R150.

171. Skaar DA, Shao Y, Haines JL, et al. Analysis of the RELN gene as a genetic risk factor for autism. Mol Psychiatry 2005; 10(6):563–571.

172. Bonora E, Beyer KS, Lamb JA, et al. Analysis of reelin as a candidate gene for autism. Mol Psychiatry 2003; 8(10):885–892.

173. Acosta MT, Pearl PL. The neurobiology of autism: new pieces of the puzzle. Curr Neurol Neurosci Rep 2003; 3(2):149–156.

174. Dutta S, Guhathakurta S, Sinha S, et al. Reelin gene polymorphisms in the Indian population: a possible paternal 5'UTR-CGG-repeat-allele effect on autism. Am J Med Genet B Neuropsychiatr Genet 2007; 144(1):106–112.

175. Zhang H, Liu X, Zhang C, et al. Reelin gene alleles and susceptibility to autism spectrum disorders. Mol Psychiatry 2002; 7(9):1012–1017.

176. Lam KS, Aman MG, Arnold LE. Neurochemical correlates of autistic disorder: a review of the literature. Res Dev Disabil 2006; 27(3):254–289.

177. Anderson GM, Freedman DX, Cohen DJ, et al. Whole blood serotonin in autistic and normal subjects. J Child Psychol Psychiatry 1987; 28(6):885–900.

178. Mulder EJ, Anderson GM, Kema IP, et al. Platelet serotonin levels in pervasive developmental disorders and mental retardation: diagnostic group differences, within-group distribution, and behavioral correlates. J Am Acad Child Adolesc Psychiatry 2004; 43(4):491–499.

179. Hranilovic D, Bujas-Petkovic Z, Vragovic R, et al. Hyperserotonemia in adults with autistic disorder. J Autism Dev Disord 2007; 37(10):1934–40. Epub 2006 Dec 13.

180. Bethea TC, Sikich L. Early pharmacological treatment of autism: a rationale for developmental treatment. Biol Psychiatry 2007; 61(4):521–537.

181. Ramamoorthy S, Bauman AL, Moore KR, et al. Antidepressant- and cocaine-sensitive human serotonin transporter: molecular cloning, expression, and chromosomal localization. Proc Natl Acad Sci U S A 1993; 90(6):2542–2546.

182. Stone JL, Merriman B, Cantor RM, et al. Evidence for sex-specific risk alleles in autism spectrum disorder. Am J Hum Genet 2004; 75(6):1117–1123.

183. Sutcliffe JS, Delahanty RJ, Prasad HC, et al. Allelic heterogeneity at the serotonin transporter locus (SLC6A4) confers susceptibility to autism and rigid-compulsive behaviors. Am J Hum Genet 2005; 77(2):265–279.

184. Bartlett CW, Goedken R, Vieland VJ. Effects of updating linkage evidence across subsets of data: reanalysis of the autism genetic resource exchange data set. Am J Hum Genet 2005; 76(4):688–695.

185. Guerini FR, Manca S, Sotgiu S, et al. A family based linkage analysis of HLA and 5-HTTLPR gene polymorphisms in Sardinian children with autism spectrum disorder. Hum Immunol 2006; 67(1–2):108–117.

186. Koishi S, Yamamoto K, Matsumoto H, et al. Serotonin transporter gene promoter polymorphism and autism: a family-based genetic association study in Japanese population. Brain Dev 2006; 28(4):257–260.

187. Yonan AL, Palmer AA, Gilliam TC. Hardy-Weinberg disequilibrium identified genotyping error of the serotonin transporter (SLC6A4) promoter polymorphism. Psychiatr Genet 2006; 16(1):31–34.

188. Zhong N, Ye L, Ju W, et al. 5-HTTLPR variants not associated with autistic spectrum disorders. Neurogenetics 1999; 2(2):129–131.

189. Ramoz N, Reichert JG, Corwin TE, et al. Lack of evidence for association of the serotonin transporter gene SLC6A4 with autism. Biol Psychiatry 2006; 60(2):186–191.

190. Brodkin ES, McDougle CJ, Naylor ST, et al. Clomipramine in adults with pervasive developmental disorders: a prospective open-label investigation. J Child Adolesc Psychopharmacol 1997; 7(2):109–121.

191. Furusho J, Matsuzaki K, Ichihashi I, et al. Alleviation of sleep disturbance and repetitive behavior by a selective serotonin re-uptake inhibitor in a boy with Asperger's syndrome. Brain Dev 2001; 23(2):135–137.

192. Kolevzon A, Mathewson KA, Hollander E. Selective serotonin reuptake inhibitors in autism: a review of efficacy and tolerability. J Clin Psychiatry 2006; 67(3): 407–414.

193. Buchsbaum MS, Hollander E, Haznedar MM et al. Effect of fluoxetine on regional cerebral metabolism in autistic spectrum disorders: a pilot study. Int J Neuropsychopharmacol 2001; 4(2):119–125.

194. Rausch JL, Johnson ME, Li J, et al. Serotonin transport kinetics correlated between human platelets and brain synaptosomes. Psychopharmacology (Berl) 2005; 180(3): 391–398.

195. Cho IH, Yoo HJ, Park M, et al. Family-based association study of 5-HTTLPR and the 5-HT2A receptor gene polymorphisms with autism spectrum disorder in Korean trios. Brain Res 2007; 1139:34–41. [Epub 2007 Jan 8]

196. Ozaki N, Goldman D, Kaye WH, et al. Serotonin transporter missense mutation associated with a complex neuropsychiatric phenotype. Mol Psychiatry 2003; 8(11): 933–936.

197. Wendland JR, DeGuzman TB, McMahon F, et al. SERT Ileu425Val in autism, Asperger syndrome and obsessive-compulsive disorder. Psychiatr Genet 2008; 18(1): 31–39.

198. Weiss LA, Veenstra-Vanderweele J, Newman DL, et al. Genome-wide association study identifies ITGB3 as a QTL for whole blood serotonin. Eur J Hum Genet 2004; 12(11):949–954.

199. Mulder EJ, Anderson GM, Kema IP, et al. Serotonin transporter intron 2 polymorphism associated with rigid-compulsive behaviors in Dutch individuals with

pervasive developmental disorder. Am J Med Genet B Neuropsychiatr Genet 2005; 133(1):93–96.

200. Naftolin F, Malaspina D. Estrogen, estrogen treatment and the post-reproductive woman's brain. Maturitas 2007; 57(1):23–26.

201. Brune CW, Kim SJ, Salt J, et al. 5-HTTLPR Genotype-Specific Phenotype in Children and Adolescents With Autism. Am J Psychiatry 2006; 163(12):2148–2156.

202. Kato MV, Shimizu T, Nagayoshi M, et al. Genomic imprinting of the human serotonin-receptor (HTR2) gene involved in development of retinoblastoma. Am J Hum Genet 1996; 59(5):1084–1090.

203. Bunzel R, Blumcke I, Cichon S, et al. Polymorphic imprinting of the serotonin-2A (5-HT2A) receptor gene in human adult brain. Brain Res Mol Brain Res 1998; 59(1): 90–92.

204. Murphy DG, Daly E, Schmitz N, et al. Cortical serotonin 5-HT2A receptor binding and social communication in adults with Asperger's syndrome: an in vivo SPECT study. Am J Psychiatry 2006; 163(5):934–936.

205. Novotny S, Hollander E, Allen A, et al. Increased growth hormone response to sumatriptan challenge in adult autistic disorders. Psychiatry Res 2000; 94(2):173–177.

206. Hollander E, Novotny S, Allen A, et al. The relationship between repetitive behaviors and growth hormone response to sumatriptan challenge in adult autistic disorder. Neuropsychopharmacology 2000; 22(2):163–167.

207. Nelson R. An Introduction to Behavioral Endocrinology. Sunderland, MA: Sinauer Associates, Inc, 1995.

208. Melke J, Goubran BH, Chaste P, et al. Abnormal melatonin synthesis in autism spectrum disorders. Mol Psychiatry 2008; 13(1):90–8. Epub 2007 May 15.

209. Paavonen EJ, Vehkalahti K, Vanhala R, et al. Sleep in Children with Asperger Syndrome. J Autism Dev Disord 2008; 38(1):41–51. Epub 2007 Mar 6.

210. Godbout R, Bergeron C, Limoges E, et al. A laboratory study of sleep in Asperger's syndrome. Neuroreport 2000; 11(1):127–130.

211. Tani P, Lindberg N, Nieminen-von WT, et al. Insomnia is a frequent finding in adults with Asperger syndrome. BMC Psychiatry 2003; 3:12.

212. Paavonen EJ, Nieminen-von WT, Vanhala R, et al. Effectiveness of melatonin in the treatment of sleep disturbances in children with Asperger disorder. J Child Adolesc Psychopharmacol 2003; 13(1):83–95.

213. Tordjman S, Anderson GM, Pichard N, et al. Nocturnal excretion of 6-sulphatoxymelatonin in children and adolescents with autistic disorder. Biol Psychiatry 2005; 57(2):134–138.

214. Felder MA. In: Klin A, Volkmar Fred R, Sparrow Sara S., eds. Asperger Syndrome. New York: The Guilford Press, 2000:xi-xii.

215. Yonan AL, Alarcon M, Cheng R, et al. A genomewide screen of 345 families for autism-susceptibility loci. Am J Hum Genet 2003; 73(4):886–897.

216. A genomewide screen for autism: strong evidence for linkage to chromosomes 2q, 7q, and 16p. Am J Hum Genet 2001; 69(3):570–581.

217. Hennah W, Varilo T, Kestila M, et al. Haplotype transmission analysis provides evidence of association for DISC1 to schizophrenia and suggests sex-dependent effects. Hum Mol Genet 2003; 12(23):3151–3159.

218. Hennah W, Thomson P, Peltonen L, et al. Genes and schizophrenia: beyond schizophrenia: the role of DISC1 in major mental illness. Schizophr Bull 2006; 32(3):409–416.

219. Sawamura N, Sawa A. Disrupted-in-schizophrenia-1 (DISC1): a key susceptibility factor for major mental illnesses. Ann N Y Acad Sci 2006; 1086:126–133.
220. Mackie S, Millar JK, Porteous DJ. Role of DISC1 in neural development and schizophrenia. Curr Opin Neurobiol 2007; 17(1):95–102.
221. Uvnas-Moberg K. Physiological and endocrine effects of social contact. Ann N Y Acad Sci 1997; 807:146–163.
222. Uvnas-Moberg K. Oxytocin may mediate the benefits of positive social interaction and emotions. Psychoneuroendocrinology 1998; 23(8):819–835.
223. Zingg HH, Grazzini E, Breton C, et al. Genomic and non-genomic mechanisms of oxytocin receptor regulation. Adv Exp Med Biol 1998; 449:287–295.
224. Gimpl G, Fahrenholz F. The oxytocin receptor system: structure, function, and regulation. Physiol Rev 2001; 81(2):629–683.
225. Bartels A, Zeki S. The neural correlates of maternal and romantic love. Neuroimage 2004; 21(3):1155–1166.
226. Takayanagi Y, Yoshida M, Bielsky IF, et al. Pervasive social deficits, but normal parturition, in oxytocin receptor-deficient mice. Proc Natl Acad Sci U S A 2005; 102(44):16096–16101.
227. Prichard ZM, Mackinnon AJ, Jorm AF, et al. AVPR1A and OXTR polymorphisms are associated with sexual and reproductive behavioral phenotypes in humans. Mutation in brief no. 981. Online. Hum Mutat 2007; 28(11):1150.
228. Champagne FA, Meaney MJ. Transgenerational effects of social environment on variations in maternal care and behavioral response to novelty. Behav Neurosci 2007; 121(6):1353–1363.
229. Pocklington AJ, Cumiskey M, Armstrong JD, et al. The proteomes of neuro-transmitter receptor complexes form modular networks with distributed functionality underlying plasticity and behaviour. Mol Syst Biol 2006; 2:2006.
230. Conciatori M, Stodgell CJ, Hyman SL, et al. Association between the HOXA1 A218G polymorphism and increased head circumference in patients with autism. Biol Psychiatry 2004; 55(4):413–419.
231. Devlin B, Bennett P, Cook EH Jr., et al. No evidence for linkage of liability to autism to HOXA1 in a sample from the CPEA network. Am J Med Genet 2002; 114(6): 667–672.
232. Ingram JL, Stodgell CJ, Hyman SL, et al. Discovery of allelic variants of HOXA1 and HOXB1: genetic susceptibility to autism spectrum disorders. Teratology 2000; 62(6):393–405.
233. Kiefer JC. Epigenetics in development. Dev Dyn 2007; 236(4):1144–1156.
234. Li J, Tabor HK, Nguyen L, et al. Lack of association between HoxA1 and HoxB1 gene variants and autism in 110 multiplex families. Am J Med Genet 2002; 114(1): 24–30.
235. Muscarella LA, Guarnieri V, Sacco R, et al. HOXA1 gene variants influence head growth rates in humans. Am J Med Genet B Neuropsychiatr Genet 2007; 144(3): 388–390.
236. Bartz JA, Hollander E. The neuroscience of affiliation: forging links between basic and clinical research on neuropeptides and social behavior. Horm Behav 2006; 50(4): 518–528.
237. Boso M, Emanuele E, Politi P, et al. Reduced plasma apelin levels in patients with autistic spectrum disorder. Arch Med Res 2007; 38(1):70–74.

238. Carter CS. Sex differences in oxytocin and vasopressin: implications for autism spectrum disorders? Behav Brain Res 2007; 176(1):170–186.

239. Cushing BS, Kramer KM. Mechanisms underlying epigenetic effects of early social experience: the role of neuropeptides and steroids. Neurosci Biobehav Rev 2005; 29(7): 1089–1105.

240. Insel TR, O'Brien DJ, Leckman JF. Oxytocin, vasopressin, and autism: is there a connection? Biol Psychiatry 1999; 45(2):145–157.

241. Knafo A, Israel S, Darvasi A, et al. Individual differences in allocation of funds in the dictator game associated with length of the arginine vasopressin 1a receptor RS3 promoter region and correlation between RS3 length and hippocampal mRNA. Genes Brain Behav 2008; 7(3):266–75. Epub 2007 Aug 13.

242. Wassink TH, Piven J, Vieland VJ, et al. Examination of AVPR1a as an autism susceptibility gene. Mol Psychiatry 2004; 9(10):968–972.

243. Yirmiya N, Rosenberg C, Levi S, et al. Association between the arginine vaso-pressin 1a receptor (AVPR1a) gene and autism in a family-based study: mediation by socialization skills. Mol Psychiatry 2006; 11(5):488–494.

244. Coutinho AM, Sousa I, Martins M, et al. Evidence for epistasis between SLC6A4 and ITGB3 in autism etiology and in the determination of platelet serotonin levels. Hum Genet 2007; 121(2):243–256. [Epub 2007, Jan 3].

245. Veenstra-Vanderweele J, Kim SJ, Lord C, et al. Transmission disequilibrium studies of the serotonin 5-HT2A receptor gene (HTR2A) in autism. Am J Med Genet 2002; 114(3):277–283.

246. Connors SL, Matteson KJ, Sega GA, et al. Plasma serotonin in autism. Pediatr Neurol 2006; 35(3):182–186.

247. Whitaker-Azmitia PM. Behavioral and cellular consequences of increasing sero-tonergic activity during brain development: a role in autism? Int J Dev Neurosci 2005; 23(1):75–83.

11

The Gene-Environment Interaction in Asperger's Disorder

Maria E. Johnson

*BrainScience Augusta and Developmental Disability Psychiatric
Consultation-Liaison, Gracewood Hospital, Augusta, Georgia, U.S.A.*

Cary Sanders

Medical College of Georgia School of Medicine, Augusta, Georgia, U.S.A.

Jeffrey L. Rausch

*BrainScience Augusta and Department of Psychiatry and Health Behavior,
Medical College of Georgia, Augusta, Georgia, U.S.A.*

COMPLEXITY OF THE GENE-ENVIRONMENT RELATIONSHIP

Although a variety of evidence points to genetic determinants of Asperger's disorder, some work points to environmental determinants in the phenotype of autism spectrum disorders (ASDs). Importantly, environmental contributions such as behavior programs are effective in modifying the expression of impairment (Chap. 14) (1). A study of how such environmental factors may impact the genotypic determination of phenotype reveal complex interactions that may provide valuable insights into etiology.

Studies of gene-environment etiologies in ASDs are complicated by the multilocus, epistatic, likely heterogeneous nature of the genetic etiology and the wide variability and changing nature of the internal and external environment. In addition, the gene-environment interaction itself is complex, both biologically and psychologically.

A synthesis of both psychological and biological gene-environment interactions is illustrated in the following model (Fig. 1). Phenotype describes the measurable manifestations of the genotype.

A. Gene expression (through programmed transcription, translation, post-translational modification, as well as epigenetic regulation of these), with an additional factor of random, probabilistic effects determines phenotype.
B. Environmental triggers affect gene expression and epigenetic regulation. For example, an environmental exposure can result in later autoimmune responses, where gene expression is turned on in response to antigen to make antibody.
C. Gene expression is determined not only by the environment but also by phenotype itself (2), since phenotype influences perception (3) and internal representation (4,5) of the environment.
D. The environment can affect phenotype, e.g., in the case where a toxin exerts a direct toxic effect on the cell.
E. Phenotype influences the environment (phenotype mediating the gene-environment correlation) (6). The gene-environment correlation describes a phenomenon where an individual's genotype through phenotype influences exposure or representation of the environment (7). Two people with

Gene Environment Interaction

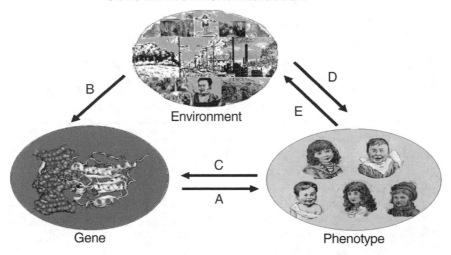

Figure 1 Gene-environment effects on phenotype are shown in the above, three-component model. Please refer to the text for a discussion of how modifiers at A, B, C, D, or E can affect phenotype. Importantly, a change at A, B, C, D, or E can cause reverberations through the circuit, making the first change not immediately discernable.

similar genetic phenotypes may experience different environments in the same way (8). They may both avoid social situations or not experience the ordinary internal representation of social experiences and so mute the effect of environmental difference.

In this way (Fig. 1), a reciprocal process unfolds, with interactions between neurodevelopment, behavior, and social function over time mediated through environmental effects on gene expression. Scarr and McCartney have also proposed a passive gene-environment correlation where one's genes would directly effect the environment. We have chosen to present our model as pictured in Figure 1. The passive gene-environment correlation is discussed in chapter 12.

The model can be used to examine potential reverberations in the circuit. Asperger's disorder, thought to be determined at least in part by heritable genetic factors (A.), may show insensitivity to external circadian cues (zeitgebers) (9). Zeitgebers determine the sleep-pattern phenotype (D.). (It is known that without external zeitgebers, sleep-pattern phenotype is such that sleep patterns run on a 25 hr/day rather than a 24 hr/day circadian pattern.) The insensitivity to external zeitgebers may lend itself to the phenotype changing the zeitgeber environment (e.g., leaving the lights on at night) (E.). External zeitgebers can induce changes in circadian clock gene expression (10,11) (B.). The sleep-pattern phenotype may also affect gene expression (C.).

Twin studies are often used to analyze the contribution of genetic versus environmental factors in complex behavioral disorders. One can study the stability of phenotype with fraternal versus identical twins in same or similar environments, or examine the effects of adverse environments on twins reared apart. Twin studies have revealed that the environment is a major source of elements that affect gene expression. While it also appears that gene expression is probabilistic rather than deterministic (12), the degree to which it is probabilistic can be minimized by examination of stimuli that interact with the realization of the genetic code potential (13). Such stimuli are challenging to precisely measure.

Important external genetic environmental circumstances (external to the organism) studied in ASDs are intrauterine conditions, obstetric events, toxins, autoimmunity, and diet.

PRENATAL AND OBSTETRIC FACTORS AS ENVIRONMENTAL DETERMINANTS

Pre- and perinatal risk factors are more common in Asperger's (14–17), autism (18–22), and ASDs (20,23,24). However, the evidence does not point to a single pre- or perinatal risk factor (14,24), and a number of other studies find no direct etiological role of obstetric complications in Asperger's or ASDs (22,24). The increased obstetric problems in ASDs may result from common, possibly genetic risk factors (22,24–27), since unaffected siblings have been shown to be more similar to affected cases in obstetric complications than they are to control subjects (24). The problems could be the manifestation of a gene-environment interaction, or simply epiphenomenological (27).

INTRAUTERINE ENVIRONMENT

The epiphenomenon could reside in the intrauterine environment, since maternal genotype (28), phenotype, psychosocial stressors (29), age, hormonal milieu (30,31), nutrition (32), medication presence (33), presence of exogenous toxic chemicals (34), and a fetal genotype-intrauterine environment interaction (35) are known to affect the development of the fetus. Gestational (fetal) programming describes permanent alterations in structure and physiology of the offspring that result from a unique intrauterine environment occurring during critical neurodevelopmental periods in certain time windows (36–41).

A growing body of evidence now implicates diverse intrauterine factors as having possible etiological effects in ASDs (18,23,42–46). Discovery and recognition of these factors is essential, since intervention during pregnancy has been shown to result in a positive long-term influence on outcome for at-risk children (47), implicating the likelihood for such benefit in ASDs or Asperger's disorder.

The evidence for intrauterine factors having potential etiological effects in Asperger's and ASDs is sizable. Markers of potential intrauterine effects in ASDs include minor physical anomalies (46), low birth weight (20), premature and postmature birth in Asperger's syndrome (15), and premature birth in autism (48). Increased maternal age both affects the intrauterine environment and increases risk for Asperger's and ASDs (20,49,50). Autistic-like behaviors have been noted in children of mothers abusing alcohol and other drugs (51), implicating such exogenous intrauterine toxins as potentially etiological. Potential intrauterine etiological factors that have been studied in ASDs include steroid hormones, thyroid hormone, teratogenic alleles, maternal neurotransmitter milieu, and maternal antibodies.

Intrauterine Steroid Hormones

A large body of evidence implicates endogenous intrauterine sex steroid androgen exposure in autism (52) and Asperger's disorder (53,54). Excess fetal testosterone may result in a magnification of the sexual dimorphism of the male brain and increased masculinization of the brain in Asperger's and ASDs. Fetal androgens as sex-dependent determinants of phenotype are discussed in full in chapter 12 (Age, Sex and Parenting).

Some data also exist implicating intrauterine stress steroid hormone (e.g., cortisol) exposure in ASDs (55–57). It has been noted that mothers of children with autism had increased psychosocial stressors during pregnancy, and an examination of the timing of prenatal stressors during pregnancy found that the mothers of children with autism were more likely than controls to experience stressors at weeks 21 to 32 of pregnancy (56). The time period was equivalent to that predicted by the authors as the embryological age where stress effects could affect neuroanatomy in a way seen in the cerebellum in autism. While these are the only studies that examined maternal prenatal stress in autism, evidence supports that maternal psychosocial stress and the resultant intrauterine gluccocorticoids can program HPA axis functions (58,59), brain neurotransmitter function (60), and long-term response to psychosocial stress (40). Maternal psychosocial stress can have sexually dimorphic biological and psychological effects (61–63), and has been shown to affect social behavior (64) and modify long-term phenotypic plasticity (59) in animals.

Intrauterine Thyroid Hormone

Intrauterine thyroid hormone has been studied in ASDs because of its essential role in neuronal migration (65) and observations of a possible relationship with ASDs to autoimmune thyroid disease.

Neuronal migration, via Reelin regulation, requires triiodothyronine (T3), and maternal hypothyroidism in early fetal brain development during the period of neuronal cell migration (weeks 8–12 of pregnancy) may produce morphological brain changes leading to ASDs (65,66). Animal models have shown that transient intrauterine deficits of thyroid hormones may result in permanent alterations of cerebral cortical architecture, architectural changes that are similar to those observed in brains of patients with autism (67). There is likely a critical period for such intrauterine thyroid hormone perturbations to have such effects (68,69), with different neuropsychological problems resulting from different critical periods (70).

Insufficient dietary iodine intake, stress (71), and a number of environmental agents [methylmercury (MeHg) (72) e.g.] can affect maternal thyroid function during pregnancy.

Intrauterine-Teratogenic Alleles

Maternal teratogenic alleles affect offspring phenotype in human disease (35,73). Some evidence exists for possible teratogenic alleles that affect the intrauterine neurotransmitter milieu, autoimmunity, and toxin metabolism in ASDs. Also, imprinted genes, important in placental growth and function (74), and fetal development (75) are implicated in ASDs and Asperger's (Chap. 10).

Maternal neurotransmitter phenotype and/or genotype may affect her intrauterine environment and thus affect her child's brain development. A deletion polymorphism in the dopa-beta-hydroxylase (DBH) gene has been identified in one study of autism mothers compared with controls. DBH catalyzes the conversion of dopamine to norepinephrine, and the authors of the study suggest that lowered maternal serum activity results in ASD in some families in part because of a uterine environment where norepinephrine is decreased relative to dopamine (76). Another study has shown evidence that maternal polymorphisms in monoamine oxidase A (MAO-A) and DBH may modify IQ in children with

were associated with lower birth weight, prematurity, and low five-minute APGAR score (93).

Differences

However, Eaton et al. did identify one difference in risk factors between the two groups—having more previous pregnancies apparently increased risk of having a child who later was diagnosed with autism, whereas having more previous pregnancies apparently decreased risk of having a child later diagnosed with Asperger's or atypical autism (93).

The Glasson study, discussed above, found that Asperger's disorder patients had a greater rate of caudal epidural anesthesia (24) compared to those with autism.

Are Obstetric Complications More Important in Lower-Functioning Autism?

Obstetric complications may play a greater role or may be a larger expression of an epiphenomenon in autism with mental retardation than in Asperger's or high-functioning autism (98). For example, in a case of triplets cited by Burgoine and Wing, the triplet with the most peri- and postnatal problems had the worst symptomatology (99). Conversely, high-functioning autism and Asperger's may not differ in obstetric risk factors (16). Consistent with this, other work has shown fewer obstetric complications in Asperger's compared with ASDs as a whole (24). However, it is interesting that one study of gifted children also found an increased rate of abnormalities during pregnancy and perinatal problems (100). It may be that extremes of human traits are reflected in prenatal and birth patterns.

XENOBIOTICS: BIOLOGICALLY ACTIVE FOREIGN ENTITIES

In the developing brain, there are critical periods of vulnerability (101) where unique susceptibilities (102) to chemical and toxic stimuli exist. The term "xenobiotic" refers to biologically active foreign entities that the genome may not be equipped to metabolize or may consider to be an antigen. At this point in time, toxic environmental risks and contributions to ASDs cannot be excluded (103), and there is a prevalent sense among many in the autism and scientific community that many environmental toxic effects have been relatively over-looked (104). For example, one report suggests that only 12 of 3000 toxins have been investigated (105). There are gaps in testing chemicals for developmental neurotoxicity (106), and sometimes a relatively stringent level of proof is required for regulation (106–108). Fortunately, a new network of pediatric environmental health specialty units has recently been commissioned to observe for such potential effects (109), and other epidemiological studies such as the Childhood Autism Risks from Genetics and Environment (CHARGE) study are underway (110).

Parents and other loved ones are concerned about potential toxic etiologies of ASDs (111) and constitute a contingency stimulating more research in the area. In a survey of 327 parents of children with ASDs, (Asperger's syndrome $N = 67$; 20.5%), parents (93%) typically blamed genetic causes if their child's autistic symptoms had been present since birth, but 70% of parents of children with regressive autistic symptoms believed in an environmental cause (112). Thus, it is often difficult to distinguish between the natural course of a disorder with delayed or regressive manifestations and that of exposure event proximal to manifestation as etiological.

Different Genetic Susceptibilities?

One potential factor that could account for the lack of evidence for toxic etiology could be whether children and parents would have a greater genetic sensitivity or vulnerability to exposure to xenobiotics (113), since different genetic susceptibility to environmental toxins can obscure both gene and environment findings.

An example of innovative control for the gene-xenobiotic confounders is seen in the work of D'Amelio et al. (114). Organophosphates (used as household and agricultural insecticides) are commonly used in North America. The authors hypothesized that the increased exposure to organophosphates in North America results in a pathogenic gene-environment interaction and identified an association in the paraoxenase (enzyme that detoxifies organophosphates) gene (PON1) to increased risk of autism in North America, but not Italy (114). It should be noted that the study didn't measure exposure levels, but estimated that exposure would be higher in North America.

There are markers to measure xenobiotic exposure that may be helpful to elucidate gene-environment interactions. Some xenobiotic exposures can be measured directly in human tissues such as blood or hair, in urine, or through urinary markers (115). Since mercury (Hg) is the most studied xenobiotic in ASDs, what follows is an examination of research to date on this toxicant.

Mercury

Mercury is one of a number of poisonous metals (e.g., lead, cadmium, radioactive metals, hexavalent chromium). These toxic metals can be changed in the environment into biologically active forms that are more toxic than the inorganic forms. The environmental modification of the metal may facilitate crossing the placenta or blood-brain barrier. Mercury can be toxic in three major classes: elemental (Hg vapor), inorganic (Hg salts), and organic forms (methyl- and ethylmercury) (116–119).

Urinary porphyrin profiles are one marker for toxic metal (i.e., mercury) exposure (120), and a number of studies measure hair levels of heavy metals to identify exposure (121–125) in the mother (126) and/or in sample cases. A metaanalysis did find a correlation between hair and blood mercury, but concluded that hair mercury should not replace blood and 24-hour urinary mercury as the gold standard for Hg poisoning (127).

Some have suggested that children with autism could possibly be genetically predisposed to heavy metal toxicity (128). While there is no conclusive evidence for such a gene-heavy metal interaction in ASDs, an epistatic gene interaction between two GST genes (GSTT1 and GSTM1) has been associated with increased levels of hair mercury in Austrian students compared with students without the double deletion present in both genes (129), implicating a genetic susceptibility to Hg poisoning. Also, rodent studies have shown genetic differences in susceptibility to autoimmunity with exposure to mercury (130).

A California public health service study linked the Environmental Protection Agency-estimated concentration of heavy metals in the ambient air around the place of birth of children diagnosed with ASDs in the California autism surveillance system and found a potential association between the heavy metals in the ambient air (mercury, cadmium, nickel) as well as the solvents trichloroethylene and vinyl chlorides (131) and the diagnosis of ASDs.

While the California public health service study did not measure any biomarkers of Hg exposure, porphyrin profiles were examined in 269 children with developmental disorders, 11 of whom were diagnosed with Asperger's disorder. Precoproporphyrin, an atypical heme molecule that is a specific indicator of heavy metal toxicity, levels were significantly increased in autism, but were not elevated in Asperger's disorder (132).

Relevant to the above discussion on potential etiological roles of a thyroidal or autoimmune nature, it is interesting to note that mercury can interfere with thyroid function during pregnancy (133) and may serve as a cofactor in human autoimmune disease (134).

Methylmercury

Biologically active Hg compounds have antifungal and antibacterial properties and so are used in organic forms in disinfectants and as preservatives in medical preparations and grain products (135). Most organic mercury is MeHg. MeHg accumulates in the aquatic food chain (136). MeHg is well established to be toxic to the human adult (137–139) and developing (102,124,140,141) nervous system.

MeHg is transported across the blood-brain barrier (142), preferentially stored in the central nervous system (CNS) (143,144) and easily transported from the pregnant mother to fetus (145). Oxidative stress (146), alterations in glutamine/glutamate cycling (146) and inhibition of protein synthesis (143) have been related to MeHg.

As may be expected, studies of low level exposure to MeHg show less clear effects (125) than do those with high dose exposures. However, low levels of MeHg have been shown to inhibit neuronal differentiation of neural stem cells (147), and cortical neural stem cells were shown to be especially sensitive to MeHg (147). Consumption of contaminated fish is the major route of exposure for humans (125,141), and most human studies have been conducted in fish-eating populations (125).

There is evidence that low levels of MeHg may produce effects on attention, sensory, and motor function (139,141). Maternal hair mercury levels have been correlated with adverse neurophysiological effects in first graders through identification of delayed brainstem-evoked potentials (148). Other studies have shown beneficial outcomes in populations exposed prenatally to mercury-containing fish, potentially attributable to the nutritional value of the essential fatty acids in the fish diet (32). Some propose, however, that pregnant women and small children should avoid eating fish because of MeHg content (149). Interestingly, there is evidence that boys may be more susceptible to the early-life neurotoxic effects of MeHg (124,145,150,151).

Ethylmercury

Thimerosal, a preservative used in medical preparation such as thimerosal (135), releases the active species of ethylmercury. Ethylmercury is not as well studied as MeHg, and it is interesting that ethylmercury has been shown to have different toxin kinetics from MeHg in animals (152–154), although policies on ethylmercury exposure are based largely from MeHg data (155). Ethylmercury has been shown to be neurotoxic in human cellular lines (156), and cases of poisoning have been identified in humans (157,158). Studies of low-dose exposure to ethylmercury have not shown large effects, and children exposed to thimerosal did not show mercury-induced autoimmunity to antimetallothionein (159).

A study published by the *New England Journal of Medicine* in otherwise normal children (age 7–10) showed mixed effects (positive and negative) of thimerosal during the prenatal period, neonatal period (birth to 28 days), and the first seven months of life on cognition (160). Higher prenatal Hg exposure was associated with better performance on one measure of language. Increasing Hg exposure from birth to 28 days was associated with better performance on one measure of fine motor coordination. Increasing Hg exposure from birth to seven months was associated with better performance on one measure of fine motor coordination and one measure of attention and executive functioning. However, higher prenatal Hg exposure was associated with poorer performance on one measure of attention and executive functioning, and increasing Hg exposure from birth to 28 days was associated with poorer performance on one measure of speech articulation (160). These results are difficult to interpret for ASDs since children with ASDs were not included in the cohort.

It has been hypothesized and supported by consumer groups that ethyl-mercury toxicity from thimerosal preservative in vaccines may have some role in the etiology of ASDs. One reason mercury-containing vaccines have been suspected is the fact that the discovery of autism in 1943 coincided with the relatively new (since the 1930s) and widespread use of thimerosal preservative in vaccines (161). In July 1999, the Food and Drug Administration (FDA) requested that companies remove the thimerosal from vaccines or justify its continued use in writing (162). Though one study identified increased Hg levels in preterm infants (163) vaccinated with hepatitis B vaccine, in population studies and continued investigations, the thimerosal hypothesis has not been proven. In fact, a large body of evidence against the hypothesis that thimerosal toxicity causes PDDs exists (127,164–167).

The observed increase in Hg levels in normal students with GST deletions (129) can potentially exemplify a gene-environment interaction on the outcome of ASD studies (e.g., in studies where equivalent Hg or thimerosal levels or exposures are found between autism groups and controls) since such an increased sensitivity could obscure the relationship. More toxicity would be expected in the autism case with equivalent exposure or levels in the less sensitive control case. Conversely, in studies where two groups differ in Hg exposure, the incidence of autistic pathology between groups could be expected to be manifest through the increased sensitivity to mercury. Interestingly, the estimated incidence of autism has continued to increase since the removal of thimerosal from vaccines.

The MMR Debate

In 1998, Wakefield et al. published a report that suggested Hg compounds contained in certain vaccines, mainly the measles-mumps-rubella (MMR) vaccine, were associated with developmental regression. A partial retraction of the results was later published (168). Dr. Wakefield's work was still under review by the UK General Medical Council at the time of this writing (169).

The design of the Wakefield study was criticized by Smeeth and colleagues, who pointed out that the study did not compare to a control group (170,171). In 2004, Smeeth et al. performed a case-control study that is particularly interesting for our purposes since it investigated "whether the MMR vaccine is associated with increased risk for autism or other PDDs" (172). The researchers found that taking the MMR vaccine as a child was not associated with an increased risk of developing a PDD. In 2001, Fombonne and colleagues investigated a possible new variant of MMR-induced autism (173). The study population contained 96 children with a PDD diagnosis, including 13 Asperger cases. Their results added "to the recent accumulation of large-scale epidemiological studies that all failed to support an association between MMR and autism at a population level" (173).

Most recently, a reasonably large ($N = 180$) study of pervasive developmental disorders (PDDs) included 28 Asperger cases. The researchers concluded that the MMR vaccine is not causally related to the PDDs based on observing that prevalence of PDDs in children exposed to the MMR vaccine increased between 1987 and 1998 even as the MMR vaccination frequency decreased (164). In 1996, when a second MMR vaccine was added to the dosing schedule, a separate analysis showed no significant change in the upward trend of PDD diagnosis. If the MMR vaccine were linked to the prevalence of PDDs, an increase in diagnosis would be expected (164). Other findings show no relationship with autism and the MMR (174–177), though the possibility of a subgroup of autism with regression and increased gastrointestinal symptoms is still being explored.

Despite these findings, the vaccination rate has decreased. Vaccine-critical Web sites frequently make serious allegations. With the burgeoning of the internet as a health information source, the public may accept this information and refuse vaccination of their children, putting children at risk for well-known communicable diseases (172). As this occurs, the incidence of vaccine-preventable diseases may rise (178). The risk/benefit ratio for various of the vaccines, for the population versus the individual continues to source lively debate.

AUTOIMMUNITY

It is possible that dietary peptides, bacterial toxins, and xenobiotics can bind to immune system receptors and enzymes resulting in autoimmune reactions in children with autism (179). Increased autoimmune disorders (180) and auto-immunity have been noted increased in families with ASDs (181).

An increased proinflammatory response to endotoxin has been identified in ASDs (182). Some autistic subjects have been shown to have antimyelin basic protein antibodies (183) and increased eosinophil and basophil reactions (183). Autoimmunity to neuronal and glial filaments was found to be elevated in subjects with autism compared to a group with mental retardation but not autism (184). Increased neuroinflammation and neuroimmunity have been identified (185). Other immune processes studied include overactivation of Th-1 cells (186), Th-2 cells (187), increased levels of cytokines IL-12 and IFN gamma (186), imbalance between Th-1and Th-2 cell activity (188), and an excessive innate immune response (189). Further, some have suggested that children with ASDs have unusual immune responses to dietary proteins (182,190) with antibodies that are cross-reactive to CNS molecules (190).

Antigliadin IgG

In 2004, Vojdani et al. measured antigliadin antibodies in 50 autistic individuals compared with 50 controls and concluded that a subgroup of autism contains individuals who have antibodies against Purkinje cells and gliadin (antigenic fragment of gluten) (190). Antigliadin IgG levels were elevated in 42% of autistic subjects and 16% of control subjects; IgM was high in 34% of autistic and 8% of controls; and IgA was elevated in 36% of autistic subjects and 14% of controls (190).

Overall, members of the autistic group also had significantly higher levels of anticerebellar antibodies in their sera. In the patients with elevated gluten antibodies, anticerebellar peptides were also elevated. Cross-reactivity of antibodies to gliadin with cerebellar proteins (specifically Purkinje cells) was demonstrated (190). There are no studies on antigliadin in Asperger's. Evidence for efficacy of diet modifications in gliadin are discussed below.

Human Leukocyte Antigen Alleles

As discussed above in the context of possible determinants of intrauterine maternal fetal autoimmune reactions, the HLA gene has polymorphic alleles, and HLA-DR4 is implicated in autoimmune thyroid dysfunction (85). A recent Collaborative Programs of Excellence in Autism (CPEA) revealed that regression in ASDs was significantly associated with a family history of autoimmune thyroid disease (191). Alleles at the HLA have been identified to be in linkage disequilibrium in some but not all (192) studies of autism (87,193,194) and ASDs (195). A transmission disequilibrium test of 107 Caucasian families showed HLA- DR4 to be increased in ASDs compared to controls and found a preferential paternal transmission of the allele (195). A family study of HLA and 5-HTTLPR genotypes in 37 ASD Sardinian families found that in 50% of these families, ASD is linked to HLA, and in the other 50% it is linked to 5-HTTLPR polymorphic genes. However, no specific alleles in the HLA or SERT were identified as significant (196).

Other Etiological Factors

Early in biological studies of autism, an increase in urinary peptides was identified and proposed to be etiological in autism (197–201), though recent work has shown no difference in urinary peptides (202–204). Increased vulnerability to oxidative stress (205) and viral hypotheses (206) have also been explored. Oxidative stress may interact with genotype in autism with the following possible gene susceptibility or protective effects: reduced folate carrier (RFC 80G > A), transcobalamin II (TCN2 776G > C), catechol-O-methyltransferase (COMT 472G > A), methylenetetrahydrofolate reductase (MTHFR 677C > T and 1298A > C), and GST (GSTM1) (205).

DIET

Parents of children with ASDs report increased use and beneficial effects of complementary and alternative medicine (primarily diet) treatments as well as dissatisfaction with the medical system in access and information regarding such approaches (207–210). Gluten (a peptide in wheat, rye, barley) and casein (a milk protein) are the two most commonly eliminated ingredients in the therapeutic diet plans.

Glutens are proteins in wheat that are important in the structure and physical properties of dough (211). The structure of gluten proteins is rich in glutamine and proline (211). Parents and autism support groups often report that the autistic episodes are exacerbated when the children eat certain foodstuffs such as dairy products, wheat, corn, sugar, apples, bananas, and chocolate. Testimonials have appeared in periodicals, Web sites, and journals. The diets may not be benign; nutrition related changes have been noted in some individuals with ASDs on restricted diets (212,213).

As immunological studies at the molecular level continue, clinical dietary intervention trials are necessary to help characterize the role of foods in the development of ASDs. However, to date, gluten and casein have not been proven causative in autoimmune or autistic disorders.

Elimination Diets

In 2006, Christison and Ivany (214) critically reviewed the scientific soundness of previous studies. At that date, there were seven published trials of gluten and/ or casein elimination in autistic children (215). Flaws included small sample sizes and short study durations and lack of monitoring for the diet restrictions.

Of those reviewed by Christison and Ivany, the 2002 trial by Knivsberg et al. (216) was the most scientifically sound. It was a single-blind randomized control-matched study and unique in its design. Subjects and controls were matched pair wise by severity of autistic symptoms, age, and cognitive level. To qualify for inclusion, subjects had a diagnosis of autism and urinary peptide abnormalities. Subjects in the experimental group were placed on a Gluten-free Casein-free (GFCF) diet for one year, and foods were evaluated by a dietician. Evaluators were blinded to the patients' treatment status; however, as pointed out by Christison and Ivany, parents, teachers, and patients were not blinded. This is one weakness of the study.

Many areas showed statistically significant improvement for the GFCF group: aloofness, routines and rituals, and responses to learning. The control group did not show significant improvement in those areas. Peer relations, anxiety levels, empathy, and physical contact traits also improved significantly in GFCF group but not in the control. Nonverbal communication, eye contact, reaction when spoken to, and language peculiarities improved significantly only in the GFCF group. Other areas with significant improvements in the GFCF group included judgment and number of interests. There were small, non-statistically significant improvements in the control group in multiple areas.

The authors summarized, "significance of difference was registered in the first four of the five areas" (216). They were referring to improvements in GFCF children in attention, social/emotional factors, communicative factors, and cognitive factors, but not sensory/motor factors.

Since the 2006 review article, Elder et al. published a 12-week randomized double-blind, repeated measures crossover trial (217). The two diets compared were GFCF and regular diet. The sample size was small ($N = 15$, with 13 subjects completing protocol). Analysis of urinary peptide levels yielded no statistically significant differences between groups. There was no statistically significant reduction in autistic symptoms by symptom scales, though parents noticed some improvement in symptoms. This study had strengths, including that all meals were provided by a central kitchen for 12 weeks. In addition, parents were educated about acceptable GFCF emergency snacks. However, the shorter duration of the trial can be considered as a weakness.

Results of GFCF diet trials have been conflicting and inconclusive. There is no empiric evidence that gluten and/or casein cause ASD. There is also no empiric evidence of the harmfulness of a GFCF diet. Parental accounts are often more positive compared to blinded raters indicating there may be some placebo effect for children with autistic disorders, in addition to any beneficial effect.

Knivsberg et al. demonstrated a successful controlled one-year trial with results supporting the possible efficacy of a GFCF diet (216). Elder et al. (217) recently demonstrated some useful methods for evaluating elimination diets. As parental testimonials continue to spread, and more families search for effective treatments for autism, it will become even more crucial that the possible role of dietary proteins in the pathogenesis of autism be elucidated.

CONCLUSIONS

The lack of resolution of etiology in ASDs and Asperger's is quite troubling. The diverse range of putative etiologies may suggest multiple potential etiologies for the phenotype. Future protection of children from unfavorable gene-environment interactions and neurodevelopmental influences is essential. Parsing out these findings for strict Asperger's disorder is difficult.

Regardless of the stance of the Asperger's and medical community over whether a "cure" is necessary, frank scientific curiosity will continue to stimulate study of this, in the words of Hans Asperger, "fascinating" personality. Environmental toxicology appears to have yielded perhaps the most provocative results in ASDs. Asperger's will become less of a mystery, with further scientific exploration of the biological basis of psychiatric disorders.

Most importantly, future genetic and environmental studies will need to address both natural phenomena contemporaneously through specific exploration of post-Mendelian environmental modifiers. The 5-HTTLPR interaction with stressful life events (2), where earlier genetic findings were inconclusive in respect to the gene-linkage to depression, can serve as a model for further visionary exploration.

REFERENCES

1. Koegel RL, Koegel LK, McNerney EK. Pivotal areas in intervention for autism. J Clin Child Psychol 2001; 30(1):19–32.
2. Caspi A, Sugden K, Moffitt TE, et al. Influence of life stress on depression: moderation by a polymorphism in the 5-HTT gene. Science 2003; 301(5631): 386–389.
3. Bachmanov AA, Beauchamp GK. Taste receptor genes. Annu Rev Nutr 2007; 27:389–414.

4. Mesulam MM. Spatial attention and neglect: parietal, frontal and cingulate contributions to the mental representation and attentional targeting of salient extrapersonal events. Philos Trans R Soc Lond B Biol Sci 1999; 354(1387):1325–1346.

5. Schore A. The Emotionally Expressive Face. Affect Regulation and the Origin of the Self. Hillsdale, NJ: Lawrence Erlbaum Associates, 1994:168–175.

6. Scarr S, McCartney K. How people make their own environments: a theory of genotype greater than environment effects. Child Dev 1983; 54(2):424–435.

7. Tsuang MT, Bar JL, Stone WS, et al. Gene-environment interactions in mental disorders. World Psychiatry 2004; 3(2):73–83.

8. Raine A, Reynolds C, Venables PH, et al. Stimulation seeking and intelligence: a prospective longitudinal study. J Pers Soc Psychol 2002; 82(4):663–674.

9. Hare DJ, Jones S, Evershed K. A comparative study of circadian rhythm functioning and sleep in people with Asperger syndrome. Autism 2006; 10(6):565–575.

10. Stratmann M, Schibler U. Properties, entrainment, and physiological functions of mammalian peripheral oscillators. J Biol Rhythms 2006; 21(6):494–506.

11. Challet E. Clock genes, circadian rhythms and food intake. Pathol Biol (Paris) 2007; 55(3–4):176–177.

12. Le CA, Bailey A, Goode S, et al. A broader phenotype of autism: the clinical spectrum in twins. J Child Psychol Psychiatry 1996; 37(7):785–801.

13. Russel P. Extensions of Mendelian genetic analysis. Genetics. 3rd ed. New York: Harper Collins, 1992:92–120.

14. Gillberg C, Cederlund M. Asperger syndrome: familial and pre- and perinatal factors. J Autism Dev Disord 2005; 35(2):159–166.

15. Cederlund M, Gillberg C. One hundred males with Asperger syndrome: a clinical study of background and associated factors. Dev Med Child Neurol 2004; 46(10): 652–660.

16. Ghaziuddin M, Shakal J, Tsai L. Obstetric factors in Asperger syndrome: comparison with high-functioning autism. J Intellect Disabil Res 1995; 39(pt 6): 538–543.

17. Rickarby G, Carruthers A, Mitchell M. Brief report: biological factors associated with Asperger syndrome. J Autism Dev Disord 1991; 21(3):341–348.

18. Gillberg C, Gillberg IC. Infantile autism: a total population study of reduced optimality in the pre-, peri-, and neonatal period. J Autism Dev Disord 1983; 13(2): 153–166.

19. Stein D, Weizman A, Ring A, et al. Obstetric complications in individuals diagnosed with autism and in healthy controls. Compr Psychiatry 2006; 47(1):69–75.

20. Kolevzon A, Gross R, Reichenberg A. Prenatal and perinatal risk factors for autism: a review and integration of findings. Arch Pediatr Adolesc Med 2007; 161(4): 326–333.

21. Matsuishi T, Yamashita Y, Ohtani Y, et al. Brief report: incidence of and risk factors for autistic disorder in neonatal intensive care unit survivors. J Autism Dev Disord 1999; 29(2):161–166.

22. Bolton PF, Murphy M, Macdonald H, et al. Obstetric complications in autism: consequences or causes of the condition? J Am Acad Child Adolesc Psychiatry 1997; 36(2):272–281.

23. Juul-Dam N, Townsend J, Courchesne E. Prenatal, perinatal, and neonatal factors in autism, pervasive developmental disorder-not otherwise specified, and the general population. Pediatrics 2001; 107(4):E63.

24. Glasson EJ, Bower C, Petterson B, et al. Perinatal factors and the development of autism: a population study. Arch Gen Psychiatry 2004; 61(6):618–627.
25. Zwaigenbaum L, Szatmari P, Jones MB, et al. Pregnancy and birth complications in autism and liability to the broader autism phenotype. J Am Acad Child Adolesc Psychiatry 2002; 41(5):572–579.
26. Zwaigenbaum L, Szatmari P, Jones MB, et al. Pregnancy and birth complications in autism and liability to the broader autism phenotype. J Am Acad Child Adolesc Psychiatry 2002; 41(5):572–579.
27. Hultman CM, Sparen P. Autism–prenatal insults or an epiphenomenon of a strongly genetic disorder? Lancet 2004; 364(9433):485–487.
28. Dunger DB, Petry CJ, Ong KK. Genetic variations and normal fetal growth. Horm Res 2006; 65(suppl 3):34–40.
29. MacLaughlin SM, McMillen IC. Impact of periconceptional undernutrition on the development of the hypothalamo-pituitary-adrenal axis: does the timing of parturition start at conception? Curr Drug Targets 2007; 8(8):880–887.
30. Gorski RA. Hypothalamic imprinting by gonadal steroid hormones. Adv Exp Med Biol 2002; 511:57–70.
31. Newbold RR, Padilla-Banks E, Snyder RJ, et al. Perinatal exposure to environmental estrogens and the development of obesity. Mol Nutr Food Res 2007; 51(7): 912–917.
32. Clarkson TW, Strain JJ. Nutritional factors may modify the toxic action of methyl mercury in fish-eating populations. J Nutr 2003; 133(5 suppl 1):S1539–S1543.
33. Ardinger HH, Atkin JF, Blackston RD, et al. Verification of the fetal valproate syndrome phenotype. Am J Med Genet 1988; 29(1):171–185.
34. Latini G, Del VA, Massaro M, et al. In utero exposure to phthalates and fetal development. Curr Med Chem 2006; 13(21):2527–2534.
35. Hummel M, Marienfeld S, Huppmann M, et al. Fetal growth is increased by maternal type 1 diabetes and HLA DR4-related gene interactions. Diabetologia 2007; 50(4):850–858.
36. Phillips DI. External influences on the fetus and their long-term consequences. Lupus 2006; 15(11):794–800.
37. Ross MG, Desai M. Gestational programming: population survival effects of drought and famine during pregnancy. Am J Physiol Regul Integr Comp Physiol 2005; 288(1):R25–R33.
38. Reusens B, Remacle C. Programming of the endocrine pancreas by the early nutritional environment. Int J Biochem Cell Biol 2006; 38(5–6):913–922.
39. Haimov-Kochman R. Fetal programming—the intrauterine origin of adult morbidity. Harefuah 2005; 144(2):97–101, 151, 150.
40. Kajantie E, Feldt K, Raikkonen K, et al. Body size at birth predicts hypothalamic-pituitary-adrenal axis response to psychosocial stress at age 60 to 70 years. J Clin Endocrinol Metab 2007; 92(11):4094–4100.
41. Ross MG, Desai M, Khorram O, et al. Gestational programming of offspring obesity: a potential contributor to Alzheimer's disease. Curr Alzheimer Res 2007; 4(2): 213–217.
42. Berger-Sweeney J, Hohmann CF. Behavioral consequences of abnormal cortical development: insights into developmental disabilities. Behav Brain Res 1997; 86(2): 121–142.

43. Connors SL, Levitt P, Matthews SG, et al. Fetal mechanisms in neurodevelopmental disorders. Pediatr Neurol 2008; 38(3):163–176.
44. Landa R, Garrett-Mayer E. Development in infants with autism spectrum disorders: a prospective study. J Child Psychol Psychiatry 2006; 47(6):629–638.
45. Tripi G, Roux S, Canziani T, et al. Minor physical anomalies in children with autism spectrum disorder. Early Hum Dev 2008; 84(4):217–223.
46. Gualtieri CT, Adams A, Shen CD, et al. Minor physical anomalies in alcoholic and schizophrenic adults and hyperactive and autistic children. Am J Psychiatry 1982; 139(5):640–643.
47. Eriksson M, Jonsson B, Steneroth G, et al. Amphetamine abuse during pregnancy: environmental factors and outcome after 14-15 years. Scand J Public Health 2000; 28(2):154–157.
48. Larsson HJ, Eaton WW, Madsen KM, et al. Risk factors for autism: perinatal factors, parental psychiatric history, and socioeconomic status. Am J Epidemiol 2005; 161(10):916–925.
49. Croen LA, Najjar DV, Fireman B, et al. Maternal and paternal age and risk of autism spectrum disorders. Arch Pediatr Adolesc Med 2007; 161(4):334–340.
50. Gillberg C. Maternal age and infantile autism. J Autism Dev Disord 1980; 10 (3):293–297.
51. Harris SR, MacKay LL, Osborn JA. Autistic behaviors in offspring of mothers abusing alcohol and other drugs: a series of case reports. Alcohol Clin Exp Res 1995; 19(3):660–665.
52. Strous RD, Golubchik P, Maayan R, et al. Lowered DHEA-S plasma levels in adult individuals with autistic disorder. Eur Neuropsychopharmacol 2005; 15(3):305–309.
53. de Bruin EI, Verheij F, Wiegman T, et al. Differences in finger length ratio between males with autism, pervasive developmental disorder-not otherwise specified, ADHD, and anxiety disorders. Dev Med Child Neurol 2006; 48(12):962–965.
54. Manning JT, Baron-Cohen S, Wheelwright S, et al. The 2nd to 4th digit ratio and autism. Dev Med Child Neurol 2001; 43(3):160–164.
55. Ward AJ. A comparison and analysis of the presence of family problems during pregnancy of mothers of "autistic" children and mothers of normal children. Child Psychiatry Hum Dev 1990; 20(4):279–288.
56. Beversdorf DQ, Manning SE, Hillier A, et al. Timing of prenatal stressors and autism. J Autism Dev Disord 2005; 35(4):471–478.
57. McGinnis WR. Could oxidative stress from psychosocial stress affect neuro-development in autism? J Autism Dev Disord 2007; 37(5):993–994.
58. Pesonen AK, Raikkonen K, Kajantie E, et al. Fetal programming of temperamental negative affectivity among children born healthy at term. Dev Psychobiol 2006; 48(8): 633–643.
59. Viltart O, Vanbesien-Mailliot CC. Impact of prenatal stress on neuroendocrine programming. ScientificWorldJournal 2007; 7:1493–1537.
60. McArthur S, McHale E, Dalley JW, et al. Altered mesencephalic dopaminergic populations in adulthood as a consequence of brief perinatal glucocorticoid expo-sure. J Neuroendocrinol 2005; 17(8):475–482.
61. Wust S, Entringer S, Federenko IS, et al. Birth weight is associated with salivary cortisol responses to psychosocial stress in adult life. Psychoneuroendocrinology 2005; 30(6):591–598.

62. Andrews MH, Kostaki A, Setiawan E, et al. Developmental regulation of 5-HT1A receptor mRNA in the fetal limbic system: response to antenatal glucocorticoid. Brain Res Dev Brain Res 2004; 149(1):39–44.

63. McArthur S, McHale E, Gillies GE. The size and distribution of midbrain dopaminergic populations are permanently altered by perinatal glucocorticoid exposure in a sex- region- and time-specific manner. Neuropsychopharmacology 2007; 32(7): 1462–1476.

64. Kofman O. The role of prenatal stress in the etiology of developmental behavioural disorders. Neurosci Biobehav Rev 2002; 26(4):457–470.

65. Roman GC. Autism: transient in utero hypothyroxinemia related to maternal flavonoid ingestion during pregnancy and to other environmental antithyroid agents. J Neurol Sci 2007; 262(1–2):15–26.

66. Gillberg IC, Gillberg C, Kopp S. Hypothyroidism and autism spectrum disorders. J Child Psychol Psychiatry 1992; 33(3):531–542.

67. Kimura-Kuroda J, Nagata I, Kuroda Y. Disrupting effects of hydroxy-polychlorinated biphenyl (PCB) congeners on neuronal development of cerebellar Purkinje cells: a possible causal factor for developmental brain disorders? Chemosphere 2007; 67(9): S412–S420.

68. Pracyk JB, Seidler FJ, McCook EC, et al. Pituitary-thyroid axis reactivity to hyper- and hypothyroidism in the perinatal period: ontogeny of regulation of regulation and long-term programming of responses. J Dev Physiol 1992; 18(3):105–109.

69. Wilcoxon JS, Redei EE. Prenatal programming of adult thyroid function by alcohol and thyroid hormones. Am J Physiol Endocrinol Metab 2004; 287(2):E318–E326.

70. Zoeller RT, Rovet J. Timing of thyroid hormone action in the developing brain: clinical observations and experimental findings. J Neuroendocrinol 2004; 16(10): 809–818.

71. Charmandari E, Kino T, Souvatzoglou E, et al. Pediatric stress: hormonal mediators and human development. Horm Res 2003; 59(4):161–179.

72. Mori K, Yoshida K, Hoshikawa S, et al. Effects of perinatal exposure to low doses of cadmium or methylmercury on thyroid hormone metabolism in metallothionein-deficient mouse neonates. Toxicology 2006; 228(1):77–84.

73. Child F, Lenney W, Clayton S, et al. The association of maternal but not paternal genetic variation in GSTP1 with asthma phenotypes in children. Respir Med 2003; 97(12):1247–1256.

74. Isles AR, Holland AJ. Imprinted genes and mother-offspring interactions. Early Hum Dev 2005; 81(1):73–77.

75. Skuse DH. Imprinting, the X-chromosome, and the male brain: explaining sex differences in the liability to autism. Pediatr Res 2000; 47(1):9–16.

76. Robinson PD, Schutz CK, Macciardi F, et al. Genetically determined low maternal serum dopamine beta-hydroxylase levels and the etiology of autism spectrum disorders. Am J Med Genet 2001; 100(1):30–36.

77. Jones MB, Palmour RM, Zwaigenbaum L, et al. Modifier effects in autism at the MAO-A and DBH loci. Am J Med Genet B Neuropsychiatr Genet 2004; 126(1):58–65.

78. Connors SL, Matteson KJ, Sega GA, et al. Plasma serotonin in autism. Pediatr Neurol 2006; 35(3):182–186.

79. Weiss LA, Abney M, Cook EH Jr., et al. Sex-specific genetic architecture of whole blood serotonin levels. Am J Hum Genet 2005; 76(1):33–41.

80. Hohmann CF, Walker EM, Boylan CB, et al. Neonatal serotonin depletion alters behavioral responses to spatial change and novelty. Brain Res 2007; 1139:163–77 (epub 2007 Jan 17:163–177).
81. Warren RP, Cole P, Odell JD, et al. Detection of maternal antibodies in infantile autism. J Am Acad Child Adolesc Psychiatry 1990; 29(6):873–877.
82. Braunschweig D, Ashwood P, Krakowiak P, et al. Autism: Maternally derived antibodies specific for fetal brain proteins. Neurotoxicology 2008; 29(2):226–231.
83. Dalton P, Deacon R, Blamire A, et al. Maternal neuronal antibodies associated with autism and a language disorder. Ann Neurol 2003; 53(4):533–537.
84. Buckner JH, Nepom GT. Genetics of rheumatoid arthritis: is there a scientific explanation for the human leukocyte antigen association? Curr Opin Rheumatol 2002; 14(3):254–259.
85. Jacobson EM, Tomer Y. The genetic basis of thyroid autoimmunity. Thyroid 2007; 17(10):949–961.
86. Vadheim CM, Rotter JI, Maclaren NK, et al. Preferential transmission of diabetic alleles within the HLA gene complex. N Engl J Med 1986; 315(21):1314–1318.
87. Lee LC, Zachary AA, Leffell MS, et al. HLA-DR4 in families with autism. Pediatr Neurol 2006; 35(5):303–307.
88. Zimmerman AW, Connors SL, Matteson KJ, et al. Maternal antibrain antibodies in autism. Brain Behav Immun 2007; 21(3):351–357.
89. Williams TA, Mars AE, Buyske SG, et al. Risk of autistic disorder in affected offspring of mothers with a glutathione S-transferase P1 haplotype. Arch Pediatr Adolesc Med 2007; 161(4):356–361.
90. Trevarthen C, Aitken KJ. Infant intersubjectivity: research, theory, and clinical applications. J Child Psychol Psychiatry 2001; 42(1):3–48.
91. Ijichi S, Ijichi N. The prenatal autistic imprinting hypothesis: developmental maladaptation to the environmental changes between womb and the social world. Med Hypotheses 2004; 62(2):188–194.
92. Attwood T. Asperger's Syndrome: A Guide for Parents and Professionals. London: Jessica Kingsley, 1998.
93. Eaton WW, Mortensen PB, Thomsen PH, et al. Obstetric complications and risk for severe psychopathology in childhood. J Autism Dev Disord 2001; 31(3):279–285.
94. Gillberg C. Clinical and neurobiological aspects of Asperger Syndrome in six family studies. In: Frith U, ed. Autism and Asperger Syndrome. Cambridge: Cambridge University Press, 1991:122–146.
95. Reichenberg A, Gross R, Weiser M, et al. Advancing paternal age and autism. Arch Gen Psychiatry 2006; 63(9):1026–1032.
96. Lauritsen MB, Pedersen CB, Mortensen PB. Effects of familial risk factors and place of birth on the risk of autism: a nationwide register-based study. J Child Psychol Psychiatry 2005; 46(9):963–971.
97. Malaspina D, Reichenberg A, Weiser M, et al. Paternal age and intelligence: implications for age-related genomic changes in male germ cells. Psychiatr Genet 2005; 15(2):117–125.
98. Lord C, Mulloy C, Wendelboe M, et al. Pre- and perinatal factors in high-functioning females and males with autism. J Autism Dev Disord 1991; 21(2):197–209.
99. Burgoine E, Wing L. Identical triplets with Asperger's syndrome. Br J Psychiatry 1983; 143:261–265.

100. Louis J, Revol O, Nemoz C, et al. Psychophysiological factors in high intellectual potential: comparative study in children aged from 8 to 11 years old. Arch Pediatr 2005; 12(5):520–525.

101. Rice D, Barone S Jr. Critical periods of vulnerability for the developing nervous system: evidence from humans and animal models. Environ Health Perspect 2000; 108(suppl 3):511–533.

102. Trask CL, Kosofsky BE. Developmental considerations of neurotoxic exposures. Neurol Clin 2000; 18(3):541–562.

103. Clements CJ. The evidence for the safety of thiomersal in newborn and infant vaccines. Vaccine 2004; 22(15–16):1854–1861.

104. Labie D. Developmental neurotoxicity of industrial chemicals. Med Sci (Paris) 2007; 23(10):868–872.

105. Stein J, Schettler T, Wallinga D, et al. In harm's way: toxic threats to child development. J Dev Behav Pediatr 2002; 23(suppl 1):S13–S22.

106. Grandjean P, Landrigan PJ. Developmental neurotoxicity of industrial chemicals. Lancet 2006; 368(9553):2167–2178.

107. Gee D. Late lessons from early warnings: Toward realism and precaution with endocrine-disrupting substances. Environ Health Perspect 2006; 114(suppl 1):152–160.

108. Jarosinska D, Gee D. Children's environmental health and the precautionary principle. Int J Hyg Environ Health 2007; 210(5):541–546.

109. Shannon M, Woolf A, Goldman R. Children's environmental health: one year in a pediatric environmental health specialty unit. Ambul Pediatr 2003; 3(1):53–56.

110. Hertz-Picciotto I, Croen LA, Hansen R, et al. The CHARGE study: an epidemiologic investigation of genetic and environmental factors contributing to autism. Environ Health Perspect 2006; 114(7):1119–1125.

111. Halsey NA, Hyman SL. Measles-mumps-rubella vaccine and autistic spectrum disorder: report from the New Challenges in Childhood Immunizations Conference convened in Oak Brook, IL, June 12–13, 2000. Pediatrics 2001; 107(5):E84.

112. Goin-Kochel RP, Mackintosh VH, Myers BJ. How many doctors does it take to make an autism spectrum diagnosis? Autism 2006; 10(5):439–451.

113. Echeverria D, Woods JS, Heyer NJ, et al. The association between a genetic polymorphism of coproporphyrinogen oxidase, dental mercury exposure and neurobehavioral response in humans. Neurotoxicol Teratol 2006; 28(1):39–48.

114. D'Amelio M, Ricci I, Sacco R, et al. Paraoxonase gene variants are associated with autism in North America, but not in Italy: possible regional specificity in gene-environment interactions. Mol Psychiatry 2005; 10(11):1006–1016.

115. Brewster MA. Biomarkers of xenobiotic exposures. Ann Clin Lab Sci 1988; 18(4): 306–317.

116. Neathery MW, Miller WJ. Metabolism and toxicity of cadmium, mercury, and lead in animals: a review. J Dairy Sci 1975; 58(12):1767–1781.

117. Mercury toxicity. Agency for Toxic Substance and Disease Registry. Am Fam Physician 1992; 46(6):1731–1741.

118. Clarkson TW. The toxicology of mercury. Crit Rev Clin Lab Sci 1997; 34(4):369–403.

119. Risher JF, De Rosa CT. Inorganic: the other mercury. J Environ Health 2007; 70(4): 9–16.

120. Woods JS, Martin MD, Naleway CA, et al. Urinary porphyrin profiles as a biomarker of mercury exposure: studies on dentists with occupational exposure to mercury vapor. J Toxicol Environ Health 1993; 40(2–3):235–246.

121. Adams JB, Holloway CE, George F, et al. Analyses of toxic metals and essential minerals in the hair of Arizona children with autism and associated conditions, and their mothers. Biol Trace Elem Res 2006; 110(3):193–209.

122. Fido A, Al-Saad S. Toxic trace elements in the hair of children with autism. Autism 2005; 9(3):290–298.

123. Ip P, Wong V, Ho M, et al. Mercury exposure in children with autistic spectrum disorder: case-control study. J Child Neurol 2004; 19(6):431–434.

124. Marsh DO, Clarkson TW, Cox C, et al. Fetal methylmercury poisoning. Relationship between concentration in single strands of maternal hair and child effects. Arch Neurol 1987; 44(10):1017–1022.

125. Myers GJ, Davidson PW. Does methylmercury have a role in causing developmental disabilities in children? Environ Health Perspect 2000; 108(suppl 3):413–420.

126. Cernichiari E, Brewer R, Myers GJ, et al. Monitoring methylmercury during pregnancy: maternal hair predicts fetal brain exposure. Neurotoxicology 1995; 16(4): 705–710.

127. Ng DK, Chan CH, Soo MT, et al. Low-level chronic mercury exposure in children and adolescents: meta-analysis. Pediatr Int 2007; 49(1):80–87.

128. Kern JK, Grannemann BD, Trivedi MH, et al. Sulfhydryl-reactive metals in autism. J Toxicol Environ Health A 2007; 70(8):715–721.

129. Gundacker C, Komarnicki G, Jagiello P, et al. Glutathione-S-transferase polymorphism, metallothionein expression, and mercury levels among students in Austria. Sci Total Environ 2007; 385(1–3):37–47.

130. Johansson U, Hansson-Georgiadis H, Hultman P. The genotype determines the B cell response in mercury-treated mice. Int Arch Allergy Immunol 1998; 116(4): 295–305.

131. Windham GC, Zhang L, Gunier R, et al. Autism spectrum disorders in relation to distribution of hazardous air pollutants in the san francisco bay area. Environ Health Perspect 2006; 114(9):1438–1444.

132. Nataf R, Skorupka C, Amet L, et al. Porphyrinuria in childhood autistic disorder: implications for environmental toxicity. Toxicol Appl Pharmacol 2006; 214(2): 99–108.

133. Takser L, Mergler D, Baldwin M, et al. Thyroid hormones in pregnancy in relation to environmental exposure to organochlorine compounds and mercury. Environ Health Perspect 2005; 113(8):1039–1045.

134. Silbergeld EK, Silva IA, Nyland JF. Mercury and autoimmunity: implications for occupational and environmental health. Toxicol Appl Pharmacol 2005; 207(suppl 2): 282–292.

135. Risher JF, Murray HE, Prince GR. Organic mercury compounds: human exposure and its relevance to public health. Toxicol Ind Health 2002; 18(3):109–160.

136. Balshaw S, Edwards J, Daughtry B, et al. Mercury in seafood: mechanisms of accumulation and consequences for consumer health. Rev Environ Health 2007; 22(2):91–113.

137. Carta P, Flore C, Alinovi R, et al. Sub-clinical neurobehavioral abnormalities associated with low level of mercury exposure through fish consumption. Neurotoxicology 2003; 24(4–5):617–623.

138. Ekino S, Susa M, Ninomiya T, et al. Minamata disease revisited: an update on the acute and chronic manifestations of methyl mercury poisoning. J Neurol Sci 2007; 262(1–2):131–144.

139. Carta P, Flore C, Alinovi R, et al. Neuroendocrine and neurobehavioral effects associated with exposure to low doses of mercury from habitual consumption of marine fish. Med Lav 2002; 93(3):215–224.

140. Johansson C, Castoldi AF, Onishchenko N, et al. Neurobehavioural and molecular changes induced by methylmercury exposure during development. Neurotox Res 2007; 11(3–4):241–260.

141. Mendola P, Selevan SG, Gutter S, et al. Environmental factors associated with a spectrum of neurodevelopmental deficits. Ment Retard Dev Disabil Res Rev 2002; 8(3):188–197.

142. Aschner M, Aschner JL. Mercury neurotoxicity: mechanisms of blood-brain barrier transport. Neurosci Biobehav Rev 1990; 14(2):169–176.

143. Philbert MA, Billingsley ML, Reuhl KR. Mechanisms of injury in the central nervous system. Toxicol Pathol 2000; 28(1):43–53.

144. Bjorkman L, Lundekvam BF, Laegreid T, et al. Mercury in human brain, blood, muscle and toenails in relation to exposure: an autopsy study. Environ Health 2007; 6:30.

145. Vahter M, Akesson A, Liden C, et al. Gender differences in the disposition and toxicity of metals. Environ Res 2007; 104(1):85–95.

146. Yin Z, Milatovic D, Aschner JL, et al. Methylmercury induces oxidative injury, alterations in permeability and glutamine transport in cultured astrocytes. Brain Res 2007; 1131(1):1–10.

147. Tamm C, Duckworth J, Hermanson O, et al. High susceptibility of neural stem cells to methylmercury toxicity: effects on cell survival and neuronal differentiation. J Neurochem 2006; 97(1):69–78.

148. Murata K, Weihe P, Renzoni A, et al. Delayed evoked potentials in children exposed to methylmercury from seafood. Neurotoxicol Teratol 1999; 21(4):343–348.

149. Ronchetti R, Zuurbier M, Jesenak M, et al. Children's health and mercury exposure. Acta Paediatr Suppl 2006; 95(453):36–44.

150. Thomas DJ, Fisher HL, Sumler MR, et al. Sexual differences in the distribution and retention of organic and inorganic mercury in methyl mercury-treated rats. Environ Res 1986; 41(1):219–234.

151. Thomas DJ, Fisher HL, Sumler MR, et al. Sexual differences in the excretion of organic and inorganic mercury by methyl mercury-treated rats. Environ Res 1987; 43(1):203–216.

152. Burbacher TM, Shen DD, Liberato N, et al. Comparison of blood and brain mercury levels in infant monkeys exposed to methylmercury or vaccines containing thimerosal. Environ Health Perspect 2005; 113(8):1015–1021.

153. Zareba G, Cernichiari E, Hojo R, et al. Thimerosal distribution and metabolism in neonatal mice: comparison with methyl mercury. J Appl Toxicol 2007; 27(5):511–518.

154. Magos L, Brown AW, Sparrow S, et al. The comparative toxicology of ethyl- and methylmercury. Arch Toxicol 1985; 57(4):260–267.

155. Harry GJ, Harris MW, Burka LT. Mercury concentrations in brain and kidney following ethylmercury, methylmercury and Thimerosal administration to neonatal mice. Toxicol Lett 2004; 154(3):183–189.

156. Humphrey ML, Cole MP, Pendergrass JC, et al. Mitochondrial mediated thimerosal-induced apoptosis in a human neuroblastoma cell line (SK-N-SH). Neurotoxicology 2005; 26(3):407–416.

157. Cinca I, Dumitrescu I, Onaca P, et al. Accidental ethyl mercury poisoning with nervous system, skeletal muscle, and myocardium injury. J Neurol Neurosurg Psychiatry 1980; 43(2):143–149.
158. Zhang J. Clinical observations in ethyl mercury chloride poisoning. Am J Ind Med 1984; 5(3):251–258.
159. Singh VK, Hanson J. Assessment of metallothionein and antibodies to metal-lothionein in normal and autistic children having exposure to vaccine-derived thimerosal. Pediatr Allergy Immunol 2006; 17(4):291–296.
160. Thompson WW, Price C, Goodson B, et al. Early thimerosal exposure and neuro-psychological outcomes at 7 to 10 years. N Engl J Med 2007; 357(13):1281–1292.
161. Bernard S, Enayati A, Roger H, et al. The role of mercury in the pathogenesis of autism. Mol Psychiatry 2002; 7(suppl 2):S42–S43.
162. Ball LK, Ball R, Pratt RD. An assessment of thimerosal use in childhood vaccines. Pediatrics 2001; 107(5):1147–1154.
163. Stajich GV, Lopez GP, Harry SW, et al. Iatrogenic exposure to mercury after hepatitis B vaccination in preterm infants. J Pediatr 2000; 136(5):679–681.
164. Fombonne E, Zakarian R, Bennett A, et al. Pervasive developmental disorders in Montreal, Quebec, Canada: prevalence and links with immunizations. Pediatrics 2006; 118(1):E139–E150.
165. Berman RF, Pessah IN, Mouton PR, et al. Low-Level Neonatal Thimerosal Exposure: Further Evaluation of Altered Neurotoxic Potential in SJL Mice. Toxicol Sci 2008; 101(2):294–309.
166. Madsen KM, Lauritsen MB, Pedersen CB, et al. Thimerosal and the occurrence of autism: negative ecological evidence from Danish population-based data. Pediatrics 2003; 112(3 pt 1):604–606.
167. Miles JH, Takahashi TN. Lack of association between Rh status, Rh immune globulin in pregnancy and autism. Am J Med Genet A 2007; 143(13):1397–1407.
168. Murch SH, Anthony A, Casson DH, et al. Retraction of an interpretation. Lancet 2004; 363(9411):750.
169. Hearing Before the General Medical Council. Press Release http://www.gmcpress office.org.uk/apps/news/events/detail.php?key=2523 .
170. Smeeth L, Hall AJ, Rodrigues LC, et al. Measles, mumps, and rubella (MMR) vaccine and autism. Ecological studies cannot answer main question. BMJ 2001; 323(7305):163.
171. Smeeth L, Rodrigues LC, Hall AJ, et al. Evaluation of adverse effects of vaccines: the case-control approach. Vaccine 2002; 20(19–20):2611–2617.
172. Smeeth L, Cook C, Fombonne E, et al. MMR vaccination and pervasive devel-opmental disorders: a case-control study. Lancet 2004; 364(9438):963–969.
173. Fombonne E, Chakrabarti S. No evidence for a new variant of measles-mumps-rubella-induced autism. Pediatrics 2001; 108(4):E58.
174. Klein KC, Diehl EB. Relationship between MMR vaccine and autism. Ann Phar-macother 2004; 38(7–8):1297–1300.
175. Madsen KM, Hviid A, Vestergaard M, et al. A population-based study of measles, mumps, and rubella vaccination and autism. N Engl J Med 2002; 347(19):1477–1482.
176. Taylor B, Miller E, Lingam R, et al. Measles, mumps, and rubella vaccination and bowel problems or developmental regression in children with autism: population study. BMJ 2002; 324(7334):393–396.

177. Richler J, Luyster R, Risi S, et al. Is there a 'regressive phenotype' of Autism Spectrum Disorder associated with the measles-mumps-rubella vaccine? A CPEA Study. J Autism Dev Disord 2006; 36(3):299–316.

178. Zimmerman RK, Wolfe RM, Fox DE, et al. Vaccine criticism on the World Wide Web. J Med Internet Res 2005; 7(2):e17.

179. Vojdani A, Pangborn JB, Vojdani E, et al. Infections, toxic chemicals and dietary peptides binding to lymphocyte receptors and tissue enzymes are major instigators of autoimmunity in autism. Int J Immunopathol Pharmacol 2003; 16(3):189–199.

180. Comi AM, Zimmerman AW, Frye VH, et al. Familial clustering of autoimmune disorders and evaluation of medical risk factors in autism. J Child Neurol 1999; 14(6):388–394.

181. Sweeten TL, Bowyer SL, Posey DJ, et al. Increased prevalence of familial autoimmunity in probands with pervasive developmental disorders. Pediatrics 2003; 112(5):e420.

182. Jyonouchi H, Sun S, Itokazu N. Innate immunity associated with inflammatory responses and cytokine production against common dietary proteins in patients with autism spectrum disorder. Neuropsychobiology 2002; 46(2):76–84.

183. Trottier G, Srivastava L, Walker CD. Etiology of infantile autism: a review of recent advances in genetic and neurobiological research. J Psychiatry Neurosci 1999; 24(2):103–115.

184. Singh VK, Warren R, Averett R, et al. Circulating autoantibodies to neuronal and glial filament proteins in autism. Pediatr Neurol 1997; 17(1):88–90.

185. Pardo CA, Vargas DL, Zimmerman AW. Immunity, neuroglia and neuro-inflammation in autism. Int Rev Psychiatry 2005; 17(6):485–495.

186. Singh VK. Plasma increase of interleukin-12 and interferon-gamma. Pathological significance in autism. J Neuroimmunol 1996; 66(1–2):143–145.

187. Molloy CA, Morrow AL, Meinzen-Derr J, et al. Elevated cytokine levels in children with autism spectrum disorder. J Neuroimmunol 2006; 172(1–2):198–205.

188. Gupta S, Aggarwal S, Rashanravan B, et al. Th1- and Th2-like cytokines in CD4+ and CD8+ T cells in autism. J Neuroimmunol 1998; 85(1):106–109.

189. Jyonouchi H, Sun S, Le H. Proinflammatory and regulatory cytokine production associated with innate and adaptive immune responses in children with autism spectrum disorders and developmental regression. J Neuroimmunol 2001; 120(1–2): 170–179.

190. Vojdani A, O'Bryan T, Green JA, et al. Immune response to dietary proteins, gliadin and cerebellar peptides in children with autism. Nutr Neurosci 2004; 7(3): 151–161.

191. Molloy CA, Morrow AL, Meinzen-Derr J, et al. Familial autoimmune thyroid disease as a risk factor for regression in children with Autism Spectrum Disorder: a CPEA Study. J Autism Dev Disord 2006; 36(3):317–324.

192. Rogers T, Kalaydjieva L, Hallmayer J, et al. Exclusion of linkage to the HLA region in ninety multiplex sibships with autism. J Autism Dev Disord 1999; 29(3):195–201.

193. Warren RP, Odell JD, Warren WL, et al. Strong association of the third hypervariable region of HLA-DR beta 1 with autism. J Neuroimmunol 1996; 67(2):97–102.

194. Torres AR, Sweeten TL, Cutler A, et al. The association and linkage of the HLA-A2 class I allele with autism. Hum Immunol 2006; 67(4–5):346–351.

195. Torres AR, Maciulis A, Stubbs EG, et al. The transmission disequilibrium test suggests that HLA-DR4 and DR13 are linked to autism spectrum disorder. Hum Immunol 2002; 63(4):311–316.
196. Guerini FR, Manca S, Sotgiu S, et al. A family based linkage analysis of HLA and 5-HTTLPR gene polymorphisms in Sardinian children with autism spectrum disorder. Hum Immunol 2006; 67(1–2):108–117.
197. Trygstad OE, Reichelt KL, Foss I, et al. Patterns of peptides and protein-associated-peptide complexes in psychiatric disorders. Br J Psychiatry 1980; 136:59–72.
198. Reichelt KL, Hole K, Hamberger A, et al. Biologically active peptide-containing fractions in schizophrenia and childhood autism. Adv Biochem Psychopharmacol 1981; 28:627–643.
199. Anderson RJ, Bendell DJ, Garnett I, et al. Identification of indolyl-3-acryloylglycine in the urine of people with autism. J Pharm Pharmacol 2002; 54(2):295–298.
200. Reichelt KL, Knivsberg AM. Can the pathophysiology of autism be explained by the nature of the discovered urine peptides? Nutr Neurosci 2003; 6(1):19–28.
201. Reichelt KL, Saelid G, Lindback T, et al. Childhood autism: a complex disorder. Biol Psychiatry 1986; 21(13):1279–1290.
202. Le CA, Trygstad O, Evered C, et al. Infantile autism and urinary excretion of peptides and protein-associated peptide complexes. J Autism Dev Disord 1988; 18(2):181–190.
203. Hunter LC, O'Hare A, Herron WJ, et al. Opioid peptides and dipeptidyl peptidase in autism. Dev Med Child Neurol 2003; 45(2):121–128.
204. Dettmer K, Hanna D, Whetstone P, et al. Autism and urinary exogenous neuro-peptides: development of an on-line SPE-HPLC-tandem mass spectrometry method to test the opioid excess theory. Anal Bioanal Chem 2007; 388(8):1643–1651.
205. James SJ, Melnyk S, Jernigan S, et al. Metabolic endophenotype and related genotypes are associated with oxidative stress in children with autism. Am J Med Genet B Neuropsychiatr Genet 2006; 141(8):947–956.
206. van GT, Heijnen CJ, Treffers PD. Autism and the immune system. J Child Psychol Psychiatry 1997; 38(3):337–349.
207. Levy SE, Hyman SL. Novel treatments for autistic spectrum disorders. Ment Retard Dev Disabil Res Rev 2005; 11(2):131–142.
208. Liptak GS, Orlando M, Yingling JT, et al. Satisfaction with primary health care received by families of children with developmental disabilities. J Pediatr Health Care 2006; 20(4):245–252.
209. Wong HH, Smith RG. Patterns of complementary and alternative medical therapy use in children diagnosed with autism spectrum disorders. J Autism Dev Disord 2006; 36(7):901–909.
210. Hanson E, Kalish LA, Bunce E, et al. Use of complementary and alternative medicine among children diagnosed with autism spectrum disorder. J Autism Dev Disord 2007; 37(4):628–636.
211. Wieser H. Chemistry of gluten proteins. Food Microbiol 2007; 24(2):115–119.
212. Arnold GL, Hyman SL, Mooney RA, et al. Plasma amino acids profiles in children with autism: potential risk of nutritional deficiencies. J Autism Dev Disord 2003; 33(4):449–454.
213. Hediger ML, England LJ, Molloy CA, et al. Reduced bone cortical thickness in boys with autism or autism spectrum disorder. J Autism Dev Disord 2007; 38(5): 848–856.

214. Christison GW, Ivany K. Elimination diets in autism spectrum disorders: any wheat amidst the chaff? J Dev Behav Pediatr 2006; 27(2 suppl):S162–S171.
215. Lucarelli S, Frediani T, Zingoni AM, et al. Food allergy and infantile autism. Panminerva Med 1995; 37(3):137–141.
216. Knivsberg AM, Reichelt KL, Hoien T, et al. A randomised, controlled study of dietary intervention in autistic syndromes. Nutr Neurosci 2002; 5(4):251–261.
217. Elder JH, Shankar M, Shuster J, et al. The gluten-free, casein-free diet in autism: results of a preliminary double blind clinical trial. J Autism Dev Disord 2006; 36(3): 413–420.

12

Age, Sex, and Parenting

Maria E. Johnson

*BrainScience Augusta and Developmental Disability Psychiatric
Consultation-Liaison, Gracewood Hospital, Augusta, Georgia, U.S.A.*

Jeffrey L. Rausch

*BrainScience Augusta and Department of Psychiatry and Health Behavior,
Medical College of Georgia, Augusta, Georgia, U.S.A.*

IMPORTANCE OF SEX AND AGE

Because of an apparent disproportionate distribution of gender prevalence and because Asperger's disorder is classified as a developmental disorder, both sex and age deserve special consideration in an understanding of its etiology. Sex and age are very much like the external environment in the way that they affect the expression of the genetic code potential. Therefore, sex and age are considered the "intrinsic" genetic environment.

AGE

Asperger's literature suggests age to be important in at least two fundamental dimensions: age in the context of development of the affected individual and parental age.

Age of Development

The genetic, epigenetic, and proteomic factors discussed in chapter 10 are age sensitive. Time, as a factor, is especially important in early brain development because of the delicate relationship of neuronal growth with discrete developmental periods, determinants of differential brain function. Time factors are known to influence brain development in several ways, including their effects on developmental timing genes, "heterochronic" genes (1). These include transcription factors (2) such as homeobox genes (3) and neurotrophic genes (4). Time factors also influence embryonic developmental proteins, known as geminin proteins (5,6), and a class of noncoding RNA molecules called micro-RNAs (7,8). Of these, only the homeobox family has been implicated to date in Asperger's.

HOXA1

HOX genes are critical to early embryogenesis where they modulate other genes (9), as discussed above. The HOXA1 gene has been implicated in head growth (10–13) and neural development (14). Unusual patterns of head growth are known to be a risk factor for Asperger's (15–23). The HOXA1 finding illustrates a non-Mendelian example of sexual dimorphism in both gene inheritance and expression. An increased frequency of a HOXA1 (7p15.3) polymorphism (A218G) has been noted in autism spectrum disorders (ASDs) (24), though not replicated (25,26).

The sex of the parent with the guanine mutation appeared to affect inheritance, and the effect of the mutation appeared to be more apparent in females (24).

Critical Periods

In pre- and postnatal development, there are discrete time windows within which there is sufficient sensitivity to developmental signaling for structural development of the brain (27). These time windows, known as critical periods, may be as short as four weeks (28,29). Amplifications or perturbations of the processes that occur in critical periods have a greater importance because the effects are organizational and enduring, and thus may last for a lifetime (30). These critical periods are known to occur before 18 years, periods during which there is greater potential for growth and differentiation. It is important to recognize that effects determined during a given critical period may not be apparent immediately and may be observed only later in life (31) when development is ready for manifestation of such functions.

A connection between ASDs and critical periods can be seen in infants with congenital cataracts. The infant must have the cataracts removed before four to six months, or blindness results (27). This occurs ostensibly because of the visual systems' need at this critical period for light patterns to develop organized visual circuits. Congenitally blind children have a high rate of ASDs, and it has been proposed that these children suffer from social impairment because of restriction in the kinds of childhood social experience that develop theory of mind (32). Also, sensory and language deprivation in early life (33–36) can affect social, visual, and language development. This would implicate visual, social, and language perceptual elements during critical periods to be contributors to Asperger's disorder.

At the same time, some parts of the brain are continuously plastic and can continue to modify function on the basis of environmental experience. Stimuli both within and outside of the brain determine structural brain changes over time. A lack of subjective experience may affect the epigenetic regulation of gene expression and activity-dependent synaptic development.

As discussed below, the activities that we engage in and the experiences that we have can determine a biological differentiation of social function in both positive and negative respects.

Activity-Dependent Development

Neuronal development is classified into activity-dependent and activity-independent processes. As discussed in chapter 10, activity-dependent process describes the process wherein a neuronal stimulus to a neuron results in "long-term potentiation," where the neuron increases the signal strength in neuronal connections because it has been activated. In prenatal brain development, neuronal differentiation from stem cells, neuronal migration, and axon growth guidance are examples of activity-independent processes; external stimulation is not required for the processes to unfold. After axon growth guidance, activity-dependent processes are important.

The infant has around 100 billion neurons at birth and produces glial cells after birth. Glial cells provide insulation for the nerve cell and increase the efficiency of signal transmission. Just as neuronal synapses change depending on experience, glial cell production can be increased by environmental stimulation. Both neuronal and nonneuronal factors can contribute to the signal strength of the neuron, and these are modified by the environment.

With respect to Asperger's disorder, activity- or experience-dependent neurodevelopment during such critical periods has been implicated. In addition, there may be effects of plasticity change potential that is available throughout life. The best examples for experience-dependent effects in Asperger's are findings regarding face categorization. Face organization in the visual cortex has been shown to be experience dependent, while cortical organization of object and place categories are similar between children and adults (37). The subjective experience of a "social gaze" has been implicated as an environmental stimulus that may determine social development in Asperger's, as an experience-dependent effect.

The Decreased Social Gaze Response

In early development, a decreased social gaze response (38), decreased attention to faces (39,40), and different face perception (41) may contribute to the development of Asperger's. The social gaze response is a measurement of the amount of time an infant looks at his mother when she is looking at him (42). The social gaze response may result in a developmental trajectory that results in the consistent deficits in face recognition reported for Asperger's (43). These include recognition of facial identity, emotion, gaze direction, gender, and lip reading (44). As noted previously in this volume, subjects with Asperger's tend to identify and process faces on the basis of attention to parts of the face rather than the whole, the global configuration of face (44–46). This cognitive style may explain evidence for altered brain localization of activity compared with controls, when processing faces (47).

Visual and language developmental perturbations during development may result from redundant connectivity of the immature brain that gradually decreases in an experience-dependent way after birth, different neural systems having different levels of redundant connectivity, and plasticity differences between different systems (48). Social experiences in early development may organize future behavior through a number of hypothetical mechanisms, including altering sensitivity to neuropeptides and steroids (49), or changing neuronal excitability or apoptosis and pruning (50). It has been proposed that mild social-cognitive processing deficits such as those seen in Asperger's (i.e., face processing and eye gaze) are usually compensated in normal development (51), and given the identification of autistic traits in the general population (52), this theory further implicates experience-dependent and epigenetic processes in the manifestation of the severity of the broader autism phenotype.

Parents and the family provide the primary social environment for the child; as such, we may thus consider parenting within the context of age and time effects on neurodevelopment.

AGE AND PARENTING

First, however, age and time have affects on the parents themselves that can be transmitted to the child. As noted in chapter 10, both increased maternal and paternal age are associated with Asperger's disorder. Reactive oxygen species, toxins, and other species accumulate with aging and may contribute to effects upon genomic determinants, as previously discussed.

Since parenting has a very important influence on early psychosocial development, particularly in children with some degree of biological risk (53–57), does advanced parental age affect parenting ability or style? Evidence shows rather that older parents may have some advantage because of greater personality and socioeconomic stability (58–60).

IMPORTANCE OF PARENTING

A foundation of psychiatry is that early child-parental interactions determine later social development. Freud's theory of psychosexual development, the object-relations theory of Melanie Klein, and the attachment theory of John

Bowlby, among others, emphasize parent-child relationships (61–64). Neuroscience research has since validated many such aspects of psychodevelopmental theory (65).

Extrinsic social environmental stimuli in the postnatal period have been shown to affect human infant phenotype (66) and neurophysiological endophenotypes (67). In the latter study, infants of depressed mothers showed greater right frontal lobe EEG asymmetry than control infants at birth. At three to six months, this asymmetry reduced in the infants of depressed mothers with intrusive interaction styles (with a shift toward greater relative left frontal EEG activation), but was increased in infants of depressed mothers with withdrawn interaction styles (67).

Animal studies have shown later gene transcription effects secondary to early social parental environmental effects (68). Parental nurturing, including the effects of touch itself, is known to affect the cortisol response (Hypothalamic Pituitary Adrenal (HPA) axis), for example, in a manner that could endow the organism with an enduring resistance to stress. This may be relevant to our subject because depression has been associated with a dysregulated HPA axis. Depressed parents, in turn, may provide less touch and nurturance to their children than nondepressed parents. Thus, we may conceptualize the potential for a reverberating circuit where the HPA response to social stress is conferred environmentally to the child. As discussed below, with respect to children with autism, those with a family history of depression have been found to demonstrate less potential for social adaptation than those without a family history of depression. Consequently, aside from depression being a heritable trait, we may conceptualize transmission of the trait from the environment as a distinct additional or separate factor.

Parent-Infant Sex Interaction

The following study implicates a further genetic contribution of the sex chromosomes in the internal representation of early parental interactions. These interactions may affect the child's social schema differently on the basis of the child's sex. In one study, mothers were instructed to play with their infants in a natural way for five minutes and then to maintain a "still-face" (neutral face with no expression) for three minutes before returning to a natural interaction style. The still-face is a stressful situation for the infant because of the violation of the expected social exchange. The infant's social and emotional responses were scored. The authors found that both male and female infants of mothers with more positive expressions in the naturalistic play situation had an increased social gaze to the still-face. However, with the same maternal positive play behavior, female infants tended to remain neutral to the still-face, whereas male infants showed positive attempts for attention, followed by negative emotions and protest (69).

Other work has shown correlations that exist between mothers and daughters but not other family members (70). These observations may underscore the need to stratify for gender in parenting studies of ASDs. In addition, these observations also suggest the possibility of gender-specific treatment outcomes.

Passive Gene-Environment Correlation

Also noted in this regard is a passive gene-environment correlation (71), as described by Scarr and McCartney, wherein, for example, a genetic vulnerability to dysregulated HPA axis response to social stress in itself constitutes an environmental variable. In other words, one's own genes (as also expressed in the parents) contribute to an environment that may determine expression of that susceptibility.

Similarly, as discussed in chapter 10, the broader autism phenotype is often noted in parent and family members of children with Asperger's. Parents of children with ASDs show low levels of autistic traits, such as local rather than global cognitive processing styles (72–74). Interestingly, within our context of sex-dependent factors, it appears that fathers are more likely than mothers to have such autistic traits (75). This may serve as a second example of how genes passively determine an environment in addition to the example discussed above for the HPA axis. The above evidence appears to support a parental contribution to autistic learning or autistic trait expression.

"Parental Causation" Hypothesis

Kanner observed cold, distant parenting in the ancestry of his cohorts. Some psychoanalysts, most notably Bruno Bettelheim, elaborated the observation further and speculated that this parenting style constituted an emotional deprivation of the child of an etiological nature (76). During the course of the mid-20th century, many parents were stigmatized, if not traumatized, by the widespread, unjustified idea that they induced the condition. It arose from Bettelheim's idea that autistic withdrawal was the result of mothers' inadequate care and responsiveness (77).

Empirical studies of the role of parenting in autism have shown little support for a "parental causation" hypothesis (77,78). Indeed, there is little evidence for any substantial etiological parenting influence in ASDs on the whole.

In a study of family interaction characteristics, parents of children with autism exhibited the same levels of marital happiness and interpersonal relationships among family members as controls (77). Parents of children with ASDs have been shown to be normal in sensitivity to their children (79) and equally synchronized with their children's focus of attention and activities (78). Such parental synchronization is an important contribution to the development of normal attachment. In fact, in a study by van Ijzendoorn and colleagues, more sensitive parents had more secure children in general, but parental sensitivity did not affect the attachment of children with ASDs (79). Thus, rather than low parental sensitivity causing ASDs, this work would imply that the presence of the ASD makes for a relative insensitivity to variance in parental sensitivity.

It is important to note as well that the genetic traits of children can mold a social environment (71). The evidence of any etiological contribution is mixed in this regard, considering one study showed that while autistic behaviors in children decreased the social behavior of their mothers (80), sociability in parents might actually enhance autistic children's avoidance (81). As discussed in chapter 11, the genetic/biological phenotype of the child mediates the perception of the experience.

Indeed, psychosocial treatments empirically supported to have therapeutic value for Asperger's disorder include behavioral therapies that stipulate firm contingencies rather than responsive senstivities (82), although not all authors agree. For example, one center reports that intensive interaction with highly emotionally responsive sensitive adult therapists could be effective for core autism symptoms (83), although the results are unclear for want of mention of a control outcome comparator.

It is clear that parental stress is increased when parenting children with ASDs, and the consequences of parental stress-coping skills could affect the child's long-term outcome. A study in children with autism found that a family history of depression and shyness negatively affected the important prognostic factor of adaptive behavior (84). Informed professional guidance can serve as an important resource for parents (72).

It is known that there are neuroanatomical differences in male and female brain as well as differences in male compared with female brain developmental trajectories (85). The differential effect of maternal emotion expression on male and female infants, as discussed above, illustrates the potential for gender-specific trajectories insofar as an identical stimulus may confer different subjective experience. Thus, environmental stimuli during development may affect males and females differently, and continue to do so throughout life because of the intrinsic environment of sex (86).

THE MALE PREDOMINANCE OF ASPERGER'S DISORDER

Sex-Linked and Sex-Limited Genes

While it has been noted that males have increased risk of ASDs compared with females with the same genetic loading otherwise (87,88), there is only a small amount of genetic evidence available to address the large discrepancy in male: female prevalence in Asperger's.

Sex-*linked* genes [coded on the sex (X or Y) chromosomes] are known to cause discrepancies in male: female prevalence in phenotypes because of the nature of Mendelian XY inheritance. Sex-*limited* genes are different because, while the same genotype may be present in both males and females, the expression of the genotype is modified by the sex of the individual in a non-Mendelian manner. For example, in a study of 8707 general population children, a polymorphism in catechol-O-methyltransferase (COMT) (22q11.2) was shown to affect executive function and IQ in boys, but not girls (89). Sex-limited genes are present not only on autosomal chromosomes but also on the sex chromosomes. Perhaps unsurprisingly, the sex chromosomes may harbor the predominance of sex-limited genes (90).

The phenomenon of sex-limited gene expression can best be explained by sex-hormone effects. Hormonal effects are known to determine different gene expression patterns (90–93), resulting in sexual dimorphism even at the microscopic level of neuronal tissue (93). Sexual dimorphism defines the measurable differences between males and females.

However, some evidence shows that the brain may develop differently in the same hormonal environment (94), implicating a possible intrinsic difference between X and Y gene expression in the brain. X chromosome loci, in particular, through a number of mechanisms, including imprinting, contribute to sexual dimorphism (95).

SEXUAL DIMORPHISM OF THE HUMAN BRAIN

Sexual dimorphism is present in the brain (85,96) and in behavior (97). Asperger's genes and neuronal synapses may be influenced by those elements that determine the sexual dimorphism of the human brain and behavior. Males tend to have more specialized, lateralized brain function, whereas females have more connectivity. There is evidence for lateralization effects in ASDs (98–100); however, one study showed lateralization effects in autism, but not Asperger's disorder (101). Good evidence for male dimorphic effects in Asperger's is the identification of a hypermasculine use of sexual dimorphic mental representations (102–105). Study of the determination of sexual dimorphism of the brain has elucidated systems that are implicated in Asperger's disorder.

DETERMINANTS OF SEXUAL DIMORPHISM

Gender

When studying sex, gender is also an important consideration. Gender takes into account the sociocultural factors in sexual dimorphic behavior, and is expressed more as attitudes. For example, parents may have different expectations of their child on the basis of sex, which could reinforce the sexually dimorphic behaviors. Parents may expect girls to be more expressive and boys to communicate less; the expectation would result in a wider discrepancy between men and women (106). Girls may be diagnosed with labels other than Asperger's because of expectations of female behavior. However, a study that compared sex differences in ASDs found that there were little differences in the core triad of symptoms, but parent reports revealed significantly more symptoms in females than males, particularly social, attention, and thought problems (107). A similar study of sex differences in toddlers with ASDs found that females were more likely to have lower scores on language, social competence, and motor skills (108).

Both of these studies raise the question of whether parent expectation for female gender behavior could result in a bias for reporting more severe symptomatology in females.

However, one study explored sexual dimorphism in the brains of children with autism (109) and showed the inverse of what would be expected with a greater reporting of symptoms based on gender. In this study, females with ASDs actually had additional sites of abnormal neuroanatomical morphology beyond those in males, supportive of a worse symptomatology in females with ASDs.

There do appear to be some core differences in personality between men and women. A study of sex differences in personality traits found that neuroticism, extraversion, agreeableness, and conscientiousness were more common in women than men (110). These personality traits could contribute to less referral for treatment.

Also, the above study identified that these gender personality differences were more pronounced in cultures where a long and healthy life, equal access to knowledge and education, and economic wealth are increased and hypothesized that the increased freedom results in less containment of behavior and a natural divergence along gender lines.

Steroid Hormones

Sexually dimorphic brain regions and behaviors may be the result of different neuroendocrine milieus (111,112), composed of gonadally and adrenal-synthesized steroid hormones (neuro*active* steroids) (111,113–115) as well as the neurosteroids synthesized locally in the central nervous system (CNS) (116–123). Neuroactive steroids and neurosteroids can act through epigenetic regulation of gene transcription as well as directly on neurotransmitter receptor activity (118,119,124–126), neural development, plasticity, and protection (117–119).

Cholesterol

Serum cholesterol has been found to be increased in Asperger's disorder (127) and in the wider group of ASDs (128,129). Cholesterol is the foundation for all steroid hormone biosynthesis (Fig. 1). Cholesterol is required for synaptogenesis, and the regulation of its metabolism is implicated in neuronal plasticity (130–132). Cholesterol also maintains the function of neuronal receptors and is important for signal transduction (133). Cholesterol modulates the oxytocin receptor and 5HT1a receptors, for example (134). The meaning of the finding of hypercholesterolemia in Asperger's is uncertain at this time, since almost all brain cholesterol is synthesized inside the blood/brain barrier. It is unknown whether changes in plasma cholesterol are related to the important effects of brain cholesterol (135).

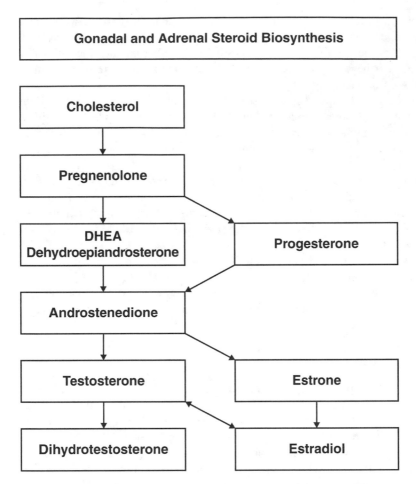

Figure 1 Cholesterol is the foundation for steroid synthesis. Estradiol, testosterone, and progesterone are the result of stepwise modification of the precursor. Androgens are metabolized to estrogens, but there is a reversible aromatization of testosterone and estradiol. *Source*: From Ref. 211.

Androgens

The cerebral cortex has androgen receptors in humans (136), and androgens play an important role in the organization and programming of brain circuits (137). Some sexual dimorphic brain regions have been shown to be androgen dependent in development (138,139).

The ratio of the size of the second digit, the index finger (2D), compared with the fourth digit, the ring finger (4D), may serve as a marker fetal testosterone (140,141), where testosterone correlates negatively with the ratio. This explains why men more commonly have a longer fourth digit (142). Studies have shown that males with Asperger's disorder have a "hypermasculinization" of this finger-length ratio compared with male controls (143,144). Additional evidence for androgen effects in ASDs is the finding of androgen hormone abnormalities in women with ASDs and their mothers (145), and higher autism scores in conditions with increased testosterone (146). Increased exposure to testosterone in utero is thought to magnify normal male traits such as "problems with communication and empathy" (145,147–150).

Estrogens

In addition to androgen receptors, estrogen receptors also mediate the actions of androgens (151). Estrogens likely have protective functions against certain diseases in men (152). Estrogens upregulate oxytocin receptors (153) and play a role in fear recognition, a system implicated in Asperger's (154,155). Estrogen is important in neurodevelopment (156), synaptic plasticity (116,157), and brain repair after injury (116,120,158,159) and is associated with increased neuronal excitability (160,161).

Estrogens modulate the sensitivity of facial expression recognition. Females at the highest-surge level of estrogen in the menstrual cycle have shown an increased ability to recognize the emotional expression of fear (162). Subjects with Asperger's show decreased recognition (163,164) and hypoactive patterns of brain function when processing fearful faces (165,166). Further work into hormonal determinants of Asperger's disorder may elucidate whether the estrogen systems contribute to the hypermasculine cognitive pattern seen in Asperger's.

Neuropeptides

Neonatal exposure to oxytocin and vasopressin (VP), necessary for aspects of normal social development, is also known to contribute to sexual dimorphism of brain and behavior (167). These two neuropeptides are structurally similar to each other, and both are important in social and affliative behavior (49,168–172). Interestingly, certain polymorphisms in genes for the receptors of VP (173,174) and oxytocin (175,176) have both been identified to occur more commonly in ASDs.

Oxytocin

The oxytocin receptor gene (OXTR) (3p 26.2) has been associated with autism (175,176) and is located in a region subject to imprinting effects (88). The oxytocin system is important in the neural circuits of social and fear processing in humans (177) and is known to have activity-dependent changes (178).

Successful treatment studies with oxytocin provide evidence for the importance of this system in Asperger's. Short-term treatment with oxytocin has been shown both to reduce repetitive behaviors and to increase social function in

Asperger's disorder and autism (179,180). Administration of intranasal oxytocin has been shown to dampen responsivity of the amygdalae to threatening social stimuli (177).

Vasopressin

There is a sex-dependent effect on VP neuron size, activity, and lateralization in males (181), and some VP effects are androgen dependent (167) and age dependent (182). Polymorphisms in the arginine-vasopressin receptor 1a (AVPR1a) gene (locus 12q14-15) have been identified in ASDs (173,174). The effect was more notable in family with less severe impairment of language (173). One study of subjects with ASD showed decreased circulating AVP and plasma apelin (183).

SEX-DEPENDENT GENE FINDINGS

Linkage and association studies can show different results when sex is studied as a unique intrinsic genetic environment (184). While the mechanism is unknown, sex-dependent effects have been noted for the serotonin system (185–187), disrupted in schizophrenia-1 (DISC-1) (188), and HOXA1 (24) (discussed above). These genes are listed in chapter 10, Table 2.

Serotonin System

A finding of a male-specific linkage peak to 17q11 (site of the 5-HT transporter) has been replicated (185,186), and a male QTL for whole blood serotonin levels ITGB3, has been associated with autism (189). Further details of the serotonin system are discussed in chapter 10 in the discussion of determinants of synaptic plasticity.

DISC 1

The DISC 1 gene located on 1q42 is important in neurodevelopment and neuronal signaling. It binds to proteins essential to neuronal migration, cytoskeletal modulation, and signal transduction (188,190–192). Polymorphisms in DISC-1 have been associated with ASDs, including Asperger's (193). The finding is stronger to date with analysis of affected males only, agreeing with a stronger association with analysis of males noted in schizophrenia (188).

CONNECTIONS BETWEEN THE SEXUALLY DIMORPHIC SYSTEMS

These sexually dimorphic systems are interrelated and likely comprise the predominant biological basis of different sex determinants of social development. Serotonin (117,194) and neuropeptides (195) are linked to each other (169,196–199) and show relationships with steroid hormones (153,200,201) and cholesterol.

Oxytocin, for example, is stimulated in response to 5HT1a and 5HT2a serotonin receptor agonism (202,203). Chronic stimulation of the 5HT2a receptor mediates the sensitivity of 5HT1a-stimulated oxytocin release (202). These observations are interesting within the context of serotonin and oxytocin's role in modulating social behavior. Serotonin 2a agonists, for example, are psychedelic drugs, compounds that may exert profound effects on social behavior.

PENETRANCE AND EXPRESSIVITY OF SEX-LIMITED TRAITS

Sex-dependent penetrance and sex-dependent expressivity of candidate Asperger's genes may be influenced by those elements that determine the sexual dimorphism of the human brain (85,96,204). Quantitative trait loci (QTL) are implicated in the inheritance of Asperger's disorder, and these QTL may be sex limited, resulting in a different penetrance and expressivity of Asperger's disorder traits.

Penetrance, a measure of the frequency with which a gene manifests itself in individuals in a population, can be limited by sex. Penetrance is complete when 100% of carriers of a particular genotype express the expected categorical phenotype, and it is incomplete when less than 100% express the expected phenotype (115,205).

Sexual limitation of penetrance usually occurs when the condition manifests in the sexual organs, as in the autosomal recessive disorder, steroid 5α-reductase deficiency (205–207). In this deficiency of the enzyme that catalyzes the conversion of testosterone to DHT, males are born with ambiguous or female genitalia, whereas females are born with female genitalia. More potent Dihydrotestosterone (DHT) is required during a critical period of embryonic development. At puberty, the males become masculinized because of the gonadal surge in testosterone. Penetrance, in this case, is sexually limited because of the complete absence of symptoms in females with the enzyme deficiency.

If one defines the phenotype of Asperger's by brain neuroanatomy, it is possible that the brain regions or QTL could experience sex-limited penetrance. It is possible that gene alleles that are triggered by androgens in androgen-dependent regions of the brain could experience sex-limited penetrance.

Also, when looking at the independent physiological features that make up the phenotype, it is possible that individual candidate genes could have sex-limited penetrance.

Sex-limited penetrance of susceptibility alleles could contribute to the clinical picture of variable expressivity. Expressivity is different from penetrance, because, with expressivity, there is a gradation of the trait expression of the phenotype between two individuals with the same genotype. This gradation can manifest as a severity of the condition or as a different clinical presentation (208). Unlike sex limitation of penetrance, it is very likely that expressivity of Asperger's disorder is sex influenced, since, rather than a limitation of the condition to males, there is only a male bias, i.e., females are subject to having Asperger's.

A wide body of literature exists regarding variable expressivity of the broader autism phenotype in ASD families, implicating a phenomenon of expressivity, but less work has examined sex determinants of expressivity. However, it is notable that a male QTL for whole blood serotonin levels has been identified (ITGB3) (184,209,210), and sex-dependent alleles of the ITGB3 gene have been implicated in autism (189). QTLs would be more likely to show a phenomenon of expressivity since they measure traits that are on a continuum.

One example of the above ideas is the inheritance of pattern baldness (92). In the condition of pattern baldness, the expression of the bald allele is influenced by the sex hormones of the individual, resulting in an increased frequency in men. In some pedigrees, two alleles of an autosomal gene b+ and b are involved in the trait, where b+/b+ gives a nonbald phenotype and b/b gives a bald phenotype in both sexes. The sex influence of these genotypes is illustrated by the heterozygous case, where the b allele manifests in Mendelian ratios as a dominant gene in males and a recessive gene in females (115). This serves as a potential example for Asperger's, where a causative gene may be more frequently observed to exhibit the phenotype concerned.

CONCLUSIONS

Asperger's disorder appears to be, at least in part, a manifestation of sexually dimorphic systems involving a role for the neuropeptides, serotonin, and steroid hormones subject to time-dependent developmental milieu. Parental effects on the development of sexually dimorphic behaviors and gender roles may be an important area of study in the examination of the developmental progression to Asperger's disorder. Since a great deal of evidence points to the sex of the individual as a major risk factor, future treatments may need to be further examined for sexually dimorphic outcomes.

REFERENCES

1. Banerjee D, Slack F. Control of developmental timing by small temporal RNAs: a paradigm for RNA-mediated regulation of gene expression. Bioessays 2002; 24(2):119–129.
2. Parks JS, Adess ME, Brown MR. Genes regulating hypothalamic and pituitary development. Acta Paediatr Suppl 1997; 423:28–32.
3. Wigle JT, Eisenstat DD. Homeobox genes in vertebrate forebrain development and disease. Clin Genet 2008; 73(3):212–226.
4. Davies AM. The role of neurotrophins during successive stages of sensory neuron development. Prog Growth Factor Res 1994; 5(3):263–289.
5. Luo L, Kessel M. Geminin coordinates cell cycle and developmental control. Cell Cycle 2004; 3(6):711–714.
6. Kroll KL. Geminin in embryonic development: coordinating transcription and the cell cycle during differentiation. Front Biosci 2007; 12:1395–1409.

7. Chen PY, Meister G. microRNA-guided posttranscriptional gene regulation. Biol Chem 2005; 386(12):1205–1218.

8. Perera RJ, Ray A. MicroRNAs in the search for understanding human diseases. BioDrugs 2007; 21(2):97–104.

9. Kiefer JC. Epigenetics in development. Dev Dyn 2007; 236(4):1144–1156.

10. Havlovicova M, Propper L, Novotna D, et al. Genetic study of 20 patients with autism disorders. Cas Lek Cesk 2002; 141(12):381–387.

11. Conciatori M, Stodgell CJ, Hyman SL, et al. Association between the HOXA1 A218G polymorphism and increased head circumference in patients with autism. Biol Psychiatry 2004; 55(4):413–419.

12. Coon H. Current perspectives on the genetic analysis of autism. Am J Med Genet C Semin Med Genet 2006; 142(1):24–32.

13. Muscarella LA, Guarnieri V, Sacco R, et al. HOXA1 gene variants influence head growth rates in humans. Am J Med Genet B Neuropsychiatr Genet 2007; 144(3): 388–390.

14. Engle EC. Oculomotility disorders arising from disruptions in brainstem motor neuron development. Arch Neurol 2007; 64(5):633–637.

15. Bailey A, Luthert P, Bolton P, et al. Autism and megalencephaly. Lancet 1993; 341(8854):1225–1226.

16. Piven J, Arndt S, Bailey J, et al. An MRI study of brain size in autism. Am J Psychiatry 1995; 152(8):1145–1149.

17. Woodhouse W, Bailey A, Rutter M, et al. Head circumference in autism and other pervasive developmental disorders. J Child Psychol Psychiatry 1996; 37(6): 665–671.

18. Courchesne E, Redcay E, Kennedy DP. The autistic brain: birth through adulthood. Curr Opin Neurol 2004; 17(4):489–496.

19. Hazlett HC, Poe M, Gerig G, et al. Magnetic resonance imaging and head circumference study of brain size in autism: birth through age 2 years. Arch Gen Psychiatry 2005; 62(12):1366–1376.

20. Lainhart JE, Bigler ED, Bocian M, et al. Head circumference and height in autism: a study by the Collaborative Program of Excellence in Autism. Am J Med Genet A 2006; 140(21):2257–2274.

21. Tripi G, Roux S, Canziani T, et al. Minor physical anomalies in children with autism spectrum disorder. Early Hum Dev 2007.

22. Mraz KD, Green J, Dumont-Mathieu T, et al. Correlates of head circumference growth in infants later diagnosed with autism spectrum disorders. J Child Neurol 2007; 22(6):700–713.

23. Gillberg C, de SL. Head circumference in autism, Asperger syndrome, and ADHD: a comparative study. Dev Med Child Neurol 2002; 44(5):296–300.

24. Ingram JL, Stodgell CJ, Hyman SL, et al. Discovery of allelic variants of HOXA1 and HOXB1: genetic susceptibility to autism spectrum disorders. Teratology 2000; 62(6):393–405.

25. Devlin B, Bennett P, Cook EH Jr., et al. No evidence for linkage of liability to autism to HOXA1 in a sample from the CPEA network. Am J Med Genet 2002; 114(6):667–672.

26. Talebizadeh Z, Bittel DC, Miles JH, et al. No association between HOXA1 and HOXB1 genes and autism spectrum disorders (ASD). J Med Genet 2002; 39(11):e70.

27. Kotrla K, Weinberger D. Developmental Neurobiology. In: Sadock BJ, Sadock VA, editors. Kaplan and Sadock's Comprehensive Textbook of Psychiatry. 7th ed. Philadelphia, PA: Lippincott, Williams and Wilkins; 2000 p. 32–40.

28. Rice D, Barone S Jr. Critical periods of vulnerability for the developing nervous system: evidence from humans and animal models. Environ Health Perspect 2000; 108(suppl 3):511–533.

29. Mendola P, Selevan SG, Gutter S, et al. Environmental factors associated with a spectrum of neurodevelopmental deficits. Ment Retard Dev Disabil Res Rev 2002; 8(3):188–197.

30. Charmandari E, Kino T, Souvatzoglou E, et al. Pediatric stress: hormonal mediators and human development. Horm Res 2003; 59(4):161–179.

31. Maurer D, Mondloch CJ, Lewis TL. Sleeper effects. Dev Sci 2007; 10(1):40–47.

32. Hobson RP, Bishop M. The pathogenesis of autism: insights from congenital blindness. Philos Trans R Soc Lond B Biol Sci 2003; 358(1430):335–344.

33. Lewis TL, Maurer D. Multiple sensitive periods in human visual development: evidence from visually deprived children. Dev Psychobiol 2005; 46(3):163–183.

34. Doupe AJ, Kuhl PK. Birdsong and human speech: common themes and mechanisms. Annu Rev Neurosci 1999; 22:567–631.

35. Kuhl PK, Tsao FM, Liu HM, et al. Language/culture/mind/brain. Progress at the margins between disciplines. Ann N Y Acad Sci 2001; 935:136–174.

36. Werker JF, Tees RC. Speech perception as a window for understanding plasticity and commitment in language systems of the brain. Dev Psychobiol 2005; 46(3): 233–251.

37. Scherf KS, Behrmann M, Humphreys K, et al. Visual category-selectivity for faces, places and objects emerges along different developmental trajectories. Dev Sci 2007; 10(4):F15–F30.

38. Tantam D. Characterizing the fundamental social handicap in autism. Acta Paedopsychiatr 1992; 55(2):83–91.

39. Dawson G, Zanolli K. Early intervention and brain plasticity in autism. Novartis Found Symp 2003; 251:266–274.

40. Tantam D, Holmes D, Cordess C. Nonverbal expression in autism of Asperger type. J Autism Dev Disord 1993; 23(1):111–133.

41. Berger M. A model of preverbal social development and its application to social dysfunctions in autism. J Child Psychol Psychiatry 2006; 47(3–4):338–371.

42. Kracke I. Developmental prosopagnosia in Asperger syndrome: presentation and discussion of an individual case. Dev Med Child Neurol 1994; 36(10):873–886.

43. Nieminen-von WT, Paavonen JE, Ylisaukko-oja T, et al. Subjective face recognition difficulties, aberrant sensibility, sleeping disturbances and aberrant eating habits in families with Asperger syndrome. BMC Psychiatry 2005; 5:20.

44. Deruelle C, Rondan C, Gepner B, et al. Spatial frequency and face processing in children with autism and Asperger syndrome. J Autism Dev Disord 2004; 34(2): 199–210.

45. Rondan C, Deruelle C. Global and configural visual processing in adults with autism and Asperger syndrome. Res Dev Disabil 2007; 28(2):197–206.

46. Deruelle C, Rondan C, Salle-Collemiche X, Bastard-Rosset D, Da FD. Attention to low- and high-spatial frequencies in categorizing facial identities, emotions and gender in children with autism. Brain Cogn 2008; 66(2):115–123.

47. Bailey AJ, Braeutigam S, Jousmaki V, et al. Abnormal activation of face processing systems at early and intermediate latency in individuals with autism spectrum disorder: a magnetoencephalographic study. Eur J Neurosci 2005; 21(9):2575–2585.
48. Neville H, Bavelier D. Human brain plasticity: evidence from sensory deprivation and altered language experience. Prog Brain Res 2002; 138:177–188.
49. Cushing BS, Kramer KM. Mechanisms underlying epigenetic effects of early social experience: the role of neuropeptides and steroids. Neurosci Biobehav Rev 2005; 29(7):1089–1105.
50. Anand KJ, Scalzo FM. Can adverse neonatal experiences alter brain development and subsequent behavior? Biol Neonate 2000; 77(2):69–82.
51. Skuse DH. Rethinking the nature of genetic vulnerability to autistic spectrum disorders. Trends Genet 2007; 23(8):387–395.
52. Constantino JN, Todd RD. Autistic traits in the general population: a twin study. Arch Gen Psychiatry 2003; 60(5):524–530.
53. Landry SH, Smith KE, Swank PR. Responsive parenting: establishing early foundations for social, communication, and independent problem-solving skills. Dev Psychol 2006; 42(4):627–642.
54. Landry SH, Smith KE, Swank PR. The importance of parenting during early childhood for school-age development. Dev Neuropsychol 2003; 24(2–3):559–591.
55. Landry SH, Smith KE, Miller-Loncar CL, et al. Predicting cognitive-language and social growth curves from early maternal behaviors in children at varying degrees of biological risk. Dev Psychol 1997; 33(6):1040–1053.
56. Knafo A, Plomin R. Parental discipline and affection and children's prosocial behavior: genetic and environmental links. J Pers Soc Psychol 2006; 90(1):147–164.
57. Eisenberg N, Wolchik SA, Goldberg L, et al. Parental values, reinforcement, and young children's prosocial behavior: a longitudinal study. J Genet Psychol 1992; 153(1):19–36.
58. Standley K, Soule AB, Copans SA, et al. Multidimensional sources of infant temperament. Genet Psychol Monogr 1978; 98(Second Half):203–231.
59. Frankel SA, Wise MJ. A view of delayed parenting: some implications of a new trend. Psychiatry 1982; 45(3):220–225.
60. van BF. Late parenthood among subfertile and fertile couples: motivations and educational goals. Patient Educ Couns 2005; 59(3):276–282.
61. Sutherland JD. The British object relations theorists: Balint, Winnicott, Fairbairn, Guntrip. J Am Psychoanal Assoc 1980; 28(4):829–860.
62. Ogden TH. On the concept of an autistic-contiguous position. Int J Psychoanal 1989; 70(Pt 1):127–140.
63. Bergmann MS. Reflections on the history of psychoanalysis. J Am Psychoanal Assoc 1993; 41(4):929–955.
64. Klein M, Tribich D. Kernberg's object-relations theory: a critical evaluation. Int J Psychoanal 1981; 62(Pt 1):27–43.
65. Schore A. The Emotionally Expressive Face. Affect Regulation and the Origin of the Self. Hillsdale, NJ: Lawrence Erlbaum Associates, Publishers, 1994:168–175.
66. Field TM, Schanberg SM, Scafidi F, et al. Tactile/kinesthetic stimulation effects on preterm neonates. Pediatrics 1986; 77(5):654–658.
67. Diego MA, Field T, Jones NA, et al. Withdrawn and intrusive maternal interaction style and infant frontal EEG asymmetry shifts in infants of depressed and non-depressed mothers. Infant Behav Dev 2006; 29(2):220–229.

68. Szyf M, Weaver I, Meaney M. Maternal care, the epigenome and phenotypic differences in behavior. Reprod Toxicol 2007; 24(1):9–19.
69. Carter AS, Mayes LC, Pajer KA. The role of dyadic affect in play and infant sex in predicting infant response to the still-face situation. Child Dev 1990; 61(3): 764–773.
70. Peterson C, Roberts C. Like mother, like daughter: similarities in narrative style. Dev Psychol 2003; 39(3):551–562.
71. Scarr S, McCartney K. How people make their own environments: a theory of genotype greater than environment effects. Child Dev 1983; 54(2):424–435.
72. Pisula E. Parents of children with autism: recent research findings. Psychiatr Pol 2002; 36(1):95–108.
73. Bolte S, Poustka F. The broader cognitive phenotype of autism in parents: how specific is the tendency for local processing and executive dysfunction? J Child Psychol Psychiatry 2006; 47(6):639–645.
74. Ruser TF, Arin D, Dowd M, et al. Communicative competence in parents of children with autism and parents of children with specific language impairment. J Autism Dev Disord 2007; 37(7):1323–1336.
75. Scheeren AM, Stauder JE. Broader autism phenotype in parents of autistic children: reality or myth? J Autism Dev Disord 2008; 38(2):276–287.
76. Volkmar FR, Klin A. Pervasive Developmental Disorders. In: Sadock BJ, Sadock VA, eds. Kaplan & Sadock's Comprehensive Textbook of Psychiatry. 7 ed. Philadelphia, PA: Lippincott Williams and Wilkins, 2000:2662–2664.
77. Koegel RL, Schreibman L, O'Neill RE, et al. The personality and family-interaction characteristics of parents of autistic children. J Consult Clin Psychol 1983; 51(5): 683–692.
78. Siller M, Sigman M. The behaviors of parents of children with autism predict the subsequent development of their children's communication. J Autism Dev Disord 2002; 32(2):77–89.
79. van Ijzendoorn MH, Rutgers AH, Bakermans-Kranenburg MJ, et al. Parental sensitivity and attachment in children with autism spectrum disorder: comparison with children with mental retardation, with language delays, and with typical development. Child Dev 2007; 78(2):597–608.
80. Dawson G, Hill D, Spencer A, et al. Affective exchanges between young autistic children and their mothers. J Abnorm Child Psychol 1990; 18(3):335–345.
81. Richer J, Richards B. Reacting to autistic children: the danger of trying too hard. Br J Psychiatry 1975; 127:526–529.
82. Stahmer AC, Ingersoll B, Carter C. Behavioral approaches to promoting play. Autism 2003; 7(4):401–413.
83. Vorgraft Y, Farbstein I, Spiegel R, et al. Retrospective evaluation of an intensive method of treatment for children with pervasive developmental disorder. Autism 2007; 11(5):413–424.
84. Mazefsky CA, Williams DL, Minshew NJ. Variability in adaptive behavior in autism: evidence for the importance of family history. J Abnorm Child Psychol 2008; 36(4):591–599.
85. Lenroot RK, Gogtay N, Greenstein DK, et al. Sexual dimorphism of brain developmental trajectories during childhood and adolescence. Neuroimage 2007; 36(4): 1065–1073.

86. Vige A, Gallou-Kabani C, Junien C. Sexual dimorphism in non-mendelian inheritance. Pediatr Res 2008; 63(4):340–347.
87. Goin-Kochel RP, Abbacchi A, Constantino JN. Lack of evidence for increased genetic loading for autism among families of affected females: A replication from family history data in two large samples. Autism 2007; 11(3):279–286.
88. Schanen NC. Epigenetics of autism spectrum disorders. Hum Mol Genet 2006; 15(spec no 2):R138–R150.
89. Barnett JH, Heron J, Ring SM, et al. Gender-specific effects of the catechol-O-methyltransferase Val108/158Met polymorphism on cognitive function in children. Am J Psychiatry 2007; 164(1):142–149.
90. Isensee J, Witt H, Pregla R, et al. Sexually dimorphic gene expression in the heart of mice and men. J Mol Med 2008; 86(1):61–74.
91. Isensee J, Ruiz NP. Sexually dimorphic gene expression in mammalian somatic tissue. Gend Med 2007; 4(suppl B):S75–S95.
92. Ellegren H, Parsch J. The evolution of sex-biased genes and sex-biased gene expression. Nat Rev Genet 2007; 8(9):689–698.
93. Vawter MP, Evans S, Choudary P, et al. Gender-specific gene expression in postmortem human brain: localization to sex chromosomes. Neuropsychopharmacology 2004; 29(2):373–384.
94. Arnold AP, Burgoyne PS. Are XX and XY brain cells intrinsically different? Trends Endocrinol Metab 2004; 15(1):6–11.
95. Skuse DH. Sexual dimorphism in cognition and behaviour: the role of X-linked genes. Eur J Endocrinol 2006; 155(suppl 1):S99–S106, S99–S106.
96. Gorski RA. Hypothalamic imprinting by gonadal steroid hormones. Adv Exp Med Biol 2002; 511:57–70.
97. Meaney MJ. The sexual differentiation of social play. Psychiatr Dev 1989; 7(3): 247–261.
98. Stroganova TA, Nygren G, Tsetlin MM, et al. Abnormal EEG lateralization in boys with autism. Clin Neurophysiol 2007; 118(8):1842–1854.
99. Escalante-Mead PR, Minshew NJ, Sweeney JA. Abnormal brain lateralization in high-functioning autism. J Autism Dev Disord 2003; 33(5):539–543.
100. Chandana SR, Behen ME, Juhasz C, et al. Significance of abnormalities in developmental trajectory and asymmetry of cortical serotonin synthesis in autism. Int J Dev Neurosci 2005; 23(2–3):171–182.
101. Rinehart NJ, Bradshaw JL, Brereton AV, et al. A clinical and neurobehavioural review of high-functioning autism and Asperger's disorder. Aust N Z J Psychiatry 2002; 36(6):762–770.
102. Baron-Cohen S. The hyper-systemizing, assortative mating theory of autism. Prog Neuropsychopharmacol Biol Psychiatry 2006; 30(5):865–872.
103. Wakabayashi A, Baron-Cohen S, Wheelwright S. Individual and gender differences in Empathizing and Systemizing: measurement of individual differences by the Empathy Quotient (EQ) and the Systemizing Quotient (SQ). Shinrigaku Kenkyu 2006; 77(3):271–277.
104. Baron-Cohen S, Wheelwright S. The empathy quotient: an investigation of adults with Asperger syndrome or high functioning autism, and normal sex differences. J Autism Dev Disord 2004; 34(2):163–175.
105. Baron-Cohen S. Autism: research into causes and intervention. Pediatr Rehabil 2004; 7(2):73–78.

106. Tordjman S. From a categorical diagnostic approach to a dimensional approach for mental disorders: interest of sex differences. Encephale 2006; 32(6 Pt 1):988–994.

107. Holtmann M, Bolte S, Poustka F. Autism spectrum disorders: sex differences in autistic behaviour domains and coexisting psychopathology. Dev Med Child Neurol 2007; 49(5):361–366.

108. Carter AS, Black DO, Tewani S, et al. Sex differences in toddlers with autism spectrum disorders. J Autism Dev Disord 2007; 37(1):86–97.

109. Bloss CS, Courchesne E. MRI neuroanatomy in young girls with autism: a preliminary study. J Am Acad Child Adolesc Psychiatry 2007; 46(4):515–523.

110. Schmitt DP, Realo A, Voracek M, et al. Why can't a man be more like a woman? Sex differences in Big Five personality traits across 55 cultures. J Pers Soc Psychol 2008; 94(1):168–182.

111. Kaminsky Z, Wang SC, Petronis A. Complex disease, gender and epigenetics. Ann Med 2006; 38(8):530–544.

112. Cutter WJ, Daly EM, Robertson DM, et al. Influence of X chromosome and hormones on human brain development: a magnetic resonance imaging and proton magnetic resonance spectroscopy study of Turner syndrome. Biol Psychiatry 2006; 59(3):273–283.

113. Negri-Cesi P, Colciago A, Celotti F, et al. Sexual differentiation of the brain: role of testosterone and its active metabolites. J Endocrinol Invest 2004; 27(6 suppl): 120–127.

114. Davies W, Wilkinson LS. It is not all hormones: alternative explanations for sexual differentiation of the brain. Brain Res 2006; 1126(1):36–45.

115. Russel P. Extensions of Mendelian Genetic Analysis. Genetics. 3rd ed. New York, NY: Harper Collins Publishers, 1992:92–120.

116. Ishii H, Tsurugizawa T, Ogiue-Ikeda M, et al. Local production of sex hormones and their modulation of hippocampal synaptic plasticity. Neuroscientist 2007; 13(4): 323–334.

117. Uzunova V, Sheline Y, Davis JM, et al. Increase in the cerebrospinal fluid content of neurosteroids in patients with unipolar major depression who are receiving fluoxetine or fluvoxamine. Proc Natl Acad Sci U S A 1998; 95(6):3239–3244.

118. Dubrovsky BO. Steroids, neuroactive steroids and neurosteroids in psychopathology. Prog Neuropsychopharmacol Biol Psychiatry 2005; 29(2):169–192.

119. Strous RD, Maayan R, Weizman A. The relevance of neurosteroids to clinical psychiatry: from the laboratory to the bedside. Eur Neuropsychopharmacol 2006; 16(3):155–169.

120. Mong JA, McCarthy MM. Steroid-induced developmental plasticity in hypothalamic astrocytes: implications for synaptic patterning. J Neurobiol 1999; 40(4): 602–619.

121. Dean SL, McCarthy MM. Steroids, sex and the cerebellar cortex: implications for human disease. Cerebellum 2007; 1–10.

122. Carrer HF, Cambiasso MJ. Sexual differentiation of the brain: genes, estrogen, and neurotrophic factors. Cell Mol Neurobiol 2002; 22(5–6):479–500.

123. Zimmerberg B, Rackow SH, George-Friedman KP. Sex-dependent behavioral effects of the neurosteroid allopregnanolone (3alpha,5alpha-THP) in neonatal and adult rats after postnatal stress. Pharmacol Biochem Behav 1999; 64(4):717–724.

124. Mellon SH, Griffin LD. Neurosteroids: biochemistry and clinical significance. Trends Endocrinol Metab 2002; 13(1):35–43.

125. Stoffel-Wagner B. Neurosteroid biosynthesis in the human brain and its clinical implications. Ann N Y Acad Sci 2003; 1007:64–78.
126. Stoffel-Wagner B. Neurosteroid metabolism in the human brain. Eur J Endocrinol 2001; 145(6):669–679.
127. Dziobek I, Gold SM, Wolf OT, et al. Hypercholesterolemia in Asperger syndrome: Independence from lifestyle, obsessive-compulsive behavior, and social anxiety. Psychiatry Res 2007; 149(1–3):321–324.
128. Tierney E, Bukelis I, Thompson RE, et al. Abnormalities of cholesterol metabolism in autism spectrum disorders. Am J Med Genet B Neuropsychiatr Genet 2006; 141(6):666–668.
129. Sikora DM, Pettit-Kekel K, Penfield J, et al. The near universal presence of autism spectrum disorders in children with Smith-Lemli-Opitz syndrome. Am J Med Genet A 2006; 140(14):1511–1518.
130. Pfrieger FW. Role of cholesterol in synapse formation and function. Biochim Biophys Acta 2003; 1610(2):271–280.
131. Guizzetti M, Costa LG. Cholesterol homeostasis in the developing brain: a possible new target for ethanol. Hum Exp Toxicol 2007; 26(4):355–360.
132. Qiu S, Korwek KM, Weeber EJ. A fresh look at an ancient receptor family: emerging roles for low density lipoprotein receptors in synaptic plasticity and memory formation. Neurobiol Learn Mem 2006; 85(1):16–29.
133. Chattopadhyay A, Paila YD. Lipid-protein interactions, regulation and dysfunction of brain cholesterol. Biochem Biophys Res Commun 2007; 354(3):627–633.
134. Aneja A, Tierney E. Autism: the role of cholesterol in treatment. Int Rev Psychiatry 2008; 20(2):165–170.
135. Dietschy JM, Turley SD. Thematic review series: brain Lipids. Cholesterol metabolism in the central nervous system during early development and in the mature animal. J Lipid Res 2004; 45(8):1375–1397.
136. DonCarlos LL, Sarkey S, Lorenz B, et al. Novel cellular phenotypes and subcellular sites for androgen action in the forebrain. Neuroscience 2006; 138(3):801–807.
137. Rubinow DR, Schmidt PJ. Androgens, brain, and behavior. Am J Psychiatry 1996; 153(8):974–984.
138. Arai Y. Sex differentiation of central nervous system–brain of man and woman. Nippon Rinsho 2004; 62(2):281–292.
139. Gilmore JH, Lin W, Prastawa MW, et al. Regional gray matter growth, sexual dimorphism, and cerebral asymmetry in the neonatal brain. J Neurosci 2007; 27(6): 1255–1260.
140. Manning JT, Scutt D, Wilson J, et al. The ratio of 2nd to 4th digit length: a predictor of sperm numbers and concentrations of testosterone, luteinizing hormone and oestrogen. Hum Reprod 1998; 13(11):3000–3004.
141. Lutchmaya S, Baron-Cohen S, Raggatt P, et al. 2nd to 4th digit ratios, fetal testosterone and estradiol. Early Hum Dev 2004; 77(1–2):23–28.
142. Peters M, Mackenzie K, Bryden P. Finger length and distal finger extent patterns in humans. Am J Phys Anthropol 2002; 117(3):209–217.
143. de Bruin EI, Verheij F, Wiegman T, et al. Differences in finger length ratio between males with autism, pervasive developmental disorder-not otherwise specified, ADHD, and anxiety disorders. Dev Med Child Neurol 2006; 48(12):962–965.
144. Manning JT, Baron-Cohen S, Wheelwright S, Sanders G. The 2nd to 4th digit ratio and autism. Dev Med Child Neurol 2001; 43(3):160–164.

145. Ingudomnukul E, Baron-Cohen S, Wheelwright S, et al. Elevated rates of testosterone-related disorders in women with autism spectrum conditions. Horm Behav 2007; 51(5):597–604.
146. Knickmeyer R, Baron-Cohen S, Fane BA, et al. Androgens and autistic traits: A study of individuals with congenital adrenal hyperplasia. Horm Behav 2006; 50(1): 148–153.
147. Baron-Cohen S, Knickmeyer RC, Belmonte MK. Sex differences in the brain: implications for explaining autism. Science 2005; 310(5749):819–823.
148. Knickmeyer RC, Baron-Cohen S. Fetal testosterone and sex differences in typical social development and in autism. J Child Neurol 2006; 21(10):825–845.
149. Knickmeyer R, Baron-Cohen S, Raggatt P, et al. Fetal testosterone and empathy. Horm Behav 2006; 49(3):282–292.
150. Baron-Cohen S, Ring H, Chitnis X, et al. fMRI of parents of children with Asperger Syndrome: a pilot study. Brain Cogn 2006; 61(1):122–130.
151. Pak TR, Chung WC, Hinds LR, et al. Estrogen receptor-beta mediates dihydrotestosterone-induced stimulation of the arginine vasopressin promoter in neuronal cells. Endocrinology 2007; 148(7):3371–3382.
152. Kula K, Slowikowska-Hilczer J, Walczak-Jedrzejowska R, et al. Physiological significance of estrogens in men–breakthrough in endocrinology. Endokrynol Pol 2005; 56(3):314–321.
153. Zingg HH, Grazzini E, Breton C, et al. Genomic and non-genomic mechanisms of oxytocin receptor regulation. Adv Exp Med Biol 1998; 449:287–295.
154. Fink G, Sumner BE, Rosie R, et al. Estrogen control of central neurotransmission: effect on mood, mental state, and memory. Cell Mol Neurobiol 1996; 16(3):325–344.
155. Fink G, Sumner BE, McQueen JK, et al. Sex steroid control of mood, mental state and memory. Clin Exp Pharmacol Physiol 1998; 25(10):764–775.
156. Naftolin F, Malaspina D. Estrogen, estrogen treatment and the post-reproductive woman's brain. Maturitas 2007; 57(1):23–26.
157. Mukai H, Tsurugizawa T, Ogiue-Ikeda M, et al. Local neurosteroid production in the hippocampus: influence on synaptic plasticity of memory. Neuroendocrinology 2006; 84(4):255–263.
158. Garcia-Segura LM, Naftolin F, Hutchison JB, et al. Role of astroglia in estrogen regulation of synaptic plasticity and brain repair. J Neurobiol 1999; 40(4):574–584.
159. Roselli CF. Brain aromatase: roles in reproduction and neuroprotection. J Steroid Biochem Mol Biol 2007; 106(1–5):143–150.
160. Beyenburg S, Stoffel-Wagner B, Bauer J, et al. Neuroactive steroids and seizure susceptibility. Epilepsy Res 2001; 44(2–3):141–153.
161. Herzog AG. Psychoneuroendocrine aspects of temporolimbic epilepsy. Part I. Brain, reproductive steroids, and emotions. Psychosomatics 1999; 40(2):95–101.
162. Pearson R, Lewis MB. Fear recognition across the menstrual cycle. Horm Behav 2005; 47(3):267–271.
163. Dawson G, Webb SJ, Carver L, et al. Young children with autism show atypical brain responses to fearful versus neutral facial expressions of emotion. Dev Sci 2004; 7(3):340–359.
164. Golan O, Baron-Cohen S, Hill J. The Cambridge Mindreading (CAM) Face-Voice Battery: Testing complex emotion recognition in adults with and without Asperger syndrome. J Autism Dev Disord 2006; 36(2):169–183.

165. Ashwin C, Baron-Cohen S, Wheelwright S, et al. Differential activation of the amygdala and the 'social brain' during fearful face-processing in Asperger Syndrome. Neuropsychologia 2007; 45(1):2–14.

166. Deeley Q, Daly EM, Surguladze S, et al. An event related functional magnetic resonance imaging study of facial emotion processing in Asperger syndrome. Biol Psychiatry 2007; 62(3):207–217.

167. Carter CS. Sex differences in oxytocin and vasopressin: implications for autism spectrum disorders? Behav Brain Res 2007; 176(1):170–186.

168. Insel TR, O'Brien DJ, Leckman JF. Oxytocin, vasopressin, and autism: is there a connection? Biol Psychiatry 1999; 45(2):145–157.

169. Insel TR, Winslow JT. Serotonin and neuropeptides in affiliative behaviors. Biol Psychiatry 1998; 44(3):207–219.

170. Carter CS, Williams JR, Witt DM, et al. Oxytocin and social bonding. Ann N Y Acad Sci 1992; 652:204–211.

171. Insel TR. Oxytocin–a neuropeptide for affiliation: evidence from behavioral, receptor autoradiographic, and comparative studies. Psychoneuroendocrinology 1992; 17(1):3–35.

172. Bartels A, Zeki S. The neural correlates of maternal and romantic love. Neuroimage 2004; 21(3):1155–1166.

173. Wassink TH, Piven J, Vieland VJ, et al. Examination of AVPR1a as an autism susceptibility gene. Mol Psychiatry 2004; 9(10):968–972.

174. Yirmiya N, Rosenberg C, Levi S, et al. Association between the arginine vasopressin 1a receptor (AVPR1a) gene and autism in a family-based study: mediation by socialization skills. Mol Psychiatry 2006; 11(5):488–494.

175. Jacob S, Brune CW, Carter CS, et al. Association of the oxytocin receptor gene (OXTR) in Caucasian children and adolescents with autism. Neurosci Lett 2007; 417(1):6–9.

176. Lerer E, Levi S, Salomon S, et al. Association between the oxytocin receptor (OXTR) gene and autism: relationship to Vineland Adaptive Behavior Scales and cognition. Mol Psychiatry 2007.

177. Kirsch P, Esslinger C, Chen Q, et al. Oxytocin modulates neural circuitry for social cognition and fear in humans. J Neurosci 2005; 25(49):11489–11493.

178. Theodosis DT, Trailin A, Poulain DA. Remodeling of astrocytes, a prerequisite for synapse turnover in the adult brain? Insights from the oxytocin system of the hypothalamus. Am J Physiol Regul Integr Comp Physiol 2006; 290(5): R1175–R1182.

179. Hollander E, Bartz J, Chaplin W, et al. Oxytocin increases retention of social cognition in autism. Biol Psychiatry 2007; 61(4):498–503.

180. Hollander E, Novotny S, Hanratty M, et al. Oxytocin infusion reduces repetitive behaviors in adults with autistic and Asperger's disorders. Neuropsychopharmacology 2003; 28(1):193–198.

181. Ishunina TA, Swaab DF. Vasopressin and oxytocin neurons of the human supraoptic and paraventricular nucleus: size changes in relation to age and sex. J Clin Endocrinol Metab 1999; 84(12):4637–4644.

182. Ishunina TA, Salehi A, Hofman MA, et al. Activity of vasopressinergic neurones of the human supraoptic nucleus is age- and sex-dependent. J Neuroendocrinol 1999; 11(4):251–258.

183. Boso M, Emanuele E, Politi P, et al. Reduced plasma apelin levels in patients with autistic spectrum disorder. Arch Med Res 2007; 38(1):70–74.

184. Weiss LA, Abney M, Cook EH, et al. Sex-specific genetic architecture of whole blood serotonin levels. Am J Hum Genet 2005; 76(1):33–41.

185. Stone JL, Merriman B, Cantor RM, et al. Evidence for sex-specific risk alleles in autism spectrum disorder. Am J Hum Genet 2004; 75(6):1117–1123.

186. Sutcliffe JS, Delahanty RJ, Prasad HC, et al. Allelic heterogeneity at the serotonin transporter locus (SLC6A4) confers susceptibility to autism and rigid-compulsive behaviors. Am J Hum Genet 2005; 77(2):265–279.

187. Hohmann CF, Walker EM, Boylan CB, et al. Neonatal serotonin depletion alters behavioral responses to spatial change and novelty. Brain Res 2007; 1139:163–77.

188. Hennah W, Varilo T, Kestila M, et al. Haplotype transmission analysis provides evidence of association for DISC1 to schizophrenia and suggests sex-dependent effects. Hum Mol Genet 2003; 12(23):3151–3159.

189. Weiss LA, Kosova G, Delahanty RJ, et al. Variation in ITGB3 is associated with whole-blood serotonin level and autism susceptibility. Eur J Hum Genet 2006; 14(8): 923–931.

190. Sawamura N, Sawa A. Disrupted-in-schizophrenia-1 (DISC1): a key susceptibility factor for major mental illnesses. Ann N Y Acad Sci 2006; 1086:126–133.

191. Mackie S, Millar JK, Porteous DJ. Role of DISC1 in neural development and schizophrenia. Curr Opin Neurobiol 2007; 17(1):95–102.

192. Hennah W, Thomson P, Peltonen L, et al. Genes and schizophrenia: beyond schizophrenia: the role of DISC1 in major mental illness. Schizophr Bull 2006; 32(3): 409–416.

193. Kilpinen H, Ylisaukko-oja T, Hennah W, et al. Association of DISC1 with autism and Asperger syndrome. Mol Psychiatry 2008; 13(2):187–196. Epub 2007 Jun 19.

194. Griffin LD, Mellon SH. Selective serotonin reuptake inhibitors directly alter activity of neurosteroidogenic enzymes. Proc Natl Acad Sci U S A 1999; 96(23): 13512–13517.

195. Gimpl G, Fahrenholz F. The oxytocin receptor system: structure, function, and regulation. Physiol Rev 2001; 81(2):629–683.

196. Raap DK, van de Kar LD. Selective serotonin reuptake inhibitors and neuro-endocrine function. Life Sci 1999; 65(12):1217–1235.

197. de WD, Diamant M, Fodor M. Central nervous system effects of the neuro-hypophyseal hormones and related peptides. Front Neuroendocrinol 1993; 14(4): 251–302.

198. Ferris CF. Vasopressin/oxytocin and aggression. Novartis Found Symp 2005; 268:190–198.

199. Coccaro EF, Kavoussi RJ, Hauger RL, et al. Cerebrospinal fluid vasopressin levels: correlates with aggression and serotonin function in personality-disordered subjects. Arch Gen Psychiatry 1998; 55(8):708–714.

200. Theodosis DT. Oxytocin-secreting neurons: A physiological model of morphological neuronal and glial plasticity in the adult hypothalamus. Front Neuroendocrinol 2002; 23(1):101–135.

201. Pak CW, Curras-Collazo MC. Expression and plasticity of glutamate receptors in the supraoptic nucleus of the hypothalamus. Microsc Res Tech 2002; 56(2):92–100.

202. Zhang Y, D'Souza D, Raap DK, et al. Characterization of the functional heterologous desensitization of hypothalamic 5-HT(1A) receptors after 5-HT(2A) receptor activation. J Neurosci 2001; 21(20):7919–7927.

203. van de Kar LD, Javed A, Zhang Y, et al. 5-HT2A receptors stimulate ACTH, corticosterone, oxytocin, renin, and prolactin release and activate hypothalamic CRF and oxytocin-expressing cells. J Neurosci 2001; 21(10):3572–3579.

204. Jancke L, Steinmetz H. Interhemispheric transfer time and corpus callosum size. Neuroreport 1994; 5(17):2385–2388.

205. Zlotogora J. Penetrance and expressivity in the molecular age. Genet Med 2003; 5(5):347–352.

206. Thigpen AE, Davis DL, Gautier T, et al. Brief report: the molecular basis of steroid 5 alpha-reductase deficiency in a large Dominican kindred. N Engl J Med 1992; 327(17):1216–1219.

207. Houk CP, Damiani D, Lee PA. Choice of gender in 5alpha-reductase deficiency: a moving target. J Pediatr Endocrinol Metab 2005; 18(4):339–345.

208. Oppenheimer EH, Esterly JR. Observations on cystic fibrosis of the pancreas. V. Developmental changes in the male genital system. J Pediatr 1969; 75(5):806–811.

209. Weiss LA, Veenstra-Vanderweele J, Newman DL, et al. Genome-wide association study identifies ITGB3 as a QTL for whole blood serotonin. Eur J Hum Genet 2004; 12(11):949–954.

210. Weiss LA, Abney M, Parry R, et al. Variation in ITGB3 has sex-specific associations with plasma lipoprotein(a) and whole blood serotonin levels in a population-based sample. Hum Genet 2005; 117(1):81–87.

211. Cenegenics Medical Institute. Gonadal and adrenal steroid biosynthesis. Available at: http://www.cenegenics.com/Library/graph2large.JPG. 2008.

13

Biological Treatment of Asperger's Disorder

Donna L. Londino and Diana Mattingly
*Department of Psychiatry and Health Behavior, Medical College of Georgia,
Augusta, Georgia, U.S.A.*

David S. Janowsky
*Department of Psychiatry, University of North Carolina, Chapel Hill,
North Carolina, U.S.A.*

INTRODUCTION

Defined in the *Diagnostic and Statistical Manual of Mental Disorders—Fourth Edition* (DSM-IV) by qualitative impairments in social interactions and restricted, repetitive, and stereotyped patterns of behavior, interest, and activities, to date there has been no specific pharmacological treatment of the "core symptoms" of Asperger syndrome, or of any of the autistic spectrum disorders. It is without argument and appropriately addressed in another chapter in this reference that the most effective treatment of Asperger's is a multidisciplinary approach, which encompasses educational needs, social relatedness with family and peers, pragmatic communicative skills, and adaptive functioning. Pharmacotherapy has predominantly been used to target problematic symptoms of maladaptive behavior, such as aggression, or comorbid disorders that occur with the syndrome such as attention deficit hyperactivity disorder (ADHD) or depression. Additionally, most clinical research in this area has focused on the treatment of individuals with autism or pervasive developmental disorder (PDD), perhaps with a small number of Asperger's subjects, but often excluding this population from the protocols. Only recently has there been attention directed toward specific treatment outcomes in individuals with Asperger syndrome. The following review of current biological treatment considerations is based on literature reviews, expert opinions, and recent research.

Despite the paucity of studies examining the efficacy or safety of psychotropic medications in this population, repeated surveys have suggested that psychotropic medication use appears to be common in persons with higher-functioning PDDs, including Asperger syndrome (1). In a 1999 survey of psychotropic medication use in children, adolescents, and adults with a diagnosis of Asperger's disorder, autism, or PDD and with documented full-scale intellect assessed as being 70 or more, Martin et al. found that 55% of 109 subjects were taking psychotropics. Of the 109 individuals in this study, 94 (86.2%) had a diagnosis of Asperger's disorder at the time of referral. Prevalence for individual classes of medications is shown in (Table 1). A survey in 1995 by Aman et al. noted that of 838 care providers of persons with autism, 42% reported the use of a psychotropic medication, anticonvulsant, or vitamin to target symptoms of the disorder (2). Subjects were categorized by severity of autism (mild, moderate, unknown, etc.), and not by diagnosis, however, 22.1% of the sample were known to have intellects that were not in the mentally retarded range. Subsequent studies following the same methodology in the states of North Carolina ($N = 417$) and Ohio ($N = 1538$) showed similar findings (3,4). In a survey specific to Asperger's disorder published in 1999, Klin and Volmar reported that 75% of

Table 1 Prevalence of Psychotropic Drug Use Among High-Functioning Pervasive Developmental Disorders, Including Asperger Syndrome

	Number	Percentage
Total subjects	109	
Current psychotropic medication use	60	55
Lifetime psychotropic medication use	75	69
Current use of 1 psychotropic medication	28	26
Current use of 2 or more medications	32	29
Drug type		
Any antidepressant	35	32
SSRI	29	27
Psychostimulant	22	20
Any neuroleptic	18	17
Atypical antipsychotic	14	13
Mood stabilizer	10	9
Anxiolytic	7	6
Antihypertensive	7	6

Abbreviation: SSRI, selective serotonin reuptake inhibitor.
Source: Modified from Ref. 1.

subjects (100 individuals awaiting screening and evaluation for Asperger's disorder through the Yale Child Study Center) had received some form of stimulant treatment either currently or in the past (5). Over 33% had received treatment with a selective serotonin reuptake inhibitor (SSRI). The authors concluded that "psychotropic medication use appears to be common among subjects with high functioning PDD, yet not generally based on the results of empirical research" (1).

At the National Institute of Mental Health in 2003, Kenneth Towbin published an extensive review, specific to the pharmacological treatment of Asperger's. (6). In this comprehensive review, Towbin addressed the logic and organization of medication treatment for symptoms of the syndrome and proposed a treatment algorithm based on these target symptoms. He reiterated that the predominant usefulness of psychotropic medications in this population is to treat behavioral problems and mood disruptions. He also noted several potential hurdles to the pharmacological treatment of a person with Asperger syndrome. These potential hurdles include resistance to medications secondary to a fear of side effects, a fixed cognition that opposes medication, and a relative lack of insight into the degree of distress that symptoms may be causing. These issues, by definition, are less applicable to children because they present for treatment accompanied by parents who give consent for and administer medications. Increasingly, however, clinicians are requiring assent by adolescents involved in treatment. These adolescents may have even less insight than adult patients with Asperger's. A thorough discussion of elicited symptoms, the comorbid diagnosis to be treated through pharmacotherapy, accompanied by a review of specific details on the expected benefits and potential side effects of medications can assist in attenuating many concerns. Adjunctive written information and integration with a plan for nonpharmacological treatments is also helpful in decreasing associated anxiety that accompanies the thought of treatment with medications.

Principles of appropriate clinical care should always guide any treatment intervention and special considerations should be given to the use of psychotropic medications in children and adolescents. Multiple reviews have noted concerns over the increased use of psychotropic medications in this population (7–9). Specific to the issue of pharmacotherapy, research addressing appropriate dosages, side effects and efficacy is limited and subsequently, treatment guidelines are often driven by extrapolation from the adult literature. Increasing reports of adverse events (i.e., risk of suicidal ideations with SSRIs, cardiac risks with psychostimulants, and metabolic abnormalities with the newer antipsychotics), warrant careful consideration prior to their use and close monitoring throughout the course of treatment (10–12). Relevant to this issue is the fact that compared with that of other disorders, studies of pharmacological treatments in Asperger syndrome are limited.

It is of utmost importance to recognize that each person with Asperger's is an individual with symptoms that may or may not necessarily cause distress or impair functioning. Is formal treatment with pharmacotherapy then indicated? A symptom that arises rarely may not be worth the risk of a side effect from a medication. The choice to use pharmacotherapy should subsequently be guided by a complete evaluation of several factors. These include (*i*) the severity of the symptom or comorbid diagnosis, (*ii*) the degree of distress or functional impairment noted by the patient and/or family, (*iii*) the person's or family's investment in other treatment recommendations, (*iv*) the success of prior behavioral interventions, and (*v*) the characteristics of the system in which the person resides. The care of an individual with Asperger's can be difficult and may be worsened by a lack of understanding of the person's differences and the syndrome itself. Caretakers may be unable to effectively implement a behavioral modification plan. A symptom may be of sufficient severity (i.e., aggression) that more immediate treatment is warranted. That being said, it is inappropriate to try and target a symptom with medications that clearly is better treated through behavioral treatment just to appease a family. Antochi and Stavrakaki describe a model useful in autism, which is here expounded to include Asperger syndrome (13). Their description of a "pluralistic approach" recognizes the "synergistic and additive effects of biological, psychological, and social factors" when considering the comorbidity between a psychiatric disorder and behavior disturbance." Behavioral difficulties may be addressed therapeutically using medications along with behavioral modifications, environmental interventions, and other strategies.

PHARMACOTHERAPY FOR SYMPTOMS AND COMORBID DIAGNOSES IN ASPERGER SYNDROME

Maladaptive and Disruptive Behavior to Include Aggression and ADHD

Aggression

The most problematic maladaptive and disruptive behavior, and the behavior most studied in relation to pharmacotherapy in all of the autistic spectrum disorders, is aggression. Aggression and violent outbursts are common in persons with autistic spectrum disorders, including Asperger's (14,15). Seen most often when asked to change activities, discontinue engagement in a task surrounding their favorite interest, or when a schedule or anticipated event does not occur, these outbursts may lead individuals to break things and hit others in frustration. Something as simple as pizza not being served on the day it is usually provided at school may be sufficient to elicit a fit of rage. Caretakers often report agitation and irritability, especially with older adolescents or adults, when they enter the person's room or rearrange items in an attempt to "clean up." At times, this agitation is sufficient enough to pose a safety risk to the patient or to others. Additionally, this symptom almost always contributes to disruption in school placement, as the educational system cannot jeopardize the well being of other students who may be harmed during an explosive tantrum. Likewise, employers will not tolerate potential aggressive behavior. One adult with Asperger syndrome was refused a permanent teaching position after the administration learned of an occasion during his substitute experience when he became irate and yelled at a student for not following his instructions. He had no intention of harm, however, his behavior was considered inappropriate and a potential liability to the school system.

As with other disorders that present with aggression, pharmacological options for this symptom include alpha-agonists, such as clonidine or guanfacine, beta-blockers, mood stabilizers, or antipsychotics. An astute clinician will also screen the individual closely for irritability associated with a mood disruption that may respond better to the implementation of an antidepressant (a review of antidepressant use in the disorder is covered in a later section). Likewise, it is useful to consider whether the aggression is a response to another heightened emotion or situational frustration that may respond better to environmental modification or a behavioral intervention. Discerning precipitating factors and potential perpetuating situations may be difficult, but these can often be carried out by the careful observation of parents, caretakers, and/or educators and will achieve the desired outcome of reducing aggressive outbursts without the use of pharmacotherapy. Acute changes in behavior almost always suggest some recent precipitant in the social environment and should be actively pursued prior to medication implementation unless safety to self or others is a concern.

Alpha-agonists. There are reports in support of using alpha-agonists (clonidine and guanfacine) in autistic disorders to target oppositional behavior, aggression, and irritability (16,17). Both studies were double-blind, placebo-controlled; however, the subject numbers were low (8 and 9, respectively), and diagnosis was made per DSM-III prior to the inclusion of Asperger syndrome. In the first study by Jaselskis et al. (16), all subjects had borderline intellect or mental retardation [mean intelligent quotient (IQ) 59 ± 16]. The ages of the subjects ranged from 5 to 13 years and the dose of clonidine ranged from 0.15 to 0.2 mg/day. Of note is that four of the six subjects in a continuation phase had a recurrence of symptoms. In the study by Fankhauser et al. (17), transdermal clonidine (5 μg/kg/day) was evaluated in children and adults (ages 5–33). The authors concluded that clonidine was effective in reducing hyperarousal behaviors. They additionally noted that several subjects had improvement in social relationships and that anxiety was reduced.

Most relevant to the specific treatment of aggression in Asperger syndrome is a retrospective review by Posey on the benefit of guanfacine (trade name Tenex) in children and adolescents with PDD (18). In addition to noting efficacy in 24% of patients, Posey reported that patients with Asperger's disorder (2 of 6 responders; 33.3%) responded even better than those with autism but only in core domains of hyperactivity, inattention, and tics. No direct benefit was seen on aggression and Posey reported that guanfacine (mean dose 2.6 mg/day) was in fact more effective for subjects that were less aggressive at baseline (3.63 ± 1.54

versus 4.33 ± 1.18; unpaired t test = 2.09, df = 78, p = 0.04) as rated by the Clinical Global Impressions Severity (CGI-S) item.

The mechanism of action of these medications is directed at central and peripheral alpha-adrenergic agonism. Clonidine and guanfacine act on pre-synaptic neurons and inhibit noradrenergic transmission at the synapse where they most likely affect norepinephrine (NE) discharge rates in the locus ceruleus and indirectly affect dopamine-firing rates. Interestingly, biological models have suggested that aggression may arise from alterations in dopaminergic reward mechanisms, and in rat models, aggression is enhanced by 6-hydroxydopamine (19,20). These animal models may suggest why these medications are potentially beneficial for aggressive symptoms in patients with different psychiatric disorders, including autism and Asperger syndrome. Adverse effects include sedation, which is quite common on initiation of treatment, but are often accommodated after a period of use, hypotension, irritability, headache, dry mouth, potential decrease in memory, and possible worsening of anxiety. Dermatological reactions have been reported in up to 50% of patients using the transdermal patch (21). In addition, gradual tolerance to the beneficial effects of clonidine were noted in studies by Jaselskis and Fankhauser et al. (16,17). Withdrawal reactions may occur after abrupt cessation of long-term therapy (>1–2 months), therefore, it is strongly recommended that patients taper the dose during drug discontinuation to prevent rebound hypertension and re-emergent tics. Guanfacine may cause less rebound and is less sedating.

Alpha-agonists should be prescribed in divided doses (most often 3 times/day). Children metabolize these medications faster than adults and thus may require more frequent dosing (4–6 times/day). The alpha-agonists should be used with caution in combination with psychostimulants because of case reports (5 to date) of sudden death with combination use (22,23). It is recommended that a baseline electrocardiogram be obtained prior to initiating treatment and that a thorough review of any family history of cardiac abnormalities be obtained and considered prior to use.

Beta-blockers. Although beta-adrenergic medications have been hypothesized to benefit persons with a wide variety of neuropsychiatric disorders, research supports their use in only three areas—anxiety disorders with prominent physiological signs, neuroleptic-induced akathisia, and impulsive aggression (24). Small case reports and pilot trials have suggested benefits on aggression and self-injurious behavior in the autistic population, however, most studies looked at benefits in individuals with some form of cognitive delay, often moderate-to-severe mental retardation (25,26). Ratey and colleagues reported almost immediate benefit from beta-blockers on aggression in eight autistic adults (25). Subjects received propanolol (dose range 100–360 mg daily) or nadolol (120 mg daily). This study also noted significant changes in both speech and social behaviors as the study progressed (27). It was hypothesized that the decrease in hyperarousal, improved anxiety, and defensiveness may have contributed to an increase in social and adaptive behavior. Pitfalls in the study were the low subject number, the open label design, and use of the beta-blocker as an adjunct to preexisting pharmacotherapy. Another report by Connor also reported benefit from nadolol (mean dose 109 mg) on aggressive behavior in an open-label study in 12 developmentally delayed individuals aged 9 to 24 years (26). Although there were no subjects who carried a specific diagnosis of Asperger syndrome, three subjects had IQs in the borderline range (IQ 71–84). Ten of the twelve subjects (83%) demonstrated improvement in overt aggression (improvement in verbal aggression and aggression to others was significant) and the medication was well tolerated with few side effects. There is some consensus that beta-blockers are best used adjunctively and are generally not efficacious as mono-therapy. Of additional interest is the suggestion by some clinicians that nadolol, a hydrophilic beta-blocker, may be preferable for anxiety symptoms, whereas propranolol and metoprolol (both of which are lipophilic) are more beneficial in treating aggression (24). Irregardless, until further studies including individuals with Asperger syndrome, or even "high-functioning" autism, are undertaken, it is difficult to suggest the use of this class of medications as first-line treatment.

Beta-blockers (i.e., propranolol, nadolol) inhibit chronotropic, inotropic, and vasodilatory physiological responses throughout the body, both selectively and nonselectively, depending on the choice of agent used. In addition, beta-blockers have membrane-stabilizing effects and GABAmimetic activity that may contribute to their benefit not only for anxiety, but also for aggressive behavior in individuals with autism, ADHD, posttraumatic stress disorder (PTSD), and organic brain dysfunction (26,28,29). The average recommended dose is 0.5 to 1.0 mg/kg/day administered in divided doses q6to 8 hours. The dose may be gradually increased to a maximum dose of 5 mg/kg/day or 120 mg/day. Full response may take up to eight weeks. Potential side effects include bradycardia, hypotension, and worsening of asthmatic symptoms. Blood pressure and pulse should be monitored and as with the alpha-agonists, a baseline electrocardiogram is generally recommended prior to initiating use. As rebound reactions have been noted on drug withdrawal, a tapering of the dose of beta-blocker is recommended upon discontinuance. Beta-blockers should be used with caution in combination with chlorpromazine and the antidepressants. Combined use of beta-blockers and chlorpromazine increases levels of both medications. Variations in metabolism and subsequent plasma levels of beta-blockers and antidepressants are seen with the combined use of these medications. Thioridazine levels may be increased by three- to fivefold in combination with beta-blockers, hence their combined use is contraindicated.

Mood stabilizers and anticonvulsants. Medications in this group include valproic acid, lithium, carbamazepine, and a host of new anticonvulsants such as lamotrigine, gabapentin, topiramate, and others. Although mood stabilizers are frequently used in other disorders for the management of aggression, data suggest that only a small percentage of individuals with autism, including Asperger's disorder, are treated with this pharmacological intervention, independent of seizure management (1,3,4). In addition, data supporting its use for this target symptom is limited. Two recently published studies reviewed the potential benefit of valproic acid to improve aggression in autistic disorders, including Asperger's disorder (30,31). Only one of these demonstrated significant benefit. In a small, open-label trial by Hollander et al., 75% of subjects demonstrated improvement in affective stability, aggression, and impulsivity (30). Two of the fourteen subjects had Asperger's disorder. One subject, an 11-year-old male (FSIQ 105) with comorbid obsessive-compulsive disorder (OCD), ADD, eating disorder—not otherwise specified (NOS), and hypotonia was ranked as "much improved" on the CGI scale after 43 months of monotherapy with divalproex sodium (dose 250–625 mg). He was described as generally functioning better and was noted to be "more pleasant." Reported side effects included mood lability and agitation. Another 17-year-old male subject (FSIQ 73) with Asperger's disorder, OCD, and seizure disorder was noted as "very much improved" on the CGI scale after 17 months of treatment with divalproex sodium (dose 500–1500 mg). He was also taking buspirone, fluvoxamine, clonazepam, and carbamazepine. Improvements were noted in his social relatedness, obsessive-compulsive symptoms, irritability, and anxiousness. Side effects included increased appetite and weight gain. In a more recent, randomized-controlled study by Hellings, however, with a cohort of 30 subjects (20 boys and 10 girls, ages 6–20 years, 2 with Asperger's disorder), no significant benefit was seen using the Aberrant Behavior Checklist–Community Version (ABC-CV) scale , irritability subscale as the outcome measure (31). Notable side effects included increased appetite and skin rash. Two subjects experienced increased serum ammonia levels accompanied by slurred speech and cognitive slowing. Interesting to consider, however, is that though the response to treatment did not differ significantly from placebo, the four individuals that maintained treatment with valproic acid after study completion experienced significant relapse in aggressive behavior after discontinuance of the medication.

Historically, the use of lithium has been common for aggression and behavioral disturbances in mentally retarded individuals (32,33) and youth with conduct disorder (34,35). Limited data is available to support lithium's specific use for aggression in autism or Asperger syndrome. In fact, early studies of lithium demonstrated limited therapeutic benefit. Lithium might be beneficial if a comorbid diagnosis of bipolar disorder is present or if the individual has a strong family history of bipolar disorder (36,37). In Kerbeshian's study, irritability (but not specifically aggression) was included as a possible predictor of lithium response in autism (36). The notation of benefit in comorbid bipolar disorder or severe mood lability is relevant, as reports have suggested a potential increased risk of bipolar disorder in Asperger patients, and a report by Duggal even suggested that disruption of amygdalar function may be a common etiology of both disorders (38,39).

A retrospective study by Hardan et al. assessed the benefit of topiramate in children and adolescents with PDDs (40). Two of the fifteen subjects were diagnosed with Asperger's disorder. These two, along with six others were considered responders [as judged by a score of 1, i.e., "very much improved" or 2 i.e., "much improved" on the Global Improvement Item of the CGI scale (CGI-GI)]. One eight-year-old male was treated for 28 weeks with 1.2 mg/kg/day of topiramate. He was also taking fluoxetine and risperidone. Improvement was noted in mood swings. The other subject, diagnosed with Asperger's disorder and disruptive behavior disorder-NOS was treated for 25 weeks with 2.9 mg/kg/day of topiramate in addition to citalopram and risperidone. Benefits on aggression and mood swings were noted.

There are no studies specific to the use of carbamazepine, gabapentin, or lamotrigine in Asperger syndrome. A 1994 open-label study by Uvebrant and Bauziene noted improvement in "non-seizure related" behavioral symptoms in children with PDDs treated with lamotrigine (41). A later study by Belsito et al., however, failed to show improvement of statistical significance in 14 children with autism treated with this same medication, despite parental reports of benefit (42). Outcome measures included the Autism Behavior Checklist, Aberrant Behavior Checklist, and Vineland Adaptive Behavior Scale. This was a double-blind, placebo-controlled trial where lamotrigine was titrated over eight weeks to a dose of 5 mg/kg/day. Although preliminary data suggest benefit on behavioral disturbance in individuals with mental retardation, brain damage, and even PTSD (43–45), these results have not translated into any specific guidelines for use in Asperger's disorder and more research is needed prior to formal recommendations.

Side effects from all of the anticonvulsants are extensive and problematic. In general, the common adverse effects include gastrointestinal distress, dose-related lethargy and behavioral change, tremor, and cognitive impairment. Children with developmental delays are more likely to experience adverse behavioral effects. Some side effects, including the risk of Stevens–Johnson rash, acute pancreatitis, hepatitis, and blood dyscrasias, are significant enough to contraindicate use unless clearly indicated and pose concern given the lack of evidence clearly supporting the benefit of these agents for the autism spectrum disorders. In summary, a retrospective review by McDougle most appropriately noted that "although there may be some benefit from the use of mood stabilizers, these agents do not appear to be as effective as other pharmacological options for the specific treatment of aggression in autism" (46). However, if more research confirms the increased co-occurrence of bipolar disorder in individuals with Asperger's disorder, the mood stabilizers will certainly play a substantial role in treatment (47).

Antipsychotics. The most extensive evidence supports the use of dopamine-blocking agents (neuroleptics) for the treatment of aggression in autistic disorders (48). Historically, haloperidol (Haldol) was the mainstay of treatment

(49), and its use has been extensively studied (50), but with the emergence of the newer second-and third-generation antipsychotics, with reportedly less risk of extrapyramidal symptoms, a shift in their use for this symptom occurred. Of the newer antipsychotics, risperidone has been most widely used. Risperidone was approved by the U.S. Food and Drugs Administration (FDA) in October 2006 for the treatment of irritability (including aggression toward others, self-injurious behavior, and mood lability) associated with autistic disorder in children and adolescents aged 5 to 16 years. In August of 2007, risperidone was FDA approved for the treatment of schizophrenia in adolescents aged 13 to 17 years. At the same time it was approved for the short-term treatment of manic or mixed episodes of bipolar I disorder in children and adolescents aged 10 to 17 years. These approvals made risperidone the first antipsychotic approved for autism, schizophrenia, or bipolar disorder in young patients (Table 2).

Substantial evidence from several rigorous studies now supports the efficacy of risperidone for the target symptoms mentioned above (51–54), as well as benefit for depression, anxiety, and stereotypic behavior (55). Prior to McDougle's 1998-published double-blind, placebo-controlled study in adults (51), support existed only in the form of open-label trials and case reports (56–58). The initial study by McDougle (51) did not include any subjects with a formal diagnosis of Asperger's disorder, however, 4 of the 15 subjects receiving medication were "high functioning" with full-scale IQs between 74 and 113. Two of these subjects were reported to be much improved, one was minimally improved, and one (with a history of multiple prior medication trials and recruited during inpatient treatment) was minimally worse. Only one of four similarly matched controls (full-scale IQ 70–92) showed any improvement. The dose of risperidone for these four subjects ranged from 2 to 4 mg daily. A subsequent large-scale multisite trial of over 100 patients (ages 5–17 years) conducted through the Research Units in Pediatric Psychopharmacology (RUPP) confirmed the benefit of risperidone in autism (52). Again, no subjects with a specific diagnosis of Asperger's disorder were included, however, 24% of this treatment group and 13% of the controls had IQs greater than 70.

A published retrospective chart review by Simeon et al. (53) reporting the benefit of risperidone in treatment-resistant children and adolescents with psychiatric disorders included eight subjects with Asperger syndrome. Results were not broken down by diagnosis; however, the authors reported moderate to marked improvement in multiple domains of functioning (reduction in aggression, psychosis, withdrawal, oversensitivity, better social skills, mood, and insight) in approximately 73% of the study cohort. The mean daily dose of risperidone was 1.2 mg and very few adverse effects were reported. It should be noted, however, that the majority of the subjects in this study were taking concomitant medications, the most common being the psychostimulants. A later study published by Shea et al. (54) specifically evaluated he benefit of risperidone on target symptoms of agitation, aggression, and severe temper outbursts in individuals with autistic spectrum disorders, including subjects with Asperger's disorder (5 of 40 in the treatment group and 5 of 39 controls). As in

Table 2 Antipsychotic Classes and FDA-Approved Indications

Antipsychotic	FDA-approved indication	
	Adults	Children
Typical high-potency		
Fluphenazine	Schizophrenia	Not approved in children
Haloperidol	Schizophrenia	Psychotic disorders ages: 3–12 yr
Perphenazine	1. Schizophrenia 2. Nausea and vomiting	Not approved in children <12
Pimozide	Tourette's syndrome	Tourette's in children >12
Thiothixene	Schizophrenia	Not approved in children <12
Trifluoperazine	1. Schizophrenia 2. Non-psychotic anxiety	Psychotic disorders ages: 3–12 yr
Typical mid-potency		
Loxapine	Schizophrenia	Not approved in children
Moban	Schizophrenia	Not approved in children
Typical low-potency		
Chlorpromazine	1. Schizophrenia 2. Nausea and vomiting 3. Postsurgical anxiety 4. Intractable hiccups 5. Bipolar disorder 6. Acute intermittent porphyria 7. Tetanus	1. Severe behavioral problems 2. Psychotic disorders ages: 6 mo.–12 yr
Thioridazine	Schizophrenia	Behavioral disorders ages: 2–12 yr
Atypical antipsychotics		
Clozapine	Refractory schizophrenia	Not approved in children
Risperidone	1. Schizophrenia 2. Short-term treatment of mixed or manic episodes in bipolar I disorder 3. Irritability associated with autism: ages 5–16 yr	1. Schizoprenia ages: 13–17 yr 2. Short term treatment of mixed or manic episodes bipolar I disorder: ages 10–17 yr
Olanzapine	1. Schizophrenia 2. Bipolar disorder acute phase and maintenance	Not approved in children
Quetiapine	1. Schizophrenia 2. Short-term treatment bipolar I disorder	Not approved in children
Ziprasidone	1. Schizophrenia 2. Short-term treatment bipolar I disorder	Not approved in children
Aripiprazole	1. Schizophrenia 2. Bipolar disorder acute phase and maintenance	1. Schizophrenia ages: 13–17 yr 2. Bipolar disorder acute phase and maintenance ages: 10–17 yr

Source: Modified from Ref. 123.

the previous study, results were not subdivided by diagnosis. Subjects taking risperidone (mean dose 0.04 mg/kg/day; 1.17 mg/day) demonstrated a significantly greater decrease ($p \leq 0.001$) on the irritability subscale of the ABC than subjects taking placebo. They also demonstrated significantly greater improvement ($p < 0.001$) on the conduct problem subscale of the parent version of the Nisonger Child Behavior Rating Form (N-CGRF) compared with placebo. Sedation and weight gain were the most commonly noted side effects. There was no difference between groups when assessed for extrapyramidal symptoms.

Olanzapine has been shown to have some positive benefit on behavior that includes aggression, irritability, and hyperactivity in individuals with autistic spectrum disorders (59–61). These early studies, however, included only children, adolescents, and adults with autistic disorder and PDD-NOS, and the majority of subjects had mental retardation. Although a study by Kemner in 2002 (62) included subjects with these same two diagnoses, the mean total IQ based on 17 of the 22 children (ages 6–16 years) was 98 with some subjects having IQs as high as 144. In this open-label, three-month trial of olanzapine (final mean dose 10.7 mg/day), all 23 subjects demonstrated significant improvement on the irritability, hyperactivity, and excessive speech subscales of the ABC. Only three of the subjects, however, demonstrated significant improvement in overall functioning as assessed by the CGI scale. Weight gain (mean 4.7 kg), increased appetite, and asthenia were the most frequent adverse effects. Three children demonstrated extrapyramidal symptoms (gait and extremity rigidity, increased salivation, psychomotor restlessness) that disappeared after the dose was decreased. A double-blind, randomized trial by Hollander published in 2006 (63) that compared olanzapine with placebo in children with PDD (one of whom had Asperger's disorder) also demonstrated the potential benefit of this agent on global functioning; however, weight gain (3.4 kg) was again a notable side effect.

In 2006, Milin and colleagues published the first, rigorous study assessing the benefit of olanzapine, specifically in individuals with Asperger's disorder (64). In this open-label, 12-week study, children and adolescents aged between 6 and 18 years with a diagnosis of Asperger's disorder were recruited for treatment with olanzapine if they had a Child Behavior Checklist Parent (CBCL-P) or Teacher (CBCL-T) total T score of 63 or more, indicating a severe behavior problem. It is notable that 5 of the 10 study completers had taken risperidone shortly before enrollment in this study, with no observable benefit. Over the 12-week treatment trial of olanzapine, significant improvements in internalizing and externalizing behavior and global functioning were observed. By the completion of the study, the primary efficacy measures on the CBCL-P had entered a nonclinical range and participant's global functioning, as determined by the CGI scale had improved "very much" ($N = 2$) or "much" ($N = 7$). All subjects were male. The mean olanzapine treatment dose was 8.25 mg/day (range 5–15 mg). The most notable side effect was weight gain with an average weight gain of 4.69 kg over the 12-week study duration. Two subjects were found to have electrocardiogram (ECG) changes. One subject was found to have sinus tachy-cardia, which was deemed unremarkable by a cardiologist. The other subject showed ECG changes consistent with ventricular hypertrophy that was no longer present at study end.

Few studies have examined the efficacy of quetiapine in autism or PDDs, and at the time of this publication, no studies were found that included subjects with Asperger's disorder. Corson et al. (65) published a retrospective chart review that examined the medical records of all patients with PDDs that had received at least four weeks of treatment with quetiapine. It is significant that the primary target symptom in the majority of subjects (15/20) was aggression. Seven of these twenty patients did not have mental retardation. Of these seven subjects, two (28.6 %) were noted to be responders as determined by improve-ment on the CGI-GI scale (Fisher exact test 0.64). Response to treatment was predicted by the duration of time that subjects took the medication, but not by age or by the dose of quetiapine. Consistent with this finding, the two responders noted above were treated for 113 weeks and 126 weeks, respectively, at doses of 375 mg and 400 mg respectively. Quetiapine demonstrated greatest efficacy for the target symptom of aggression. Two of the seven subjects with a target symptom of impulsivity (as opposed to aggression) demonstrated only minimal improvement or worsening. Side effects were seen in half of the patients and included weight gain (mean 5.7 kg), sedation, and insomnia. One patient dis-continued treatment because of tardive dyskinesia. Additionally, 7 of the 20 subjects discontinued treatment secondary to lack of efficacy.

As with quetiapine, there are no published controlled studies examining the efficacy of the two newest antipsychotics, ziprasidone and aripiprazole, for aggression or other symptoms seen in the autistic spectrum disorders. A case series by McDougle et al. (66) examining the efficacy of ziprasidone (mean dose 59.2 ± 34.8 mg/day) in children and adolescents with autism of PDD-NOS, included one subject without mental retardation; however, this patient also had comorbid psychosis and Tourette's disorder, and the targeted symptoms were delusions, mood instability, and tics. A prospective, pilot, open-label trial of aripiprazole by Stigler et al. (67) in five adolescents with PDDs (including one with Asperger's disorder) demonstrated the efficacy of this medication on symptoms of aggression, self-injurious behavior, and irritability. Subjects were treated for a minimum of eight weeks (mean 12.8 weeks) at a mean dose of 12 mg/day. All five participants demonstrated significant improvement as determined by changes on the CGI. Sedation was the only side effect. No extrapyramidal symptoms or changes in cardiac status were observed.

Initial findings of a 14-week, open-label study of aripiprazole in youth with Asperger's disorder and PDD-NOS (68,69), support early findings of the potential benefit of this agent on symptoms of irritability and aggression in this population. Twelve of the first thirteen study participants were reported to be responders as determined by a 25% reduction in ABC irritability subscale scores. These subjects also were rated as "very much improved" or "much improved" on the CGI-GI. The mean dose of aripiprazole used during the study was 7.5 mg/day. The most common side effect was sedation (77%). Seven of the thirteen subjects gained weight, although two subjects lost weight. The mean weight change over the duration of the study was 1.23 kg.

Unfortunately, ideal antipsychotics do not exist and the potential side effects of treatment with these agents should be thoroughly reviewed prior to the decision to use them. Treatment with the high potency older antipsychotics was problematic for the potential development of tardive dyskinesia. Low potency antipsychotics carried moderate cardiac risks. Although initially thought to be free of concerns regarding extrapyramidal effects, even the newer antipsychotics have demonstrated the potential to also cause dyskinesias (62,65,70,71). Children have increased dopamine receptors (72) and may be at increased risk with prolonged treatment to develop irreversible movement disorders. Likewise, there is now substantial concern regarding metabolic abnormalities that occur with the use of the newer antipsychotics, both in adults and in children and adolescents (73,74). Insulin resistance may increase the chances of developing premature diabetes. Prolactin elevation following dopamine antagonism in the tuberoinfundibular pathway of the anterior pituitary gland can potentially lead to amenorrhea, galactorrhea, sexual dysfunction, reduced fertility, and decreased bone density (75). Weight gain associated with almost all of the newer antipsychotics carries a number of substantial health problems, including fatigue, sleep disorders, and cardiovascular risks (76,77). Other problematic side effects vary with the choice of agent but include considerations surrounding QTc (corrected QT) prolongation (i.e., ziprasidone), hepatic abnormalities (risperidone, olanzapine), anticholinergic effects, electroencephalogram abnormalities, "obsessive-compulsive-like" behavior, dysthymia, and nocturnal enuresis.

Attentional Problems and Hyperactivity

According to the DSM-IV, ADHD cannot be diagnosed if it only "occurs exclusively during the course of a pervasive developmental disorder" (78). Although this qualification exists for diagnostic consideration, it has been well documented that symptoms of hyperactivity and inattention are highly prevalent in PDDs, including Asperger syndrome (79,80). Ghaziuddin et al. published a report noting that in 35 patients with Asperger syndrome, two-thirds had an additional psychiatric diagnosis (79). Children with Asperger syndrome were most likely to have comorbid ADHD, whereas adolescents and adults were more likely to have depression. Additionally, studies by Ehlers et al. and Nyden et al. demonstrated that autism and Asperger syndrome are characterized by similar neuropsychological deficits as seen in individuals with ADHD (81,82). Despite this data, few placebo-controlled studies have examined the benefit of psychostimulant use, the standard treatment for these symptoms, in this population.

In a naturalistic retrospective analysis of psychostimulants in PDDs, Stigler et al. reported that use of these medications for ADHD symptoms in autism was overall ineffective and poorly tolerated for the majority of patients (83). Her group, however, did note that patients with Asperger's disorder, in contrast to those with autistic disorder or PDD-NOS, were significantly more likely to have a beneficial response to a stimulant trial ($p < 0.01$). Children with Asperger's disorder were 4.04 times more likely to respond to a stimulant than those with autism, and 2.98 times more likely to respond than patients with PDD-NOS. Adverse effects, including agitation, dysphoria, and irritability, were common; however, agitation was more frequently noted in children with autism and PDD-NOS than in those with Asperger syndrome. A follow-up study by the Research Units on Pediatric Psychopharmacology (RUPP) Autism Network published in 2005 also demonstrated a trend, although nonsignificant, for the diagnosis of Asperger syndrome to have a moderating effect on the response of ADHD symptoms to the use of methylphenidate (84). The subjects diagnosed with Asperger's disorder (5 of 66) and PDD-NOS (14 of 66) were more likely to be responders to both placebo and stimulant treatment than those subjects with autism ($p = 0.07$). Side effects were similar to those seen in other studies and included irritability, decreased appetite, insomnia, and emotional outbursts.

The most commonly used stimulants for the treatment of ADHD include methylphenidate, dextroamphetamine, and the mixed preparation of d,l-amphetamine. All are now available in short- and long-acting forms and all have efficacy and safety profiles that are comparable to each other. Differences between the agents include potency, onset and duration of action, and preparation forms. The empiric basis for the use of stimulants for symptoms of hyperactivity, impulsivity, and inattention rests on findings from multitudes of short-term, randomized, placebo-controlled studies conducted over the past 30 years, although their specific mechanism of action is not clearly understood. Methylphenidate products promote the release of stored dopamine and block the return of dopamine at presynaptic dopamine transporter sites. Amphetamine products also block dopamine reuptake at the transporter, but appear to promote the release of newly synthesized dopamine more selectively. The ultimate effect is that dopamine function in the striatum, and at least indirectly, in the prefrontal cortex is enhanced. In addition, both agents appear to decrease the firing rate of neurons in the locus ceruleus, although it is unclear whether this has a facilitative or inhibitory effect on the NE system. Notably, drugs with more selective action on either dopamine (guanfacine) or NE (imipramine) have smaller clinical effects than the nonselective psychostimulant medications.

Short-acting stimulants are readily absorbed and demonstrate benefit on behavior within 30 to 60 minutes after ingestion. Peak levels are obtained within one to three hours and the duration of action of most immediate release formulations is three to five hours. Both methylphenidate and amphetamine are broken down in the liver, and the parent compound and its metabolites are excreted in the urine within 24 hours. Dosing is generally determined on a weight per kilogram basis with the methylphenidate products being dosed from 1 to 1.5 mg/kg/day either in divided doses or in one dose of a sustained-release product. Dextroamphetamine products are grossly twice as potent and general guidelines for dosing are 0.5 to 0.7 mg/kg/day again in divided doses or one daily dose of a long-acting agent administered in the AM. If short-acting preparations are used, they are most effective when dosed in the morning and at lunchtime, with considerations of a 3 to 4 p.m. dose if needed to assist with attention during homework, sports, or management of early afternoon and evening behavior. It is generally recommended that the later dose of stimulant be of a lower potency (half or less of the morning dose) to minimize rebound effects and possible interference with sleep. Optimal dosing is achieved by obtaining feedback from caretakers and teachers and can be acquired by formal rating scales such as SNAP-IV rating scale [a revision of the Swanson, Nolan and Pelham (SNAP) questionnaire], Connor forms or CBCL-P and CBCL-T (Achenbachs). Normalization of symptoms is desirable, but dosing should be determined in balance with a consideration of potential side effects.

Side effects of psychostimulant use are often problematic, and studies have suggested that individuals with autism are more sensitive to these adverse effects (85). It is still unclear whether this is true for persons with Asperger syndrome. Adverse effects associated with stimulant use include appetite suppression, sleep disturbance, mood changes including irritability and depression, gastrointestinal distress, tics and other stereotypical behavior, and growth delay.

A relatively new option for the treatment of attentional problems, impulsivity, and hyperactivity is the selective NE reuptake inhibitor, atomoxetine, approved by the FDA in 2002 for the treatment of ADHD in children older than 6 years, adolescents, and adults. Since atomoxetine's approval, one retrospective review (86), two open-label studies (87,88) and one placebo-controlled study (89) have examined its benefit in individuals with autistic spectrum disorders. In the study by Jou et al. (86), 20 subjects, including two with Asperger's disorder and 8 without mental retardation, were identified as having received atomoxetine within the 12 months prior to study onset. These subjects were assessed for treatment response on the basis of improvement in the CGI-GI and the Connors Parent Rating Scale (CPRS). One of the two subjects (treated with 25 mg for 30 weeks) with Asperger's disorder was judged to be a responder on the basis of a score of "much improved" on the CGI-GI. Both subjects demonstrated improvements in CPRS scores (–4 and –12, respectively). In the first open-label study of atomoxetine conducted by Posey et al. (87), all subjects had nonverbal IQs of less than 70. In comparison, an open-label study by Troost et al. (88) included only participants with an IQ greater than 70, including one with a diagnosis of Asperger's disorder. Although atomoxetine (mean dose 1.19 ± 0.41 mg/kg/day) was associated with significant improvement in scores on the ADHD-Rating Scale-IV, Parent Version, and the CPRS-R, only 7 of the 12 original participants completed the study. The other five discontinued atomoxetine because of adverse effects, including increased aggression, anxiety, and gastrointestinal distress. It is unclear whether the subject with Asperger's disorder was a completer or discontinued treatment early. A double-blind, placebo-controlled crossover study (89) that included one subject with Asperger's disorder also demonstrated efficacy of atomoxetine (mean highest dose 44.1 ± 21.9 mg/day) on symptoms of hyperactivity. Compared with the open-label studies, side effects were more tolerable. Only one participant terminated the study prematurely, however, this subject had a recurrence of violence and hallucinations that required hospitalization. Limitations include the fact that results were not subdivided for subclasses of the PDDs and concomitant medications were allowed.

Mood Disruption to Include Depression and Anxiety

There are multiple references to the development of mood disruption to include depression and anxiety in persons with Asperger syndrome, particularly as they get older (79,90,91). In a study designed to assess the prevalence of anxiety and mood problems among children with the disorder, Kim et al. (92) followed the emotional outcomes of 59 children initially diagnosed with autism ($N = 40$) or Asperger syndrome ($N = 19$). Compared with a sample of 1751 community children, children and young adolescents (ages 9–14) with Asperger syndrome and autism were assessed as having a greater rate of anxiety and depression. Families endorsed that the presence of either of these mood disruptions had a significant impact on their overall functioning and adaptation. In this study, there were no differences in the number of mood problems between the subjects with autism (high-functioning) and those with Asperger syndrome, although other studies have reported a higher incidence of emotional disturbance in those with the syndrome (93).

The findings that indicate a high comorbidity of Asperger syndrome with mood symptoms are of considerable interest. Links between affective disorders and autism have been suggested for decades and depression as well as social anxiety appears to be overrepresented in close relatives of individuals suffering from autistic spectrum disorders (94). It is unclear whether these associations are intrinsic to the disorder. It is likewise unclear as to whether the hypothesized neurochemical or neuroanatomical differences that may predispose individuals with these disorders to mood disruption are inheritable. Proposed mechanisms of action have included theories surrounding the role of serotonin and the serotonin transporter gene (95,96). Others have hypothesized that dysfunction of the prefrontal cortex and the amygdala may be responsible for the high incidence of depressive and anxious symptoms (97,98). Psychosocial contributants to the development of depression and anxiety in individuals with Asperger syndrome certainly include the frustration associated with difficulties in negotiating appropriate responses to others and to the environment. As opposed to the more aloof presentation of individuals with more severe autism, persons with Asperger syndrome express a desire to fit in socially and have friends, but appear to lack effectiveness in skills that might assist in meeting these goals. Wanting to make friends and fit in, but unable to, these individuals may withdraw. This can lead to increasing anxiety, behavioral disruption, and depression, which further impair opportunities to form new relationships and engage in new experiences, thereby perpetuating the problem.

It is often difficult to distinguish symptoms consistent with the Asperger syndrome from those seen in anxiety or depression. Prior to choosing to treat with pharmacotherapy, Towbin (6) stresses the importance of a clinical history, indicating that symptoms are a change from baseline, that they impair function, and that they arise together as a syndrome consistent with the criteria of a particular disorder. The clinician should be aware that the individual with Asperger syndrome may have more difficulty understanding the meaning of emotional disturbance and subsequently fail to report symptoms unless specifically questioned. He may not exhibit a sad or anxious affect, and suicidal statements may be stated in such a manner that clinicians or others underestimate their significance. All of these considerations contribute to difficulties with diagnosis and determination of treatment needs.

The generally accepted pharmacological treatment of depression and anxiety in Asperger syndrome is the same as the pharmacological treatment of these symptoms in individuals without the syndrome. This includes the use of SSRIs, NE dopamine reuptake inhibitors (NDRI's), selective serotonin NE reuptake inhibitors (SNRIs), noradrenergic specific serotonergic antidepressants (NaSSAs), tricyclic antidepressants (TCAs), and serotonin-2 antagonists reuptake inhibitors (SARIs). None of these agents have been found to be more beneficial than the others for depression and anxiety either in Asperger syndrome or in those without Asperger's (6). Additionally, FDA indications in the pediatric population are limited to a narrow range of therapeutic uses (Table 3).

The best evidence to date for the treatment of symptoms of anxiety and depression supports the use of SSRIs although, as with pharmacotherapy for aggression, the scope of controlled trials and evidence-based literature is limited. There have been case reports and retrospective studies of several SSRIs in the autistic spectrum disorders; however, placebo-controlled studies have involved only fluvoxamine and fluoxetine. (99). Additionally, most of the studies examined the benefit of these medications on a multitude of symptoms, including aggression, social interactions, and obsessive stereotypical behavior, making it difficult to specifically determine the effectiveness of these medications on the specific symptoms of anxiety and/or depression. Outcome measures (CGI, ABC) most commonly assessed global functioning and not depression or anxiety in particular. Two published studies (100,101) used anxiety instruments (Hamilton Anxiety Scale and the Screen for Child Anxiety–Related Emotional Disorders, or SCARED, respectively). Several studies used the Yale-Brown Obsessive-Compulsive Scale (Y-BOCS); however, the literature concerning pharmacological treatment of obsessive and stereotypic behavior will follow in the next section.

A retrospective study by Couturier et al. (102) of citalopram in children and adolescents (ages 4–15 years) included three subjects with Asperger syndrome with target symptoms of anxiety. Two of these three were reported as very

Table 3 Antidepressants in Children and Adolescents

Class of drug	Generic name	Trade name	Dosage form and strength	Pediatric approval status
SSRI	Citalopram	Celexa	Tablets: 20 mg, 40 mg Oral solution: 10 mg/5 mL	Safety and efficacy not established in children <18 yr old
	Escitalopram	Lexapro	Tablets: 5 mg, 10 mg, 20 mg Oral solution: 5 mg/5 mL	
SSRI	Fluoxetine	Prozac	Capsules: 10 mg, 20 mg Enteric-coated tablets: 90 mg Delayed release pellets: 90 mg Oral solution 20 mg/5 mL	Approved in the USA for children >8 yr old (depression and OCD)
SSRI	Fluvoxamine	Luvox	Tablets: 25 mg, 50 mg, 100 mg	Approved in the USA for children >8 yr old (OCD)
SSRI	Paroxetine	Paxil Paxil CR	Tablets: 10 mg, 20 mg, 30 mg, 40 mg Oral suspension: 10 mg/5 mL Controlled-release tablets: 12.5 mg, 25 mg	Not indicated in children <18 old—potential increased risk of self harm and SIs
SSRI	Sertraline	Zoloft	Oral solution: 20 mg/mL Capsules/tablets: 25 mg, 50 mg, 100 mg	Approved in the United States for children >7 yr old(OCD)
NDRI	Bupropion	Wellbutrin Wellbutrin-SR, Zyban Wellbutrin XL	Tablets: 75 mg, 100 mg Sustained-release tablets: 100 mg, 150 mg Extended-release tablets: 150 mg, 300 mg	Safety and efficacy not established in children <18 yr old Often used as augmentation in children with ADHD
SNRI	Venlafaxine	Effexor Effexor XR	Tablets: 25 mg, 27.5 mg, 50 mg, 75 mg, 100 mg Sustained-release tablets: 37.5 mg, 75 mg, 150 mg	Not indicated for children <18 yr old Potential increased risk of self harm and SIs

(Continued)

Table 3 Antidepressants in Children and Adolescents (*Continued*)

Class of drug	Generic name	Trade name	Dosage form and strength	Pediatric approval status
NaSSA	Mirtazapine	Remeron Remeron SolTAb	Tablets: 15 mg, 30 mg, 45 mg Oral disintegrating tablets: 15 mg, 30 mg, 45 mg	Safety and efficacy has not been established in pediatric patients Clinically used as adjunct for appetite stimulation and sleep aid in children treated with psychostimulants
TCA	Clomipramine	Anafranil	Tablets: 10 mg, 25 mg, 50 mg, 75 mg	Approved for use in children >10 yr old for OCD
TCA	Imipramine	Tofranil Tofranil PM	Tablets: 10 mg, 25 mg, 50 mg, 75 mg Capsules: 75 mg, 100 mg, 125 mg, 150 mg Injection: 12.5 mg/mL	Approved for children >5 yr old, for enuresis
SARI	Trazodone	Desyrel	Tablets: 50 mg, 100 mg, 150 mg, 300 mg	Safety and efficacy not established in children >18 yr old Often used as a sleep aid in children and teenagers with insomnia

Abbreviations: SSRI, selective serotonin reuptake inhibitor; NDRI, norepinephrine dopamine reuptake inhibitor; SNRI, selective serotonin norepinephrine reuptake inhibitor; NaSSA: noradrenergic/specific serotonergic antidepressants; TCA, tricyclic antidepressants; SARI, serotonin-2 antagonists/reuptake inhibitors.

much improved after 10 to 14 months of treatment at dosages of 20 and 40 mg/ day, respectively. The third subject with Asperger's disorder discontinued treatment after one month and was reported to have an increase in tics with citalopram treatment. Another retrospective study by Namerow et al. (103) confirmed the potential benefits of citalopram, especially in individuals with Asperger's disorder. All subjects with Asperger's (6 of 15) demonstrated improvement in mood symptoms, as was determined by scores on the CGI-GI scale. Anxiety symptoms were most responsive. The mean duration of treatment for subjects with Asperger's disorder was 409 days (range 63–588 days) at a mean dose of 19.2 mg/day (range 10–30 mg/day).

Obsessive and Stereotypic Cognitions and Behavior Patterns

In addition to the core social impairments (failure to develop age-appropriate relationships, lack of reciprocity, impaired use of nonverbal gestures, lack of eye contact) currently defined as necessary for the diagnosis of an autistic spectrum disorder, including Asperger's disorder, individuals diagnosed with these conditions must also demonstrate at least one of the following criteria: (*i*) restricted, circumscribed interests, (*ii*) rigid adherence to schedules or rituals, (*iii*) interest in small parts of objects, and (*iv*) hand flapping. The first two criteria in particular are commonly seen in persons with Asperger syndrome. These symptoms often contribute to nonfunctional behavioral patterns that are inflexible, and if disrupted, frequently lead to anxiety, irritability, frustration, and even aggression. These obsessive and stereotypic cognitions and behavior patterns have historically been considered as similar to the recurrent obsessions and compulsions seen in OCD, although research in this area has suggested that there are notable differences (104). In autism, including Asperger syndrome, individuals are more likely to demonstrate "compulsive" preoccupation with their particular interest and ruminations on specific timing and occurrences of scheduled activities in contrast to the distressful intrusive thoughts and subsequent behavioral compulsions seen in OCD. These obsessions tend to be more distressful to families and friends of individuals with Asperger syndrome than to the person himself.

Despite these noted differences, similarities between the obsessions and compulsions in OCD and the "obsessional" characteristics seen in autism have driven efforts to determine whether pharmacological choices in OCD (serotonergic agents) may be of benefit in autistic disorders. Early studies (105,106) suggested that indeed clomipramine (a tricyclic antidepressant agent with potent serotonin reuptake–blocking action) was effective in autism. Gordon et al. (106) demonstrated the efficacy of clomipramine over placebo and desipramine in treating obsessive-compulsive and stereotyped motor behaviors in children and adults (ages 6–23 years) with autism. Although the diagnosis of autism was made by DSM-III-R criteria (before the addition of Asperger syndrome in DSM-IV), 9 of 24 subjects had IQs in the nonretarded range of 70 to 107. Side effects were considered severe and included seizures (grand mal), tachycardia (resting heart rate 160 to 170 beats per minute), and conduction delays (QTc interval increased 0.45 seconds). Subsequent studies noted similar findings and poor tolerability (107,108). Because of these potentially serious side effects, clomipramine is not widely recommended as first-line treatment in autism and its use should be implemented with caution and close monitoring.

Advancing from the noted benefit of clomipramine on repetitive behaviors, research began with other serotonergic agents, specifically the SSRIs. The first controlled study by McDouble et al. examined fluvoxamine in 30 adults with autistic disorder (109). As noted in the clomipramine study, the diagnosis was made by the DSM-III-R criteria; however, 10 of the 15 subjects receiving medication had IQs over 70 (range 71–114). In this 12-week, double-blind study, fluvoxamine (mean dose 276.7 mg/day) was superior to placebo for repetitive thoughts and behavior ($F = 11.48$, $p < 0.001$) as measured by Y-BOCS scores. Side effects included mild sedation and nausea, but overall fluvoxamine was well tolerated.

Although well tolerated and efficacious in the adult population, a later study by McDougle et al. (110) failed to show any benefit of fluvoxamine in children and adolescents with autistic spectrum disorder, including Asperger syndrome (8 of 34). In a 12-week double-blind, placebo-controlled study, only one subject showed some significant improvement with the medication. Two subjects experienced worsening of their ritualistic behavior. Other side effects included hyperactivity, agitation, insomnia, aggression, anxiety, and anorexia. Fluvoxamine dosing began at 25 mg every other day and was increased by 25 mg every three to seven days as tolerated. Final mean dose was 106.9 mg/day. A later study by Martin et al. also failed to show significant efficacy (on repetitive behavior, mood, or overall functioning) in subjects (mean age 11.3 ± 3.6 years) treated with fluvoxamine (mean dose, 66.7 mg/day) in a 10-week prospective, open-label study (111). Seven of eighteen subjects had a diagnosis of Asperger syndrome. Only 14 subjects completed the study. Four subjects discontinued because of behavioral activation. Eight of the fourteen (including all 4 females in the study) were partial responders, but results were not significant. Only three subjects were reported to be full responders, as noted by improvements in the Children's version of the Y-BOCS, SCARED, or the CGI-S scale. The authors concluded that fluvoxamine should not be used for the routine treatment of anxiety or OCD-like symptoms for most children and adolescents with autistic spectrum disorders because of the potential of behavioral activation.

Early studies have suggested that fluoxetine may be beneficial for stereotypical and obsessive behavior in persons with autistic spectrum disorders, including Asperger syndrome. Hollander et al. demonstrated the benefit of fluoxetine in children and adolescents (ages 5–16 years) with PDDs (112). Five of the 39 children were diagnosed with Asperger's disorder. In this 20-week, placebo-controlled crossover study, fluoxetine (mean dose 9.9 mg/day, range 2.4–20 mg/day) was significantly better than placebo for reducing repetitive behaviors on the Children's Yale-Brown Obsessive-Compulsive Scale (CY-BOCS). Likewise, a study by Buschbaum et al. (100) noted improvement in Y-BOCS scores in five adults with high-functioning autism (IQ range 74–119) and one adult with Asperger's disorder treated in a 16-week, placebo-controlled, cross-over trial of fluoxetine (average dose 40 mg/day). Three of these same adults were considered responders as determined by improvement in CGI scores. The one adult with Asperger's had a decrease in Y-BOCS scores from 31 to 8 and a score of "much improved" on the CGI. This study also used functional imaging to examine differences in metabolic rates before and after fluoxetine treatment. Individuals who had relatively high metabolic rates in the anterior cingulate cortex prior to treatment were more likely to show a clinical response. This is notable considering reports suggesting that the anterior cingulate cortex and the medial frontal region, specifically Brodmann's area 25, may modulate internal emotional response (113). In both studies, side effects from fluoxetine were minimal.

No controlled studies have examined the benefit or tolerability of the other SSRIs (sertraline, paroxetine, escitalopram, or citalopram) in autistic spectrum disorders. In a 12-week, prospective, open-label study of 42 adults with PDDs, McDougle et al. (114) found sertraline effective in improving aggression and repetitive behavior, however, none of the subjects with Asperger's disorder (6 of 42) were considered responders. In the retrospective study of citalopram by Couturier et al. (102), stereotypies and preoccupations were reported to be only minimally improved with treatment, however, the retrospective study by Namerow et al. (103) examining the same medication found notable improvements particularly in "preoccupations with nonfunctional routines, repetitive behaviors or stereotypies, and deviations in daily routines." A 10-week, open-label, prospective study by Owley et al. (115) found escitalopram (mean dose 11.1 ± 6.5 mg/day) effective in multiple domains assessed by the ABC-CV. These included stereotypical behaviors, lethargy, hyperactivity, and irritability ($p = 0.001$) and inappropriate speech ($p = 0.35$). Results were not subdivided by diagnosis, making it difficult to ascertain whether the response of persons with Asperger's was any different than the group as a whole. In addition, tolerability was a concern. Ten of twenty-eight (36%) of subjects were unable to tolerate even a 10-mg/day dose.

In addition to being efficacious for aggression in autistic spectrum disorders, the atypical antipsychotics, especially risperidone, have been shown to improve repetitive behavior. McDougle et al. have published multiple reports of the benefit of risperidone for this target symptom (51,55). In the early 1998 study of risperidone in adults with PDDs, repetitive behavior was found to be improved with risperidone use ($p < 0.001$) as was depression ($p < 0.03$) and anxiety ($p < 0.02$). These findings were replicated in the later study evaluating the effect of risperidone in children with PDDs. In the 49 children treated with medication for eight weeks, scores on the Children's Version of the Y-BOCS decreased from 15.51 (SD = 2.73) to 11.65 (SD = 4.02). Neither of these studies included

Syndrome Diagnostic Scale (ASDS). Of 13 subjects, 9 completed the 12-week trial. Final risperidone dose ranged from 0.5 mg/day to 1.5 mg/day. A statistically significant improvement from baseline in SANS score was found for the 12-week completers ($F = 13.41$, $p < 0.0001$) and subjects terminating early as assessed by 12-week last observation carried forward (LOCF) ($F = 9.54$, $p < 0.0001$). Statistically significant improvement was also observed in the total ASDS score for both groups ($F = 8.41$, $p < 0.0001$ and $F = 7.45$, $p < 0.001$, respectively) and for each of the six individual components of the ASDS (language dysfunction, social behavior, maladaptive behavior, cognitive dysfunction, sensorimotor dysfunction, and general dysfunction). Our analysis suggested that improvement in social behavior as assessed by the ASDS was not simply a derivative of the improvement in maladaptive behavior with risperidone. Maladaptive behavior was a significant covariate on the improvement of social behavior ($t = 3.68$, $p < 0.005$), but improvement of social behavior was still significant ($F = 3.14$, $p < 0.023$) after accounting for maladaptive behavior improvement. A subsequent study (122) using the same research design, but also inclusive of a magnetic spectroscopy imaging (MRS) before and after starting risperidone, replicated previous findings of improvements in social functioning as measured by the ASDS and SANS scores. Additionally, examination of the brain metabolite MRS data indicated a treatment effect on normalization of choline asymmetry seen prior to treatment. We additionally saw a trend for improvement in SANS scores to significantly interact with normalization of choline ratios ($F = 12.05$, $p < 0.075$).

CONCLUSIONS

Clearly, more research is needed before specific recommendations can be made with confidence about the tolerability and efficacy of pharmacological interventions specifically for individuals with Asperger syndrome. The available literature is limited by low subject numbers and by the inclusion of this subpopulation with more severely impaired individuals with autism and other PDDs. Few studies exist that only examined psychotropic use in persons with this diagnosis. As noted by Milin et al. (64), this is significant considering "preliminary evidence to suggest Asperger may be a subgroup within the PDD population who respond differently to pharmacotherapy and who are not identified in studies where results for subgroups are reported together." Most current research (118) regarding pharmacotherapy in autistic disorders, including research into nontraditional agents (i.e., N-acetylcysteine, hyperbaric oxygen therapy) continues to include Asperger syndrome with other PDDs.

Since its inception into the DSM-IV, we have broadened our understanding of this specific diagnosis. This expanded knowledge will assist in determining where further efforts should be targeted to optimize the outcomes of our therapeutic interventions. As Towbin concluded, "pharmacotherapy is not the ultimate treatment for Asperger syndrome, but it has a definite place." Professionals that have the privilege of working with these unique individuals wait expectantly for more specific recommendations on how to best use medications as part of the overall treatment plan. Until that time, clinicians should be guided by standards of care that encompass a thorough understanding of Asperger syndrome. This includes knowledge surrounding the specific nature of symptoms, their contribution to impairment of functioning, and how amenable these symptoms are to a biologically driven treatment through the use of pharmacotherapy.

REFERENCES

1. Martin A, Scahill L, Klin A, et al. Higher-functioning pervasive developmental disorders: rates and patterns of psychotropic drug use. J Am Acad Child Adolesc Psychiatry 1999; 38(7):992–931.
2. Aman MG, VanBourgondien ME, Wolford PL, et al. Psychotropic and anticonvulsant drugs in subjects with autism: prevalence and patterns of use. J Am Acad Child Adolesc Psychiatry 1995; 34(12):1672–1681.
3. Langworthy-Lam MA, Aman MG, VanBourgondien ME. Prevalence and patterns of use of psychoactive medicines in individuals with autism in the Autism Society of North Carolina. J Child Adolesc Psychopharmacol 2002; 12(4):311–321.
4. Aman MG, Lam KS, Collier-Crespin A. Prevalence and patterns of use of psychoactive medicines among individuals with autism in the autism society of Ohio. J Autism Dev Disord 2003; 33(5):527–534.
5. Klin A, Volkmar FR. Asperger's syndrome. In: Cohen DJ, Volkmar FR, eds. Handbook of Autism and Pervasive Developmental Disorders, 2nd ed. New York, NY: Wiley, 1997:94–112.
6. Towbin KE. Strategies for pharmacologic treatment of high functioning autism and Asperger syndrome. Child Adolesc Psychiatric Clin N Am 2003; 12:23–45.
7. Jensen PS, Bhatara VS, Bitiello B, et al. Psychoactive medication prescribing practices for U.S. children: gaps between research and clinical practice. J Am Acad Child Adolesc Psychiatry 1999; 38(5):557–565.
8. Thomas CP, Conrad P, Casler R, et al. Trends in the Use of Psychotropic Medications Among Adolescents, 1994-2001. Psychiatr Serv 2006; 57(1):63–69.
9. Olfson M, Blance C, Liu L, et al. National trends in the outpatient treatment of children and adolescents with antipsychotic drugs. Arch Gen Psychiatry 2006; 63(6):679–685.
10. Hammad TA, Laughren T, Racoosin J, et al. Suicidality in pediatric patients treated with antidepressant drugs. Arch Gen Psychiatry 2006; 63(3):332–229.
11. U.S. Food and Drug Administration. Available at: http://www.fda.gov/cder/drug/infopage/ADHD. Accessed September 2007.
12. Newcomer JW. Second generation (atypical) antipsychotics and metabolic effects: a comprehensive literature review. CNS Drugs 2005; 19(suppl 1):1–93.
13. Antochi RM, Stavrakaki C. Determining pharmacotherapy options for behavioral disturbances in patients with developmental disabilities. Psychiatric Annals 2004; 34(3):205–212.
14. Harris JC. Developmental Neuropsychiatry: Assessment, Diagnosis, and Treatment of Developmental Disorders. Oxford, UK: Oxford University Press, 1995:463–484.

15. Jensen PS, Youngstrom EA, Steiner H, et al. Consensus report on impulsive aggression as a symptom across diagnostic categories in child psychiatry: implications for medication studies. J Am Acad Child Adolesc Psychiatry 2007; 46(3): 309–322.

16. Jaselskis CA, Cook EH Jr., Fletcher KE, et al. Clonidine treatment of hyperactive and impulsive children with autistic disorder. J Clin Psychopharmacol 1992; 12(5): 322–327.

17. Fankhauser MR, Karumanchi VC, German ML et al. A double-blind, placebo-controlled study of the efficacy of transdermal clonidine in autism. J Clin Psychiatry 1992; 53(3):77–82.

18. Posey DJ, Puntney JI, Sasher TM, et al. Guanfacine treatment of hyperactivity and inattention in pervasive developmental disorders: a retrospective analysis of 80 cases. J Child Adolesc Psychopharmacol 2004; 14(2):233–241.

19. Schultz W. Reward signaling by dopamine neurons. Neuroscientist 2001, 7(4): 293–302 (review).

20. Leavitt ML, Yudofsky SC, Maroon JC, et al. Effect of intraventricular nadolol infusion on shock-induced aggression in 6-hydroxydopamine-treated rats. J Neuropsychiatry Clin Neurosci 1989; 1:167–172.

21. Holdiness MR. A review of contact dermatitis associated with transdermal therapeutic systems. Contact Dermatitis 1989; 20(1):3–9.

22. Swanson JM, Flockhart D, Udrea D, et al. Clonidine and the treatment of ADHD: questions about safety and efficacy. J Child Adolesc Psychopharmacol 1995; 5:301–304.

23. Cantwell DP, Swanson J, Connor DF. Case study: adverse response to clonidine. J Am Acad Child Adolesc Psychiatry 1997; 36(4):539–544.

24. Ruedrich S, Erhardt L. Beta-adrenergic blockers in mental retardation and developmental disabilities. Mental Retard Dev Disabil Res Rev 1999; 5(4):290–298.

25. Ratey JJ, Mikkelsen E, Sorgi P, et al. Autism: the treatment of aggressive behaviors. J Clin Psychopharmacol 1987; 7:35–41.

26. Connor DF, Ozbayrak KR, Benjamin S, et al. A pilot study of nadolol for overt aggression in developmentally delayed individuals. J Am Acad Child Adolesc Psychiatry 1997; 36(6):826–834.

27. Ratey JJ, Bemporad J, Sorgi P, et al. Open trial effects of beta-blockers on speech and social behaviors in 8 autistic adults. J Autism Dev Disord 1987; 17(3):439–436.

28. Buitelaar JK, van der Gaag RJ, Swaab-Barneveld H, et al. Pindolol and methylphenidate in children with attention-deficit hyperactivity disorder: clinical efficacy and side-effects. J Child Psychol Psychiatry 1996; 37:587–595.

29. Connor DF. Beta-blockers for aggression: a review of the pediatric experience. J Child Adolesc Psychopharmacol 1993; 13:99–114.

30. Hollander E, Dolgoff-Kaspar R, Cartwright C, et al. An open trial of divalproex sodium in autism spectrum disorders. J Clin Psychiatry 2001; 62(7):530–534.

31. Hellings JA, Weckbaugh M, Nickel EF, et al. A double-blind, placebo-controlled study of valproate for aggression in youth with pervasive developmental disorders. J Child Adolesc Psychopharmacol 2005; 15(4):682–692.

32. Craft M, Ismail IA, Krishnamurti D, et al. Lithium in the treatment of aggression in mentally handicapped patients: a double blind trial. Br J of Psychiatry 1987; 150: 685–689.

33. Langee HR. Retrospective study of lithium use for institutionalized mentally retarded individuals with behavior disorders. Am J Ment Retard 1990; 94:448–452.

34. Campbell M, Adams PB, Small AM, et al. Lithium in hospitalized aggressive children with conduct disorder: a double-blind and placebo-controlled study. J Am Acad Child Adolesc Psychiatry 1995; 34(4):445–453.
35. Malone RP, Delaney MA, Luebbert JF, et al. A double-blind placebo-controlled study of lithium in hospitalized aggressive children and adolescents with conduct disorder. Arch Gen Psychiatry 2000; 57(7):649–654.
36. Kerbeshian J, Burd L, Fisher W. Lithium carbonate in the treatment of two patients with infantile autism and atypical bipolar symptomatology. J Clin Psychopharmacol 1987; 7:401–405.
37. Steingard R, Biederman J. Lithium responsive manic-like symptoms in two individual with autism. J Am Acad Child Adolesc Psychiatry 1987; 26:932–935.
38. Delong RG. Correlation of family history with specific subgroups: Asperger's syndrome and bipolar affective disease. J Autism Dev Disord 1988; 18(4):593–600.
39. Duggal HS. Bipolar disorder with asperger's disorder. Am J Psychiatry 2003; 160:184–185.
40. Hardan AY, Jou RJ, Handen BL. A retrospective assessment of topiramate in children and adolescents with pervasive developmental disorders. J Child Adolesc Psychopharmacol 2004; 14(3):426–432.
41. Uvebrant P, Bauziene R. Intractable epilepsy in children. The efficacy of lamotrigine treatment, including nonseizure-related benefits. Neuropediatrics 1994; 25:284–289.
42. Belsito KM, Law PA, Kirk KS, et al. Lamotrigine therapy for autistic disorder: a randomized double-blind, placebo-controlled trial. J Autism Dev Disord 2001; 31(2): 175–181.
43. Bozikas V, Bascialla F, Yulis P, et al. Gabapentin for behavioral dyscontrol with mental retardation. Am J Psychiatry 2001; 158:965–966.
44. Davanzo PA, King BH. Open trial lamotrigine in the treatment of self-injurious behavior in an adolescent with profound mental retardation. J Child Adolesc Psychopharmacol 1996; 6(4):273–279.
45. Berlant J, van Kammen DP. Open-label topiramate as primary or adjunctive therapy in chronic civilian post-traumatic stress disorder: a preliminary report. J Clin Psychiatry 2002; 63:15–20.
46. McDougle CJ, Stigler KA, Posey DJ. Treatment of aggression in children and adolescents with autism and conduct disorder. J Clin Psychiatry 2003; 64(4):16–25.
47. Duggal HS. Mood stabilizers in Asperger's syndrome. Aust N Z J Psychiatry 2001; 35(3):390–391.
48. King BH. Pharmacological treatment of mood disturbances, aggression, and self-injury in persons with pervasive developmental disorders. J Autism Dev Disorder 2000; 30(5):439–445.
49. Campbell M, Anderson LT, Meier M, et al. A comparison of haloperidol and behavior therapy and their interaction in autistic children. J Am Acad Child Adolesc Psychiatry 1978; 17(4):640–655.
50. Scahill L, Martin A. Psychopharmacology. In: Volkmar FR, Klin A, Paul R, et al., eds. Handbook of Autism and Pervasive Developmental Disorders. Hoboken, NJ: Wiley, 2005:1102–1122.
51. McDougle CJ, Holmes JP, Carlson DC, et al. A double-blind, placebo-controlled study of risperidone in adults with autistic disorder and other pervasive developmental disorders. Arch Gen Psychiatry 1998; 55(7):633–641.

52. McCracken JT, McGough J, Shah B, et al. for Research Units on Pediatric Psychopharmacology (RUPP) Autism Network. Risperidone in children with autism and serious behavioral problems. N Engl J Med 2002; 347(5):314–321.

53. Simeon J, Milin R, Walker S. A retrospective chart review of risperidone use in treatment-resistant children and adolescents with psychiatric disorders. Prog Neuropsychopharmacol Biol Psychiatry 2002; 26(2):267–275.

54. Shea s, Turgay A, Carroll A, et al. Risperidone treatment of disruptive behavioral symptoms in children with autistic and other pervasive developmental disorders. Pediatrics 2004; 114(5):634–641.

55. McDougle C, Scahill L, Ama M, et al. Risperidone for the core symptoms domains of autism: results from the study by the Autism Network of the Research Units of Pediatric Psychopharmacology. Am J Psychiatry 2005; 162:1142–1148.

56. Fisman S, Steele M. Use of risperidone in pervasive developmental disorders: a case series. J Child Adolesc Psychopharmacol 1996; 6:177–190.

57. Hardan A, Johnson K, Johnson C, et al. Case study: risperidone treatment of children and adolescents with developmental disorders. J Am Acad Child Adolesc Psychiatry 1996; 35:1551–1556.

58. McDougle CJ, Holmes JP, Bronson MR, et al. Risperidone treatment of children and adolescents with pervasive developmental disorders: a prospective open-label study. J Am Acad Child Adolesc Psychiatry 1997; 36:685–693.

59. Potenza M, Holmes J, Kanes S, et al. Olanzapine treatment of children, adolescents, and adults with pervasive developmental disorders: an open-label pilot study. J Clin Psychopharmacol 1999; 19:37–44.

60. Demb HB, Roychoudhury K. Comments on "Olanzapine treatment of children, adolescents, and adults with pervasive developmental disorders: an open-label pilot study". J Clin Psychopharmacol 2000; 20:580–581 (letter).

61. Stavrakaki C, Antochi R, Emery P. Olanzapine in the treatment of pervasive developmental disorders: a case series analysis. J Psychiatry Neurosci 2004; 29(1):57–60.

62. Kemner C, Willemsen-Swinkets S, DeJonge M, et al. Open-label study of olanzapine in children with pervasive developmental disorder. J Clin Psychopharmacol 2002; 22(5):455–460.

63. Hollander E, Wasserman S, Swanson M, et al. A double-blind placebo-controlled pilot study of olanzapine in childhood/adolescent pervasive developmental disorder. J Child Adolesc Psychopharmacol 2006; 16(5):541–548.

64. Milin R, Simeon JG, Batth S, et al. An open trial of olanzapine in children and adolescents with Asperger disorder. J Clin Psychopharmacol 2006; 26(1):90–92.

65. Corson AH, Barkenbus JE, Posey DJ, et al. A retrospective analysis of quetiapine in the treatment of pervasive developmental disorders. J Clin Psychiatry 2004; 65(11):1531–1536.

66. McDougle CJ, Kem DL, Posey DJ. Case series: use of ziprasidone for maladaptive symptoms in youths with autism. J AM Acad Child Adolesc Psychiatry 2002; 41(8):921–927.

67. Stigler KA, Posey DJ, McDougle CJ. Aripiprazole for maladaptive behavior in pervasive developmental disorders. J Child Adolesc Psychopharmacol 2004; 14(3):445–463.

68. Stigler KA, Diener JT, Kohn AE, et al. A prospective, open-label study of aripiprazole in youth with Asperger's disorder and pervasive developmental disorder not

otherwise specified. Presented at: American Academy of Child and Adolescent Psychiatry Annual Meeting; October 28, 2006; San Diego, CA.

69. Erickson CA, Posey DJ, Stigler KA, et al. Pharmacotherapy of autism and related disorders. Psychiatric Annals 2007; 37(7):490–500.

70. Feeney DJ, Klykylo W. Risperidone and tardive dyskinesia. J Am Acad Child Adolesc Psychiatry 1995; 56:484–485.

71. Keck ME, Muller MB, Binder EB, et al. Ziprasidone-related tardive dyskinesia. Am J Psychiatry 2004; 161:175–176.

72. Seeman P, Bzowej NH, Guan HC, et al. Human brain dopamine receptors in children and aging adults. Synapese 1987; 1:399–404.

73. Straker D, Correll CU, Kramer-Ginsburg E, et al. Cost-effective screening for the metabolic syndrome in patients treated with second-generation antipsychotic medications. Am J Psychiatry 2005; 162:1217–1221.

74. Fedorowicz VJ. Metabolic side effects of atypical antipsychotics in children: a literature review. J Psychopharmacol 2005; 19(5):533–550.

75. Petty RG. Prolactin and antipsychotic medications: mechanism of action. Schizophr Res 1999; 35:67–73.

76. National Institutes of Health. Clinical guidelines on the identification, evaluation, and treatment of overweight and obesity in adults – the evidence report. Obes Res 1998; 6(suppl2), 51S–209S.

77. Stigler KA, Potenza MN, Posey DJ, et al. Weight gain associated with atypical antipsychotic use in children and adolescents: prevalence, clinical relevance, and management. Paediatr Drugs 2004; 6(1):33–44.

78. American Psychiatric Association. Diagnostic and Statistical Manual of Mental Disorders. 4th ed. Wahington, DC: American Psychiatric Press, 1994.

79. Ghaziuddin M, Weidmer-Mikhail E, Ghaziuddin N. Comorbidity of Asperger syndrome: a preliminary report. J Intellect Disabil Res 1998; 42(pt 4):279–283.

80. Gilchrist A, Green J, Cox A, et al. Development and current functioning in adolescents with Asperger syndrome: a comparative study. J Child Psychol Psychiatry 2001; 42(2):227–240.

81. Ehlers S, Nyden A, Gillberg C et al. Asperger syndrome, autism and attention disorders: a comparative study of the cognitive profile of 120 children. J Child Psychol Psychiatry 1997; 38:207–217.

82. Nyden A, Gillberg C, Hjelmquist E, et al. Executive function/attention in boys with Asperger syndrome, attention disorders and reading/writing disorder. Autism 1999; 3:213–228.

83. Stigler KA, Desmond LA, Posey DJ, et al. A naturalistic retrospective analysis of psychostimulants in pervasive developmental disorders. J Child Adolesc Psychopharmacol 2004; 14(1):49–56.

84. Research Units on Pediatric Psychopharmacology Autism Network. Randomized, controlled, crossover trial of methylphenidate in pervasive developmental disorders with hyperactivity. Arch Gen Psychiatry 2005; 62(11):1266–1274.

85. Aman MG. Stimulant drug effects in developmental disorders and hyperactivity-toward a resolution of disparate findings. J Autism Dev Disord 1982; 12(4):385–398.

86. Jou RJ, Handen BL, Harden AY. Retrospective assessment of atomoxetine in children and adolescents with pervasive developmental disorders. J Child Adolesc Psychopharmacol 2005; 15(2):325–330.

87. Posey DJ, Wiegand RE, Wilkerson J, et al. Open-label atomoxetine for attention-deficit/hyperactivity disorder symptoms associated with high-functioning pervasive development disorder. J Child Adolesc Psychopharmacol 2006; 16(5):599–610.

88. Troost PW, Steenhuis MP, Tuynman-Qua HG, et al. Atomoxetine for attention deficit/hyperactivity disorder symptoms in children with pervasive developmental disorders: a pilot study. J Child Adolesc Psychopharmacol 2006; 16(5):611–619.

89. Arnold LE, Aman MG, Cook AM, et al. Atomoxetine for hyperactivity in autism spectrum disorder: placebo-controlled crossover pilot trial. J Am Acad Child Adolesc Psychiatry 2006; 45(10):1196–1205.

90. Gillott A, Furniss F, Walter A. Anxiety in high-functioning children with autism. Autism 2001; 5:277–286.

91. Ghaziuddin M, Alessi N, Greden JF. Life events and depression in children with pervasive developmental disorders. J Autism Dev Disord 1995; 25(5):495–502.

92. Kim JA, Szatmari P, Bryson SE, et al. The prevalence of anxiety and mood problems among children with autism and Asperger syndrome. Autism 2000; 4(2): 117–132.

93. Tongue BJ, Brereton AV, Gray KM, et al. Behavioural and emotional disturbance in high-functioning autism and Asperger syndrome. Autism 1999; 3(2):117–130.

94. Piven J, Palmer P. Psychiatric disorder and the broad autism phenotype: evidence from a family study of multiple-incidence autism families. Am J Psychiatry 1999; 156(4):557–563.

95. Cook EH, Leventhal BL. The serotonin system in autism. Curr Opin Pediatr 1996; 8(4):348–354.

96. Tordjman S, Gutknecht L, Carlier M, et al. Role of the serotonin transporter gene in the behavioral expression of autism. Mol Psychiatry 2001; 6(4):434–439.

97. George MS, Ketter TA, Post RM. Prefrontal cortex dysfunction in clinical depression. Depression 1994; 2:59–72.

98. Sweeten TL, Posey DJ, Shekhar A, et al. The amygdala and related structures in the pathophysiology of autism. Pharmacol Biochem Behav 2002; 71(3):449–455.

99. Posey DJ, Erickson CA, Stigler KA, et al. The use of selective serotonin reuptake inhibitors in autism and related disorders. J Child Adolesc Psychopharmacol 2006; 16(1):181–186.

100. Buschbaum MS, Hollander E, Haznedar MM, et al. Effect of fluoxetine on regional cerebral metabolism in autistic spectrum disorders: a pilot study. Ing J Neuro-psychopharmacol 2001; 4(2):119–125.

101. Martin A, Koenig K, Anderson GM, et al. Low-dose fluvoxamine treatment of children and adolescents with pervasive developmental disorders: a prospective, open-label study. J Autism Dev Disord 2003; 33(1):77–85.

102. Couturier JL, Nicholson R. A retrospective assessment of citalopram in children and adolescents with pervasive developmental disorders. J Child Adolesc Psycho-pharmacol 2002; 12(3):243–248.

103. Namerow LB, Thomas P, Bostic JQ, et al. Use of citalopram in pervasive devel-opmental disorders. J Dev Behav Pediatr 2003; 24(2):104–108.

104. McDougle CJ, Kresch LE, Goodman WK, et al. A case-controlled study of repet-itive thoughts and behavior in adults with autistic disorder and obsessive-compul-sive disorder. Am J Psychiatry 1995; 152(5):772–777.

105. McDougle CJ, Price LH, Volkmar FR, et al. Clomipramine in autism: preliminary evidence of efficacy. J Am Acad Child Adolesc Psychiatry 1992; 31(4):746–750.

106. Gordon CT, State RC, Nelson JE, et al. A double-blind comparison of clomipramine, desipramine, and placebo in the treatment of autistic disorder. Arch Gen Psychiatry 1993; 50(6):441–447.

107. Brasic JR, Barnett JY, Sheitman BB, et al. Behavioral effects of clomipramine on prepubertal boys with autistic disorder and severe mental retardation. CNS Spectr 1998; 3:39–46.

108. Remmington G, Sloman L, Konstantareas M, et al. Clomipramine versus haloperidol in the treatment of autistic disorder: a double-blind, placebo-controlled, crossover study. J Clin Psychopharmacol 2001; 21(4):440–444.

109. McDougle CJ, Naylor ST, Cohen DJ, et al. A double-blind, placebo-controlled study of fluvoxamine in adults with autistic disorder. Arch Gen Psychiatry 1996; 53:1001–1008.

110. McDougle CJ, Kresch LE, Posey DJ. Repetitive thoughts and behavior in pervasive developmental disorders: treatment with serotonin reuptake inhibitors. J Autism Dev Disord 2000; 30(5):427–435.

111. Martin A, Koenig K, Anderson G, et al. Low-dose fluvoxamine treatment of children and adolescents with pervasive developmental disorders: a prospective, open-label study. J Child Adolesc Psychopharmacol 2002; 12(4):311–321.

112. Hollander E, Phillips A, Chaplin W, et al. A placebo-controlled crossover trial of liquid fluoxetine on repetitive behaviors in childhood and adolescent autism. Neuropsychopharmacology 2005; 30:582–589.

113. Devinsky O, Morrell MJ, Vogt BA. Contributions of anterior cingulate cortex to behavior. Brain 1995; 118:279–306.

114. McDougle CJ, Brodkin ES, Naylor ST, et al. Sertraline in adults with pervasive developmental disorders: A prospective, open-label investigation. J Clin Psychopharmacol 1998; 18:62–66.

115. Owley T, Walton L, Salt J, et al. An open-label trial of escitalopram in pervasive developmental disorders. J Am Acad Child Adolesc Psychiatry 2005; 44(4):343–348.

116. Hollander E, Novotny S, Hanratty M, et al. Oxytocin infusion reduces repetitive behaviors in adults with autistic and Asperger's disorders. Neuropsychopharmacology 2003; 28:193–198.

117. Insel TR, O'Brien DJ, Leckman JF. Oxytocin, vasopressin, and autism: is there a connection. Biol Psychiatry 1999; 45:145–157.

118. National Institutes of Health. Search for clinical trials. Available at: http://www.clinicaltrials.gov. Accessed October 2007.

119. Delong GR, Teaque LA, Kamran MM. Effects of fluoxetine treatment in young children with idiopathic autism. Dev Med Child Neurol 1998; 40:551–562.

120. Fukuda T, Sugie H, Ito M, et al. Clinical evaluation of treatment with fluvoxamine, a selective serotonin reuptake inhibitor in children with autistic disorder. No To Hattatsu 2001; 33(4):314–318.

121. Rausch JL, Sirota EL, Londino DL, et al. Open-label risperidone for Asperger's disorder: negative symptoms spectrum response. J Clin Psychiatry 2005; 66:1592–1597.

122. Londino DL, Sirota EL, Hessenthaler M, et al. Magnetic Spectroscopy in Asperger's syndrome before and after risperidone treatment. Presented at: American Academy of Child and Adolescent Psychiatry Annual Meeting; October 28, 2006; San Diego, CA.

123. 2008 Physician's Desk Reference (PDR). 62nd ed. Belmont, CA: Wadsworth/ITP, 2007.

14

Psychosocial Interventions for Asperger's Disorder

Lisa A. Ruble

*Department of Educational and Counseling Psychology,
University of Kentucky, Lexington, Kentucky, U.S.A.*

Grace Mathai

Department of Pediatrics, University of Louisville, Louisville, Kentucky, U.S.A.

Peter Tanguay and Allan M. Josephson

*Division of Child and Adolescent Psychiatry, Department of Psychiatry and
Behavioral Sciences, University of Louisville, Louisville, Kentucky, U.S.A.*

INTRODUCTION

Although cases of autism may have been reported in the literature more than 100 years ago (1), it was not until 1943 that descriptions of what would become known as autism and Asperger's disorder (AD) were popularized (2). In contrast to Kanner, Asperger (3,4) believed that the syndrome was a personality trait rather than a developmental disorder. AD was added to the American Psychiatric Association's Diagnostic and Statistical Manual (DSM-IV, 4th Edition) (5,6) to integrate those individuals who could not be diagnosed as "classically" autistic, but who had impairment in social relationships.

Since that time, the solution of adding categories to encompass more subjects has been challenged, with various authors being unable to find clear-cut differences between the various groups (7–12). It has been suggested by some authors that while some of the disorders classified under PDD (such as fragile X and Rett's) are associated with specific genetic abnormalities and symptoms complexes, it may be more appropriate to consider the disorders of autism, AD, and PDD-Not Otherwise Specified (PDD-NOS), as representing a "spectrum" of social and language impairment. Although the idea may appear clinically persuasive to some, it can be argued that it is far from proven and the spectrum may be no more than a concatenation of symptoms representing a range of genetically influenced defects. However, as a clinicians specializing in diagnosing individuals with autism and autistic-like conditions, we have found the concept of a social communication spectrum disorder to be useful, at least until a scientifically more sophisticated model comes along. This, however, begs the question, "A spectrum of what?" In the next section, we will attempt to answer this as well as to touch on other models that may help explain some of the fundamental deficits seen in persons with autism.

THE DEFICITS IN AUTISM SPECTRUM DISORDER

Failure to Develop Social Communication Skills and Knowledge

Infants come into the world with innate behavioral propensities that serve to maximize their interaction with caretakers. Like some higher primates, very young children emit various innate, universal, facial expressions (13,14), and can discriminate their mother's face from that of a stranger (15). "Affect attunement" (16) is a term that characterizes the manner in which an infant and her mother spontaneously interact crossmodally, matching duration, intensity, and rhythm signals. Mothers talk to their infants in "motherese," using exaggerated tone of voice, body language, gestures, and facial expressions to which their infants learn to respond with their own set of nonverbal behaviors. At two to four months of age, 30% of children automatically follow their mother's line of sight to an object, but by 14 months of age, all children do so without verbal prompting or gesture on the part of their mother (17). Faced with an experimental "visual cliff," 12-month-old infants learn to look to their mother's face to determine what they should do (18). If their mothers pose joy or interest, the children will cross; if the mothers pose fear or anger few infants cross.

Persons with autism fail to engage in the nonverbal social communication interactions typically seen in young children (19,20). It is not that autistic children fail to attach to their caretakers or that they avoid proximity. Like normal children and as well as children with Down syndrome, children with autism are clearly attached to their mothers, and they attempt to remain close to them. (21). In the Ainsworth Strange Situation, they seek contact with their mothers as much as normal children matched on age and IQ (22). They do not, however, show attention-sharing behaviors, such as pointing to objects (23), despite being able to distinguish between pictures of objects and various sounds as well as age- and IQ-matched nonautistic subjects (24), nor do they show deficits in perception of faces as stimulus objects (25). They do not seem to recognize the emotional and contextual meaning of facial expression, gesture, and the nonverbal vocalizations of emotion (24). In comparison to children with "mental handicap" matched on mental age (MA), autistic children fail to use the speaker's direction of gaze to orient themselves to objects (26). In comparison to children with Down syndrome (27), they rarely used emotional gestures, even though they usually could initiate them upon request. Autistic children do not chat, nor do they become proficient at give-and-take conversation, even when they develop language.

The earliest development of social interaction, marked by sending social signals and learning to recognize signals, has been generally called "affective reciprocity," to which is gradually added, starting at six to eight months of age, "joint attention," in which the infant appears to interact with the mother in order to gain a response. Later, in the second year of life, typical children develop a theory of mind, in which they act as if they understand, nonverbally, that the "minds" of other people are different from their own, and that these minds can be sources of important information. Later, by three years of age, children begin to develop two new and diverging sets of skills, which have been called "intuitive psychology" and "intuitive physics" (28). Intuitive psychology denotes understanding that a person's behavior can be driven by inner motives, while intuitive physics is about learning how things work, about facts, and about inanimate objects. Young children learn to guess the motives of others by reading their nonverbal cues within the social context. This ability has also been called "mind-reading," and its absence "mind-blindness." Most children develop equal skills as mind-reading and understanding the world of objects, but occasionally one may see a child with much greater skill in understanding the world of objects than the world of psychological motives. While the concepts of intuitive psychology and intuitive physics are intriguing as explanation for perceived dissociations between social intelligence and factual knowledge, its value must be proven through more extensive research.

Using two popular research instruments, the Autism Diagnostic Interview-Revised (ADI-R) (29) and the Autism Diagnostic Observation Schedule (ADOS) (30) we have endeavored to classify persons with autism, AD, and PDD-NOS along a spectrum of communication disorder. This approach has been clinically useful to us (31,32). The most severely autistic persons have deficits in affective reciprocity, joint attention, and social knowledge; those with moderate social communication deficits tend to have mostly joint attention and social knowledge deficits, while the mildest forms have a lack of social knowledge. Whether this will prove useful to others remains to be seen.

Executive Function Deficits

Although the definition of executive functions may vary between investigators, it generally includes the ability to form abstract concepts, to develop a flexible plan of action aimed at solving problems, and to monitor and self-correct one's responses. Because persons with autism have been thought to have weaknesses in tasks involving cognitive flexibility, verbal reasoning, and complex social memory, it has been proposed that executive-functioning deficits are a core cognitive deficiency of the syndrome. While some studies have supported executive-functioning deficits in autism (33,34), studies by Liss et al. (35) report that impaired executive-functioning is not unique to autism and may also be found in developmental language disorders. Russell et al. (36) concluded that children with autism are challenged by executive tasks because they are unlikely to encode rules in a verbal form.

Weak Central Coherence in Autism

Many years ago, it was noted that autistic persons were relatively adept at solving block design tests and imbedded figure tasks, doing so with even greater skill than shown by typical controls (37). It was proposed that this superior performance might be due to the their use of a local processing strategy coupled with an ability to ignore global cues. Such a strategy might be consistent with their failing to focus on the overall social implications of interpersonal encounters while attending to irrelevant nonsocial cues.

   Although it is not encoded in the DSM-IV, it has been proposed that the term "autism" represents the most severe forms of social communication disorder, while "AD" represents a less severe degree of social communication failure.

A CONCEPTUAL FRAMEWORK FOR TREATMENT PLANNING

The purpose of this chapter is to describe psychosocial interventions for individuals with AD that take into account impaired theory of mind, executive function, and central coherence. Before discussing specific interventions, an overview of expectations of therapy is provided as well as a conceptual framework to consider for treatment planning. When counseling families about outcomes from psychosocial treatments, one should help them develop appropriate and helpful expectations. Research shows that while psychosocial interventions are able to facilitate the person's understanding, skill development, and cognitive beliefs, they are not able to make a person "normal." For example, interventions targeted for social skills are reported as extremely important by parents and often a reason for referral (38). The clinician's task is to educate families in the understanding that although social skill differences are lifelong, social skills can be influenced by environmental input. The most important aspect of a therapeutic relationship is to be an informed clinician first, who understands both the state of the science as well as the limited research behind interventions, and second is to be able to translate this information into efficacious therapeutic services.

   Although AD is a lifelong disability, many adults with AD lead extremely productive, fulfilling, and successful lives. One would ask: "How can an individual such as this be considered 'disabled' or 'handicapped?'" To help sort out answers to this question, a review of terminology is provided. In 1980, The

World Health Organization (39) adopted an international classification of impairment, disability, and handicap, which is proposed to occur along a continuum. Impairment is defined as "any loss or abnormality of psychological, physiological, or anatomical structure or function." Impairment would relate to the diagnosis of AD on the basis of the disordered development of socialization and restricted repertoire of interests. Disability is "any restriction or lack (resulting from an impairment) of ability to perform an activity in the manner or within the range considered normal for a human being." For example, the person with AD is "disabled" when unable to participate in a role or function typically expected, such as a member of a social club at school. Handicap, on the other hand, is similarly defined as "a disadvantage for a given individual, resulting from impairment or a disability that limits or prevents the fulfillment of a role that is normal (depending on age, sex, and social and cultural factors) for that individual." Emphasized in this definition is the concept of "disadvantage." The person with AD is handicapped when not allowed to participate because of the disadvantage imposed by the attitudes or perceptions from others about AD. For example, if a child is excluded from taking part on a little league baseball team because children with AD are not allowed, then the child is handicapped on the basis of the attitude of others rather than the child's actual skill.

Using the WHO definition of impairment, disability, and handicap as a conceptual framework allows for the analysis of the bidirectional influence of the person and the environment, a consideration that is important for setting expectations and developing interventions. It implies that therapeutic strategies are part of the enhancement of environmental supports, which are designed to offset personal challenges or impairments that may result in disability or even handicap (40). Psychosocial interventions take a two-pronged approach: one aimed at the individual and the other directed toward the environment. Interventions that focus on the individual include psychoeducational and developmental approaches, as well as more standard cognitive behavioral methods to address core features that result from impaired development in theory of mind, executive function, and central coherence. Interventions directed toward the environment include psychoeducational consultation with people (family members, teachers, employers) regarding environmental supports for the individual. The ultimate goal is for the individual to be able to participate as fully as possible and achieve maximum potential. To begin to build environmental supports, clinicians must be cognizant of evidence-based practices.

EVIDENCE-BASED PRACTICES

Evidence-based practices refer to "a body of scientific knowledge about service practices . . . or about the impact of clinical treatments or services" (41, p. 1179) on outcomes. The evidence behind a treatment is determined by demonstrating a relationship between the independent variable (treatment) and the dependent variable (outcome). Described as indicators of quality, robustness, or validity of scientific evidence (41, p. 1180), evidence-based practice allows for the comparison of treatments on the basis of the degree of scientific rigor. Typically, a narrowly defined and homogeneous target group is used in such treatment studies (42) as well as comparison groups, randomization procedures, and established outcome measures (41). Studies that are employed within the context of highly controlled conditions such as these are often referred to as "efficacy" studies (43), which are concerned with internal validity and ask the question whether a particular treatment works under optimal conditions.

Much to our chagrin, however, results gained from efficacy studies do not always translate directly to clinical practice. And although efficacy studies are necessary for demonstrating whether a treatment works, such studies are insufficient for demonstrating effectiveness (42,44). Treatment effectiveness, in contrast to treatment efficacy, refers to the clinical utility of a treatment and asks how well a treatment will work within the context of service delivery and under different conditions using less homogeneous participants. Effectiveness research involves issues of external validity, such as generalization to a more broadly defined population, and has varying implementation and levels of participation on the basis of real-world conditions (42). Effectiveness studies must be robust enough to take these factors and other less controlled variables into account. Clinicians have to deal with factors that efficacy research ignores and considers as nuisance variables. Examples include practitioner, client, service delivery, organization, and service system characteristics (44).

Although research support for psychosocial interventions is emerging for individuals with AD (45–54), the amount of evidence available to guide treatment selection and implementation is limited (38,47,55), and a gap in the translation of laboratory-based efficacy studies and effectiveness studies specifically in autism spectrum disorder (ASD) is recognized (56,57). Efficacy studies on social skills groups for individuals with ASD, for example, have been reported (58–63); however, data on "effectiveness" of outpatient social skills groups are limited (56,64). To further complicate matters, as with research on individuals with autism, research on AD is also lacking. Therefore, given the relatively weak distinction between AD and high-functioning autism and the shared overlap of impaired social development and restricted interests, information learned from interventions for individuals with high-functioning autism can be applied to AD (55).

PLANNING PSYCHOSOCIAL INTERVENTIONS

Effective psychosocial interventions are individualized for persons with AD as well as adapted. Because of the limited information available to guide treatment selection and implementation, clinicians who are better able to understand the consequences of impaired theory of mind, executive function, and central coherence are better prepared to create, adapt, apply, evaluate, and monitor psychosocial interventions. These skills are important because research indicates that individuals with AD do not benefit from traditional insight-oriented or talk therapy (55). Further, studies suggest that individuals with AD may not respond to strategies used for individuals with other disorders such as attention deficit hyperactivity disorder (ADHD) (47,65). Instead, evidence does suggest that a more directive approach helps focus the individual on the salient aspects of the targeted skill/concept by breaking down the skill/concept into concrete terms that can be explained visually as well as verbally (45,56). Gresham (66) offers a useful heuristic for the components of social behavior impairments that include social skill deficits, social skill performance deficit, self-control skill deficits, and self-control performance deficits. In additional to behavioral deficits described by Gresham, differences in social cognition and social thinking in persons with AD (55) must be taken into account as well as motivation to learn specific skills . If the person prefers to be solitary, then learning how to get along better with others, how to have conversations, and how to make friends may not be meaningful. Reasons for addressing the targeted skill/concept must be on the basis of the person's interests and motivations and made clear to the person.

Treatment Evaluation

Research suggests that a skill-specific approach is more successful (67) than a more general approach. Therefore, identifying specific skills to target can occur as part of a treatment evaluation. The use of interviews from multiple informants (e.g., parent, child, and teacher), rating scales, and criterion-referenced assessments facilitate goal selection. For social skills, most assessments are standardized and not as helpful in treatment planning or outcome monitoring because they are not broken down to the degree necessary for individuals with AD. Examples of criterion-referenced assessments are available and include the Skillstreaming program (68) and the Treatment and Research Institute for Autism Spectrum Disorders (TRIAD) Social Skills Assessment (TSSA) (69) as examples. Both assessments provide multi-informant rating scales. The TSSA, however, was developed specifically for individuals with ASD and also consists of a multimethod approach. Direct child interactions and parent and teacher report/ratings are included. The direct child interactions involve evaluation of the child's ability to label emotions of self and others and to attribute causes for various emotions; to identify solutions to social problems; to take the perspective of others; and to initiate, respond, and maintain interactions. Skills such as role-playing and using rating scales are also assessed, which is important for treatment strategies. The teacher and parent forms can help evaluate problem behaviors that interfere with friendships, the child's understanding of emotions and perspectives of others, and skills reflecting initiating, maintaining, and responding to others. Research suggests that the multi-informant approach is important because children do not consistently exhibit the same behaviors across environments (70). Examples of parental concerns identified by the TSSA are provided in Table 1. These concerns, which were generated from six parents of children with ASD,

Table 1   An Example of Social Concerns Reported by Parents/Caregivers of Individuals with AD

Conversation skills	Social problem solving/flexibility skills
Have more meaningful relationships	Be more flexible and have less need to have things their own way
Be less blunt during conversations	React less strongly to minor things
Not stand too close to or too far from people during interactions	Be less compulsive about having stuffed objects with them wherever they goes
Be more able (willing) to maintain complex conversations	Have less fear and frustration with people, especially unfamiliar ones
Use socially appropriate behavior during conversations	Be less perfectionist in themselves and others
Stop asking others repeated questions	Be less impulsive
Respond to others in a friendly manner	Stop touching others inappropriately
Spend more time interacting with family, rather than time alone in room	Decrease socially unacceptable behaviors (nose picking, licking hands and arms, etc.)
Learn to talk and listen for equal amounts of time	Decrease compulsive behavior (showering, washing hands)

Abbreviation: AD, Asperger's disorder.

were reported as part of the evaluation and also used to organize the content and outcomes of a social skills group. To establish the group goals, the concerns were analyzed and categorized into two categories: (*i*) increasing conversational skills and (*ii*) increasing social problem solving/flexibility skills.

Choosing a Treatment Approach

After a treatment evaluation/assessment and goal selection, it is necessary to establish specific strategies designed for increasing social cognitive understanding, prosocial behaviors, and other skills identified by the assessment. Because of combined effects of disordered development of theory of mind, executive function, and central coherence, therapeutic techniques must be adapted, individualized, and specific to AD to teach complex skills such as social behaviors (48). No specific single treatment approach is, however, effective for all skills and for all individuals. Instead, a combination of therapeutic methods is suggested. Some methods have more research support than others. Fortunately, several examples of treatment approaches are reported in the literature. Interventions vary according to (*i*) the theoretical underpinnings of the approach (e.g., behavioral, cognitive behavioral, relationship-based), (*ii*) the delivery of intervention (e.g., direct instruction, peer-mediated instruction), (*iii*) the context of intervention, (e.g., school, clinic), (*iv*) the composition of instruction (e.g., individual, group), (*v*) the instructional strategy (e.g., social stories, video self-modeling, social scripts), (*vi*) the age of the participants (e.g., preschool, middle school), and (*vii*) the level of behavior (e.g., micro, molar). For in-depth reviews of therapeutic strategies for social interventions, see Kransny et al. (56), McConnell (71), Odom et al. (72), and Rogers (57).

Further, standard techniques often applied to other populations, such as didactic instruction, role-plays, and feedback, are effective (59) when also accompanied by specific strategies for individuals with ASD. Emerging support for social skills interventions come from several sources (48,49,51). A caution is that individuals with AD have difficulty generalizing information from a clinical context to home, school, and community settings. Treatment plans, therefore, should include activities that address problems with generalization (48,52,73).

Several specific interventions for individuals with AD are reported as successful in increasing prosocial and communication skills as well as decreasing problematic or interfering behaviors. The common element of these interventions is the match between the strategy and the learning style of persons with AD as discussed earlier. Visually depicted information is essential for providing more in-depth definitions or task analysis of the skills (i.e., drawings to depict social situations) that enhance concept learning and application. Visual cuing also serves as a prompt to help the person organize his/her thoughts and initiate interactions. Social stories and comic strip conversations (74) are strategies used to help explain perspectives of self and others. Cognitive scripts (75) assist in teaching the person to initiate and maintain conversations independently, while video self-modeling (76) teaches positive behaviors and reduces unwanted behaviors by allowing persons to view themselves in situations where they are performing at a more advanced level than they typically function. Power cards (77) incorporate special interests of the person with AD as part of the teaching and reinforcement of academic, behavior, and social skills. The common element of all these strategies is that they take into account the need for concrete information that is not abstract and is based on visual learning.

Social interventions may also focus on discrete skills/abilities or on a set of comprehensive skills. Specific skills include self-esteem building (78), self-awareness (79), reading nonverbal body cues and language (59), and understanding emotions (80). A more comprehensive approach focuses on basic interaction skills, conversation skills, play and friendship skills, emotional processing skills, and social problem–solving skills (56,81). An example of a 12-week social skills group or individual curriculum is provided in Table 2.

Three studies, which were conducted within the context of an outpatient clinic setting, were reviewed as examples that most mirror clinical practice (58,82,83). Howlin and Yates (82) reported the outcomes of a social skills group held in a hospital setting over one year. Ten males with autism or AD who were aged between 19 and 44 years (mean age 28.4 years) participated. The overall goals of the program were to increase conversational skills and independence in work and living environments. The group met monthly for 2.5 hours and the agenda for the group was developed during the first session. Initiating and maintaining conversations and problem solving were skills addressed throughout the sessions. Various methods were used to collect outcomes, including self and

Table 2 Example of a 12-Week Social Skills Curriculum

Session	General content
1	"Making friends" (why it is important, how to do it)
	Introduction to "self-monitoring" using problem solving as an example
2	Problem solving (why it is important, the steps involved)
3	Consequences of different solutions
4	Social problem solving including "tattling" and bullying
5	Understanding and expressing emotions (anger, anxiety, and sadness)
6	Social thinking (perspective taking)
7	Compliments and greetings
8	Components that make up conversations
9	Starting and ending conversations
10	Staying on topic during conversations
11	Having conversations: putting it all together
12	Pizza party that incorporates skills

caregiver reports and direct observation. Family members observed improvements in several areas such as conversational and social skills, appearance, self-confidence, independence, decision-making ability, problem-solving skills, and making and keeping friends. The self-report measure also noted improvements. Conversational outcomes were evaluated by coding of videotapes of role-plays. Role-plays consisted of social situations, such as pretending to be at a wedding, and required to introduce oneself to someone and talk to a guest. The other situation consisted of a telephone conversation about an employment opportunity. The coding categories, which were selected on the basis of the skills taught over the year, had good interrater reliability. For conversations during the wedding scenario, a significant change was noted in the percent time initiating or maintaining conversation. For conversations during the telephone scenario, significant changes in percent appropriate responses versus inappropriate utterances were observed.

In the second study, Barry et al. (58) evaluated the effectiveness of a social skills group for elementary-age children with autism in an outpatient psychology department clinic for children with PDDs at a university. Four children aged between six and nine years were recruited. Seven typical peers also were recruited. A licensed psychologist, two graduate students, and one undergraduate research assistant implemented the groups. Several data collection methods were used including standardized and observation tools and parent report. Live coding of greetings, conversation, and play skills was done during five-minute play sessions with a typical peer using a 43-item inventory with good interrater reliability. Weekly phone calls to parents were conducted using the same inventory to assess generalization of skills. Two self-report measures of perception of social support and loneliness were administered. Peer training was also conducted. Treatment consisted of eight two-hour sessions with the children with autism only. Assessment of play skills was included with a typical peer. Parents observed a role-play and received worksheets. Post measures as well as a six-week follow-up obser-vational assessment were collected. Notable improvement in greeting and play skills were found as well as self-report of increased feelings of social support from peers. Parent report identified improvements in greeting skills only.

In the third example, we provide a description of outcomes of a social skills group program delivered in a naturalistic clinical setting (83). Six boys who were clinically referred rather than research-recruited and aged between 9 and 11 years participated in a 12-week intervention. Each session occurred weekly and lasted 75 minutes. Two licensed psychologists, one with expertize in ASD, implemented the group. The curriculum described in Table 2 was applied, and emphasized conversational skills and problem solving skills. Pre- and posttreatment assess-ment tools were selected on the basis of their feasibility; ease of administration, scoring, and interpretation in a clinical setting; sensitivity to treatment effects; and social validity. Improvement in conversational skills was assessed using the method described by Howlin and Yates (82). The boys were asked to role-play a five-minute conversation scenario of meeting a new classmate at school. Improvement in problem-solving skills was evaluated by asking the boys to read a scenario involving being teased or bullied and completing questions regarding the situation (e.g., what was the problem; how did each person think and feel; what are some solutions; what is the best solution). In addition to direct child assessment, parental report was also provided regarding their observations of changes in behavior at home and in the community. Generalization of skills into settings outside the clinic was addressed by allowing the parents to observe the group sessions from behind a mirror and completing a rating scale of the quality of their child's engagement. Children were also required to complete homework assignments outside the clinical setting on a weekly basis. A coder unaware of the content of the intervention coded the conversational role-plays and problem solving questionnaires. At follow up, children were reported by their parents to have improved in 75% of skills observed during the session by the parent. On the basis of coding of direct child behavior, improvements in conversation skills were observed for all areas assessed (getting the person's attention, asking a question or making a statement, and ending the conversation) except for staying on the topic. No changes were observed for topic maintenance. For problem-solving skills, all boys were able to accurately identify problems at baseline. The most noted improvement was in the number of solutions generated for problems. Over half of the boys at the end of the group were able to generate multiple solutions to problems. The following information provides more details on implementing the curriculum used in this study.

For every skill that is addressed, a general, four-step procedure is useful (Table 3) when introducing a topic. First, a Social Story[TM] (53,74,84,85) is used to introduce the importance of the skill from another's perspective. Social Stories provide written information that describes situations, other's perspectives about the situation, skills, and responses. Next, a sorting activity that breaks down the skill into its component parts (i.e., a task analysis) or depicts the correct versus

Table 3 Four-Step Procedure for Skills Teaching

1. Define the skill and explain why it is important
2. Demonstrate what the skill looks like (the right way vs. the wrong way)
3. Perform role-plays demonstrating the skill
4. Provide homework to practice the skills

incorrect way to perform the skill is implemented. The use of picture cards (e.g., pictures from magazines, hand drawings on 3″ × 5″ cards) helps individuals develop a concrete depiction of the positive skill being taught (86). Third, role-plays are used for the specific skill and, when possible, based on issues described by the individual or by parents/significant others. Fourth, homework for skill practice is provided. If parents, caregivers, or significant others are not part of the treatment session, either through observation or as part of family therapy, it is necessary that as much information as possible be shared with them. Because of the significant issues in individuals with AD generalizing information from one context to another, it is necessary that plans for generalization, such as homework and family communication about the session, be in place.

To promote active and attentive engagement during the session, it is helpful that visual schedules and self-monitoring/regulation strategies are used (87). A goal is established at the beginning of the session. If needed, a reward is also identified for goal accomplishment (e.g., answer questions, stay calm).

As mentioned previously, structuring the therapeutic relationship requires a more directive approach (45) wherein expectations of the therapy process and goals are clearly established. Often individuals with AD have significant organizational problems and difficulties following through with assignments or homework. Lack of compliance does not necessarily mean resistance. Explicit examples and assistance with scheduling is needed and often teaching problem solving can be used to identify solutions to disorganization. Bloomquist (88) has examples of handouts that can be used to visually guide the process of problem solving. Goal setting should also be explicit. Because of the difficulty individuals with AD have generating solutions to problems, they often have difficulty conceptualizing the benefit of therapy across many areas (e.g., building relationships, dealing with frustration, etc).

Another unique aspect that must be emphasized when applying cognitive behavior therapy to individuals with AD is that more time often needs to be spent on emotion education and learning the relationships between emotions, thoughts, and behaviors. Although not specific to AD, Bloomquist (88) has several visually aided resources on emotion education and helpful and unhelpful thoughts.

ADDRESSING COMORBID PSYCHIATRIC DISORDERS

Individuals with AD are at risk for comorbid psychiatric disorders (89–91), which includes depression, anxiety, obsessive-compulsive disorder, bipolar disorder, and, to a much lesser extent, schizophrenia (89,92–95). Of the comorbid disorders, depression is reported as the most frequently occurring secondary condition (89).

Emerging research suggests that individuals with AD can benefit from psychosocial interventions, such as cognitive behavioral strategies, to ameliorate anxiety, depression, self-injurious behavior, and obsessive-compulsive disorder (45,50,52,54). The diagnosis of AD cannot be ignored as part of treatment, however, as research also suggests that problems of anxiety or depression may be influenced by the social perceptions and behaviors of individuals with AD (98). Anderson and Morris (45) provided a detailed overview of the strategies to adapt the components of cognitive behavioral therapy for individuals with AD. Modifications include use of visual-based systems as discussed earlier for establishing baseline symptoms and goal monitoring. Such a symptom can be a visual "emotion thermometer." An example of a thermometer that was created by a 10-year-old is provided as part of the case study example later in this chapter (see Figure 1).

FAMILY THERAPY

Family therapy has traditionally meant a clinical intervention, which alters the interaction of family members to benefit a symptomatic member and all other family members. For most, it implies a clinician meeting with all family members and working to understand and alter thoughts, feelings, and behaviors for therapeutic benefit. This restricted definition has given way to a broader, more integrated way of viewing family intervention (99), which now includes psychoeducation, parent management training (100), home services, and the integration of family therapy with psychotherapy and pharmacotherapy (101). There is limited research on family therapy in AD. The multiplicity of ways of intervening with families has precluded studying a specific modality of family therapy.

There is, however, an emerging clinical literature and experience, which gives guidance in working with families (102,103). Some of the literature focuses on the significant management problems when AD is complicated by problematic family dynamics (104). A recent theoretical paper on social attribution processes has implications for family therapy (98). Social attribution refers to ways in which children assign meaning to life events, a process that leads to the internalization of mental representations or social perception. These processes are likely affected by neurological underpinnings of AD, yet this literature supports that they may also be powerfully shaped by family interaction requiring intervention.

Themes in Family Therapy

Many families deal with issues that are common to families with a child with some chronic medical or psychiatric illness. Any clinician working with a family with a member who has AD needs to be aware of these issues to aid their identification and management.

Sadness

Parents can experience sadness, as well as grief, when they observe their child's deficits. The fact that these deficits can be subtle, yet powerfully impact social relationships, makes it all the more difficult. In describing her son's poor social sense, one parent commented, "It makes me sad to see my son 'not getting it'" and seeing this played out in that "He doesn't want to do things with other kids."

Fatigue and Lack of Patience

When children do not respond to parental limit setting, it tests a parent's patience. One parent said, "I ask nicely, repeatedly, but only when I explode will he do what I want. I wish it didn't get to this."

Guilt

At the core of many parents' frustrations is the feeling, often unspoken, that "I don't want to be around my own kid." It is extremely guilt inducing when caring parents are driven to distraction by their child's behavior and have thoughts such as these.

Confusion Regarding Symptoms

The irrational nature of many symptoms of AD makes it difficult for parents to know when to hold their children accountable for problematic behavior. One father's statement, "It goes in one ear and out the other," was complicated by the fact he felt his son had some control over his behavior but was not sure "where this control ends and the Asperger's begins."

Sibling Embarrassment

Siblings are frequently embarrassed by the child's behavior. They are reluctant to have friends around when their sibling with AD is present. Actions such as indiscriminate touching others, perseveration, and poor social sense (e.g., talking within 12 inches of an individual's face) are examples of embarrassment-inducing behaviors.

Acceptance of the Difference

Many parents and families have a constant struggle regarding acceptance of AD. Once they have accepted that their child's behavior is different, these families still must expect some behavioral compliance and responsivity to parental expectations.

MODELS OF FAMILY INTERVENTION

The psychoeducational model, used widely with other major mental illnesses, is the commonest model of family intervention in AD. In this model, parents are supported in dealing with the disorder, given information on treatment, and offered approaches to manage the disorder.

The Anderson family had six children. David, aged 10 years, presented for psychiatric treatment after being diagnosed with a learning disorder and ADHD. Further evaluation revealed that he met criteria for AD. His problems included physical aggression with siblings, perseveration, and the need for sameness in his environment. At home, he was oppositional and aggressive, while at school he withdrew from others. His lack of affective variability led his family to call him "the judge" because he always seemed stern and foreboding. The Andersons' other five children had remarkably good social adaptation. The parents, the father an educator and the mother a nurse, had been married for 19 years. They responded well to instruction in behavioral modification techniques, yet often expressed their frustration over David's inability to "make connections." Family intervention offered support, help to arrange for a respite from parenting David, and educating the other children about his deficits.

Yet, clinical families are often not as well functioning as the Andersons and symptoms of AD induce stress in those less sturdy. Eric Rolland was a 12-year-old, first-born son diagnosed with AD as a three-year-old. One of the first symptoms the family noticed was that he would panic when he would see an exit sign in any building, requiring his parents to remove him from the room. His sister, three years younger, had excellent social skills and commented to her parents that "Eric should have friends over more often." When Eric was seven, his parents amicably divorced; afterward they continued to share a great deal of time with him. His obsessive behaviors, such as always insisting on visiting the same fast food restaurant, drained the family of patience. The family enjoyed humor and father stated, "We laugh as a family but we can't laugh with Eric. He doesn't understand laughter. He thinks every time we laugh, we are laughing at him. He doesn't get it." Mother, on her part, tried to help him with his homework but experienced that "all Eric wants to do is for me to give him the answers."

The Blade family had very different stresses induced by AD. Sam was the second of four children, diagnosed with AD at the age of eight. Marked family conflict, particularly aggressive competition between Sam and his two-year-older brother Mark, led to clinical consultation when Sam was 13. This conflict worsened when his father had to travel frequently for his job. Mother then spent extra time with Sam to facilitate his needs, and this alienated the other children. Father ultimately quit his job and took a salary decrease. He came to see that he needed to support his wife in monitoring many aspects of Sam's care, including multiple school changes and attending school conferences.

The directional influence is not only in the direction of the effect of symptoms on the family. Families do not cause AD, as was once thought with autism, but most assuredly problematic family function can exacerbate the symptoms of AD. Managing a child with AD and dealing with intense family conflict is a potent combination, with the stress of each potentiating the other.

In the Rolland family, an important marital factor leading to parental divorce was Mr. Rolland's lackadaisical attitude toward employment. Eric's mother, who was a hard working insurance agent, angered that his father, an artist, was often unemployed. While good natured and caring toward his son, Mr. Rolland did not financially provide for his family. At times the mother said, "It's like raising three kids." Eric's social attribution was such that he expected his mother to take care of things, just as mother took care of the family during father's frequent unemployment. When Eric was rigid, uncompromising, and resisting mother's request for responsibility, she wondered whether "this was Asperger's disorder" or Eric merely "acting like his father."

The Blade family had significant structural problems. Mr. Blade's absence led Mrs. Blade, a somewhat passive woman, to be indulgent with her children. She had difficulty setting limits, and both Mark and Sam became entitled. Their conflicts led to physical conflict and Mark's entitlement and lack of empathy were associated with critical comments regarding Sam's behavior. When 15-year-old Sam would touch his mother, hug her, and say, "I love you mommy," Mark would mock his immaturity. When the father quit his job and became more involved with the family, his inadequacy and impulsive anger further exacerbated the problematic interactions between his sons.

Therapeutic interventions in these families included directing Mr. Rolland to become more active in family life. He was encouraged to support Eric's mother in expecting more accountability from Eric for his behavior. He ultimately became gainfully employed. Mr. Blade, on the other hand, left his traveling job and was home more often. He became more assertive, took charge of some of his son's behavior, and attempted to be a peacemaker, taking the pressure off Mrs. Blade. Marital work ensued; Sam's mother desired more intimacy and support from her husband from whom she felt estranged, "as a single mother for all those years."

In assessing family dynamics, it is difficult to know when to intervene in interactions deemed problematic or when to educate a family about symptoms of AD. Children with AD who present with social alienation, obsessions, resistance to change, and rages are not easy to parent. Stress in the family may be a response to troubling symptoms and this should be initially assumed. Yet, a careful family evaluation may reveal areas where family distress and functioning leads to a worsening of symptoms. How to determine whether a family is responding to disorder or predisposing to a disorder is a complex evaluation, fully discussed elsewhere (105,106). Some areas that help this delineation include an assessment of parents' knowledge of developmental norms, parental support of each other, success outside the parenting world, and stability of the other children.

CASE STUDIES

Given the frameworks offered thus far for individual, group, and family therapy, case studies are offered, including specific details of therapeutic strategies introduced earlier.

Case Study 1

Bob was diagnosed with AD at the age of seven years by an experienced developmental pediatrician in the area of ASD. Bob had fluent language and average intellectual abilities. He was referred for outpatient therapy for behavioral and social difficulties.

Treatment Assessment

The Collaborative Model for Promoting Competence and Success (COMPASS) framework (40) was used to guide the treatment assessment/planning process (see Table 4). COMPASS is a process approach that assists in identifying inherent strengths and weaknesses as well as environmental supports and challenges that compound or have an impact upon the individual's ability to be resilient in his or her environment. The COMPASS assessment revealed the following information for Bob.

Table 4 Description of Bob's Challenges and Supports

Personal challenges	Personal strengths
Behavioral	• Very interested in rocks
• Accepting "no"	• Knowledgeable about rock types and formations
• Accepting correction	• Affectionate
• Frustration tolerance	• Wants to hang out with peers and have friends
• Transitions/changes in routine	• Likes going to the park
Social	• Listening to music
• Initiating	• Reading
• Responding to social bids	• Computers
• Maintaining interactions	
• Repetitive interests that dominate conversations	
• Reciprocity	
Emotional	
• Worries excessively	
• Obsessive preoccupations	
Sensory	
• Sensitivities to sound and textures	
Environmental challenges	Environmental strengths
• Consistency between people and places	• Is praised verbally
• Noisy environments	• Positive supports used to shape behavior
• Adequate knowledge and information regarding Asperger disorder with faculty at school	• Has a place where he can be alone and uninterrupted
• Kids who tease	• Mom is a strong advocate
	• 60 min of speech therapy a week

Background Information

Parent/teacher priorities. Bob's mom, Mrs. Morris, reported that her major concerns regarding Bob were difficulties in recognizing and expressing his feelings appropriately; social difficulties with regard to initiating and interacting with peers were also reported. Proximity to others was a major issue as Bob often intruded on others' personal space by hugging others inappropriately and appearing to be unaware that he was causing significant discomfort to his communicative partners.

His teacher, Mrs. Simpson reported that her major concerns were Bob's inability to read the body language of his peers and respond appropriately. Bob appeared to be quite desperate in wanting to be accepted by his peers, but was often intrusive, insistent, and oblivious to subtle hints of rejection. In his attempts to be accepted, he often imitated actions of others whom he believed to be popular, often resulting in trouble. Certain classmates took advantage of this vulnerability, teasing him, and setting him up.

Both his parent and his teacher agreed that Bob had difficulty managing and expressing his feelings, which resulted in him having several outbursts a week. Small incidents seemed to set him off leading to full-blown outbursts.

Child Assessment

The TSSA (69) was administered to gain specific information on Bob's affective understanding, social cognitive understanding (perspective taking and problem solving skills), and behavioral skills of initiating, maintaining, and terminating interactions as well as responding to social bids.

Assessment of affective understanding and perspective taking. Bob was shown several pictures of children's faces and given various pictorial scenarios that contained a problem involving two or more people. When shown the pictures, Bob was able to accurately identify the emotions on the children's faces and relate a time when he might have experienced the emotion. When asked what would make a significant other (Mom, Dad, or brother) experience the similar emotion, responses were often tied in with his own behavior; for example, he replied, "Dad is happy when I do well in school." When shown pictures of problem situations, Bob was able to identify most problems and given an accurate account of what thoughts and feelings the characters involved might be experiencing. Generating solutions to the problems appeared to be more of a challenge; for example, if someone younger is being teased, the solution was for the victim to retaliate in a manner that would further escalate the problem situation. Overall, Bob's perspective-taking and problem-solving skills appeared to be limited.

Assessment of preferred activities. This task involved presenting Bob with a list of "things to do" and "places to go" and asking him how much he liked each one (i.e., not at all, a little, a lot). Overall, Bob reported he liked to play board games, sports, build things with Legos, play on the computer, play Nintendo/ videogames, and go to the park. He preferred to do all activities with other kids, indicating motivation for social skills instruction.

Assessment of role-play skills. Role-play skills were evaluated to see if he understood how to do a role-play which is helpful for treatment purposes, as well as to see how well he initiates and responds to others. Bob interacted with the examiner in role-plays that dealt with possible daily interactions. During the role-plays, Bob often avoided greetings going straight to the point; eye contact and direction of facial expressions were not always consistently directed to others. Conversations tended to be on his terms, and he showed very little interest in his partner's interests and themes.

Treatment Goals

The COMPASS evaluation combined with the TSSA revealed two major areas of concern: (*i*) awareness of internal/extrinsic triggers and appropriate expression of his emotions and (*ii*) initiating appropriately with peers and adults.

Treatment Plan

Increasing understanding and expression of emotions. A social story (74) (www.thegray center.org) was used to explain to Bob the importance of expressing emotions appropriately and staying calm. The story started by explaining that it was okay to experience feelings. It clearly indicated what some appropriate alternatives were when Bob got upset, such as breathing and counting or taking a break. The story also described the benefits of staying calm and expressing feelings in appropriate ways such as being able to do better at home and school and being able to make friends easier. The benefits were clearly motivating for Bob as making friends was important to him.

The next step involved construction of an "anger thermometer" (107). An anger thermometer helped Bob in quantifying his emotions and grading it along a continuum visually. It also helped him identify his body responses to various levels of emotion. Becoming aware of his triggers helped him to monitor his responses more effectively. Bob also wrote down what he could do at different levels on his thermometer to calm down. An example of his thermometer (Fig. 1) shows the strategies Bob could adopt given the triggers or stressors in his environment. He was given a number of scripts that would give him the words to use when in the situation such as "I need help" or "I need a break." Next, $3'' \times 5''$ cards were used to depict activities, thoughts, and responses. He sorted the activities on the basis of what was helpful and what was unhelpful as well as what would be a more appropriate alternative/replacement behavior. This activity helped him identify thoughts that triggered a body response and precipitated an action. A visual graphic was also used to show him the relationship between these different concepts (Fig. 2). These activities enhanced Bob's

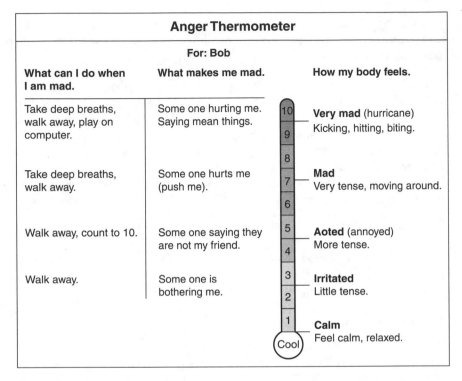

Figure 1 Bob's anger thermometer.

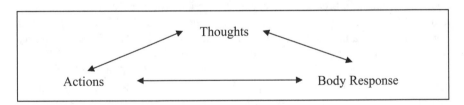

Figure 2 Visual graphic used to demonstrate relationships between thoughts, actions, and responses.

awareness of body responses to triggers and provided a visual cue that helped him visualize his thermometer and choose the appropriate response. Once he realized that thoughts played a major role in how he felt and acted, Bob also participated in activities that helped him identify unhelpful thoughts that triggered certain exaggerated or inappropriate actions. With the help of his therapist, Bob wrote down some typical unhelpful thoughts that he routinely experienced. A common example was "he did it on purpose" which was often retaliated by hitting back. A counter or "helpful" thought was then identified—"this was an accident." Role-play demonstrations helped Bob understand the significance of "helpful" thoughts and their impact on his behavior. Sorting activities that involved sorting "helpful" thoughts from "unhelpful" thoughts helped increase his awareness of thoughts as triggers.

A self-monitoring system was introduced where at regular intervals a parent or teacher checked with Bob if he was calm. The absence of inappropriate reactive responses led to tokens that could be exchanged for a reward. The reinforcements encouraged Bob to respond in a calm manner rather than a reactive manner.

Increasing initiating appropriately. The first step involved explaining through the use of a social story why initiating appropriately was important. The benefits discussed were creating a good impression that would help lead to making more friends. Bob then matched scripts with a variety of adults and peers he knew in his environment. For example, he could greet a classmate with a "Hi" and his teacher with a "Good morning." Other scripts that could be used for initiating in a number of different contexts were also discussed and taught, such as asking to join his classmates at play, asking another classmate to join in his play, offering to share toys or snacks, and offering to help when needed. Visuals incorporating the appropriate body language were used to emphasize eye contact, facial expressions, posture, and proximity to others. The Social Skills Picture book (108) was a resource that was used to give Bob step-by-step instructions on how to successfully initiate within the different contexts.

Several opportunities to practice using role-plays first with a therapist and then other peers within a group setting gave him more confidence to practice in real-world settings. Each role-play was followed by feedback. Bob also had the opportunity to view video recordings of his attempts to initiate where he could observe and discuss how his behavior impacted on others. Right and wrong ways were also role-played to demonstrate the impact each had on making connections with peers. Different scenarios were also modeled for Bob when an attempt to initiate play with another peer was rejected, such as asking someone else.

Bob's teacher continued to have concerns about his proximity to others during greetings. He still greeted his teachers and certain other adults in school with a big hug. A "social circles" visual was used to address this problem. Bob drew his own "social circle." In the middle of the page was his name followed by concentric circles, each circle with a different color. The first concentric circle consisted of "family" which he color coded in blue. He could greet all the people in the blue circle with a hug. The next concentric circle was green, this circle consisted of "best friends;" he could sit next them or pat them on the back. The third concentric circle was yellow, which comprised other classmates and teachers. Bob could greet the folks in yellow with a smile, nod, "high five" or "good morning" but needed to be at arms length from them. The visual depiction clearly indicated whom he could have close proximity with and whom he could not. Teachers and others in his environment were instructed to redirect Bob to the visual social circle if he responded otherwise.

Verbal praise and other material rewards were used to encourage appropriate responses. All therapy sessions were observed by Bob's parents. They played a major role in helping Bob carry over his treatment plan to naturalistic settings, giving him opportunities to practice in real-life settings and making sure his teachers were aware of the strategies in place so that they could help implement them and reinforce accordingly.

Follow-Up

A six-month follow-up with parents and teachers revealed that Bob was consistently initiating appropriately. Teachers reported that hugs were a nonissue, all school personnel and others in his environment were consistently responding to him regarding physical proximity. Outbursts had decreased from a daily occurrence to a couple of times a week. Every time a stressful event occurred, Bob was observed to verbalize to himself the number he was at on his anger thermometer. Occasionally he needed redirection from another adult as to what the number implied that he should do, for example, a six and above meant take deep breaths and ask for a break.

Case Study 2

Dave Fuller was 17 years old when referred to our outpatient program. He had received a diagnosis of AD at the age of 11 years from a local developmental clinic. He was a straight A student, with superior IQ and presented as socially awkward, pedantic, and having trouble with organizational skills.

Treatment Assessment

The COMPASS assessment is summarized below and includes information from Dave, his parents, and teachers (Table 5).

Background Information

Parent/teacher priorities. Dave's parents, Mr. and Mrs. Fuller, reported that their major concern regarding Dave was that he was increasingly becoming a social isolate. Dave was spending much of his time in things that he was good at such as reading, academics, and his volunteer work with the kids. Dave's only friend was his cousin. Unlike other boys his age, he did not hang out with his peers or date and spent nearly all of his time at home after school. Parents were also concerned that Dave relied tremendously on them to get his work done. His dad pretty much took charge of his planner and school calendar and reminded him when his assignments were due and what needed to be completed when.

Dave's teacher spoke very highly of Dave's academic excellence. She was more concerned about his social awkwardness and shyness. Dave never attended any social activity such as school dances or other social events.

Table 5 Description of Dave's Challenges and Supports

Personal challenges	Personal strengths
Behavioral	• Intelligent
• Hard time losing	• Modest
• Planning and organizational skills	• Creative
• Avoids social opportunities	• Plays piano
Social	• Desires to be social
• Socially isolated	• Positive attitude
• Maintaining interactions	• Very polite
• Awkwardness such as fidgetiness	• Helpful
and grimacing during interactions	• Volunteers with children
Emotional	with disabilities
• Anxiety during interactions	• Quick recall team
• Expressing worry about many things	• Chemistry club
Sensory	• Math team
• Sensitivity to noise, crowds,	
and being touched	
Environmental challenges	Environmental strengths
• Not many peers in neighborhood	• Supportive peers in school
• Lack of understanding regarding	• Supportive teachers
Asperger syndrome	• Supportive family
• All male school	• Extended family support
• Does not fit in with majority of peers	• Cousin is a good friend
	• Treatment with anxiolytics

Individual Assessment

The TSSA (69) was administered. Dave was dressed very maturely and appeared to be slightly apprehensive. He was pleasant and friendly throughout the assessment. His use of language was also very mature. Eye contact was adequate. There was a tendency to speak too fast, and Dave was observed to be quite fidgety. Certain odd mannerisms were observed with how Dave used his hands and facial expressions.

Assessment of affective understanding and perspective taking. Dave was shown several pictures of children's faces and picture of various situations that contained a problem involving two or more people. When shown the pictures, he was able to label each emotion presented, tell a time when he had felt the emotion, as well as relate what would cause a significant other to experience the similar emotion. When given the scenarios, Dave was able to identify the problem, explain the possible thoughts and feelings of the people involved, as well as generate multiple solutions to each problem. Overall, he demonstrated good perspective taking and affective understanding skills.

Assessment of preferred activities. Dave reported that he liked to do many activities with friends or family, as well as some alone. With friends, Dave reported enjoying going to a movie, going out to eat, going bowling, and going to a swimming pool. In reality, however, Dave hardly indulged in any of these pursuits with friends.

Assessment of role-play skills. During role-plays, Dave was able to initiate greetings and interactions. Although he was very pleasant, conversations comprised uneasy long pauses. Dave did not contribute very much, neither did he show much interest in the examiner's topic of interest. A strength was his positive response to social bids from others.

Treatment Goals

The COMPASS evaluation combined with the TSSA revealed two major areas of concern: (*i*) planning and organizational skills and (*ii*) reciprocal interactions with peers.

Treatment Plan

Improving Dave's planning and organizational skills. The first step involved having Dave understand the importance of planning and organizational skills and its overall impact on his life. A semantic organizer approach (109) or flow chart was used to illustrate in a concrete manner the implications of planning and organization (Fig. 3). The organizer presented the information in a visual/spatial mode highlighting relationships, sequences, and outcomes.

The next step involved having Dave develop an awareness of what type of environments were most conducive to his learning and what some strategies were that contributed to being organized. It became apparent that Dave was very often caught up in the moment; he would often sit at his computer and research something that piqued his interest for hours, losing all sense of time. His dad often had to redirect him to assignments and tests that were due. Parents were constantly in touch with his teachers and were on top of his due dates. Parents could also access some homework assignments online.

An individualized organization system was developed for Dave along with parent and teacher support. Dave was very motivated to do well in school and go to university to pursue science and psychology; he now understood that planning and organization played a huge role in his academic performance. Rather than relying on his parents for help, he also understood the importance of taking on this responsibility himself.

Since Dave was a visual learner, he did better with information when it was written than when presented auditorily. The first step in this process required Dave to meet with all his teachers individually and write down assignments, tests, and dates in his planner. He then created an assignment folder for each

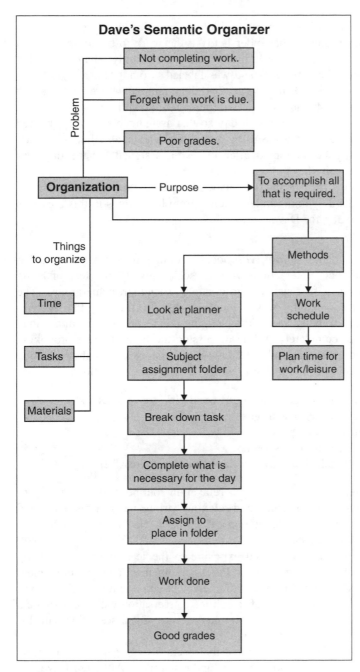

Figure 3 Dave's flow chart for organization.

subject. This folder held assignment guidelines and due dates for the given subject. The front pocket of the folder held all the work to be completed and what he was working on currently and was labeled accordingly. The back pocket held all the completed assignments and was labeled "Completed."

Assignments were broken down so that all assignments were completed at least two days prior to the due date. Dave then wrote down in his planner what amount of work he needed to do each day so that assignments were completed and handed in on the given dates. Surfing on the Internet and all other nonrelated activities could only be attempted after the work assigned for the day was completed and checked off.

His attempts to organize and plan his work were monitored by both parents and teachers. Gradually gaining independence from his parents in this area was intrinsically motivating for Dave.

Increasing reciprocal interactions with peers. A huge roadblock for Dave that got in the way of social interactions was his social anxiety and fear of being rejected or ridiculed. A first step was to create a "social-stress hierarchy." The construction of this hierarchy was a breakthrough for Dave in that he was expressing his fears verbally and acknowledging this to be stressful rather than avoiding the matter completely. While discussing the highest stress-provoking item, he dissolved into tears and it took several sessions to put the hierarchy together. A simplistic version of the hierarchy is presented as follows:

- Attending a dance or party with guys and girls (most stressful)
- Being at a social event with guys and girls
- Hanging out with the guys
- Being introduced to a new peer
- Talking on the telephone with a classmate (least stressful)

The next step involved learning a relaxation routine. Dave learned progressive muscle relaxation, tensing, and relaxing various parts of his body, and began to practice using this technique on a daily basis. He found that deliberate attempts to relax his body calmed him down.

The next step involved graded exposure to the least anxiety-producing stressor and gradually working upwards. Parent involvement and encouragement was much required during this phase of the intervention. Initially, Dave was encouraged to have at least one brief telephone conversation with a classmate a week. During sessions, he began to role-play various social scenarios with his therapist especially on having a reciprocal conversation.

A number of topics were generated that peers his age generally converse about, such as music, sports, video games, and restaurants. Although Dave had no interest in some of these topics, he was required to stay current, show interest, ask questions, and make comments when his communicative partner was on the topic.

Visual cues and modeling was used to demonstrate active listening skills, such as maintaining eye contact, nodding, making comments, and asking questions.

Video self-modeling was a strategy that was used to help Dave identify how he could improve his posture and use of gestures to enhance his conversational skills. He figured that putting his hands in his pockets or holding them behind his back reduced the possibility of fidgeting.

Gradually, new people were introduced to do role-plays with Dave, first a young intern and then other team members. Meanwhile, Dave had moved on to the next step on his anxiety hierarchy and was required to have one social outing a week with his cousin or other classmates at school. Soon, Dave's small network of guy friends began to increase and quite unexpectedly a few girls began to join the social outings. His parents also created opportunities for Dave to meet new friends, including girls from their neighborhood. Dave's mom recalled an incident when she was driving Dave back from school; she stopped to give a female peer who lived in their neighborhood a ride. These tactful opportunities gave Dave more confidence in interacting with his peers. As exposures to anxiety-producing social situations increased, Dave reported decreasing anxiety in these situations. His new confidence and praise from parents were reinforcing to continue exploring social opportunities with peers.

Follow-Up

A two-month follow-up indicated that Dave was independently planning and organizing his work with minimal supervision from parents and teachers. It appeared that the key ingredients to success in this area was becoming aware of what methods and learning strategies worked for Dave. Parent-teacher collaboration was another important factor as well as the additional support from teachers initially to set the plan in motion.

As for increasing reciprocal interactions, Dave enthusiastically reported attending his senior prom with a date. Parents reported that Dave was involved in social outings with his peers at least twice a week.

SUMMARY

Although evidence-based practices in psychosocial treatments for AD are lacking, clinicians are providing an increasing range of mental and behavioral health services to this underserved population. AD is one of the most complex disorders to treat because a combination of theoretical approaches (e.g., developmental, cognitive behavioral) are most likely the most effective. Many clinicians must seek out additional training opportunities in AD to appreciate the unique learning styles and specialized therapeutic approaches for individuals with AD. Examples of therapeutic strategies designed to offset the personal challenges associated with AD as well as a conceptual framework for intervention planning were provided.

Several examples of case studies for family therapy and individual outpatient therapy were also provided.

REFERENCES

1. Barr MW. Some notes on echolalia, with the report of an extraordinary case. J Nerv Ment Dis 1898; 25:21–30.
2. Kanner L. Autistic disturbances of affective contact. Nerv Child 1943; 2:217–250.
3. Wing L. Asperger's syndrome: a clinical account. Psychol Med 1981; 11:115–129.
4. Asperger H. "Autistic psychopathology" in childhood. In: Frith Uta, ed. Autism and Asperger Syndrome. Cambridge, UK: Cambridge University Press, 1991:37–92.
5. American Psychiatric Association. Diagnostic and Statistical Manual of mental Disorders. 3rd ed. Washington, DC: American Psychiatric Association, 1980.
6. American Psychiatric Association. Diagnostic and Statistical Manual of Mental Disorders. 4th ed. Washington, DC: American Psychiatric Association, 1994.
7. Ghaziuddin M, Butler E, Tsai L, et al. Is clumsiness a marker for Asperger syndrome? J Intellect Disabil Res 1994; 38:519–527.
8. Manjiviona J, Prior M. Comparison of Asperger syndrome and high-functioning autistic children on a test of motor impairment. J Autism Dev Disord 1995; 25:23–39.
9. Ehlers S, Nyden A, Gillberg C, et al. Asperger syndrome, autism and attention disorders: a comparative study of the cognitive profiles of 120 children. J Child Psychol Psychiatry 1997; 38:207–217.
10. Klin A, Volkmar FR, Sparrow SS, et al. Validity and neuropsychological characterization of Asperger syndrome: convergence with nonverbal learning disabilities syndrome. J Child Psychol Psychiatry 1995; 36:1127–1140.
11. Eisenmajer R, Prior M, Leekam S, et al. Comparison of clinical symptoms in autism and Asperger's disorder. J Am Acad Child Adolesc Psychiatry 1996; 35:1523–1531.
12. Sevin JA, Matson JL, Coe D, et al. Empirically derived subtypes of pervasive developmental disorders: a cluster analytic study. J Autism Dev Disord 1995; 25: 561–578.
13. Izard C. Innate and universal facial expressions: Evidence from developmental and cross-cultural research. Psychol Bull 1994; 115:288–299.
14. Malatesta C, Izard CE. The ontogenesis of human social signals: from biological imperative to symbolic utilization. In: Fox N, Davidson R, eds. The Psychobiology of Affective Development. Hillsdale, NJ: Erlbaum, 1984:161–206.
15. Field TM, Cohen D, Garcia R, et al. Mother-stranger face discrimination by the newborn. Infant Behav Dev 1984; 7:19–25.
16. Szajnberg NM, Skrinjaric J, Moore A. Affect attunement, attachment, temperament, and zygosity: a twin study. J Am Acad Child Adolesc Psychiatry 1989; 28:249–253.
17. Scaife M, Bruner J. The capacity for joint visual attention in the infant. Nature 1975; 253:265–266.
18. Sorce J, Emde R, Campos J, et al. Maternal emotional signaling: its effect on the visual cliff behavior of 1-year olds. Dev Psychol 1985; 21:195–200.
19. Baron-Cohen S, Tager-Flusberg H, Cohen D. Understanding Other Minds. New York, NY: Oxford University Press, 1993.
20. Sigman M, Capps L. Children with Autism—A Developmental Perspective. Cambridge, MA: Harvard University Press, 1997; pp 34–60.

21. Dissanayake C, Crossley SA. Proximity and sociable behaviours in autism: evidence for attachment. J Child Psychol Psychiatry 1996; 37:149–156.
22. Rogers SJ, Ozonoff S, Maslin-Cole C. A comparative study of attachment behavior in young children with autism or other psychiatric disorder. J Am Acad Child Adolesc Psychiatry 1991; 30:483–488.
23. Sigman M, Mundy P, Sherman T, et al. Social interactions of autistic, mentally retarded and normal children and their caregivers. J Child Psychol Psychiatry 1986; 27: 647–656.
24. Hobson P. The autistic child's appraisal of emotion. J Child Psychol Psychiatry 1986; 27:321–342.
25. Volkmar FR, Sparrow SS, Rende RD, et al. Facial perception in autism. J Child Psychol Psychiatry 1989; 30:391–398.
26. Baron-Cohen S, Baldwin DA, Crowson M. Do children with autism use the speaker's direction of gaze strategy to crack the code of language? Child Dev 1997; 68:48–57.
27. Attwood A, Frith U, Hermelin B. The understanding and use of interpersonal gestures by autistic and Down's Syndrome children. J Autism Dev Disord 1988; 18: 241–257.
28. Baron-Cohen S, Wheelwright S, Spong A, et al. Studies of theory of mind: Are intuitive physics and intuitive psychology independent? J Dev Learning Disord 2001; 5:47–78.
29. Lord C, Rutter M, Le Couteur A. Autism Diagnostic Interview-Revised: A revised version of a diagnostic interview for caregivers of individuals with possible pervasive developmental disorder. J Autism Dev Disord 1994; 24:659–685.
30. Lord C, Rutter M, Goode S, et al. Autism Diagnostic Observation Schedule: a standardized observation of communicative and social behavior. J Autism Dev Disord 1989; 19:185–212.
31. Tanguay PE, Robertson J, Derrick A. A dimensional classification of autism spectrum disorder by social communication domains. J Am Acad Child Adolesc Psychiatry 1998; 37:271–277.
32. Robertson J, Tanguay P, L'Ecuyer S, et al. Domains of social communication handicap in autism spectrum disorder. J Am Acad Child Adolesc Psychiatry 1999; 38: 738–745.
33. Ozonoff S, Strayer DL, McMahon WM, et al. Executive function abilities in autism and Tourette syndrome: an information processing approach. J Child Psychol Psychiatry 1994; 35:1015–1032.
34. Hughes C, Russell J, Robbins TW. Evidence for executive dysfunction in autism. Neuropsychologia 1994; 32:477–492.
35. Liss M, Fein D, Allen D, et al. Executive functioning in high-functioning children with autism. J Child Psychol Psychiatry 2001; 42:261–270.
36. Russell J, Jarrold C, Hood B. Two intact executive capacities in children with autism: implications for the core executive dysfunctions in the disorder. J Autism Dev Disord 1999; 29:103–112.
37. Shah A, Frith U. Why do autistic individuals show superior performance on the block design task? J Child Psychol Psychiatry 1993; 34:1351–1364.
38. Little L. Maternal perceptions of the importance of needs and resources for children with Asperger syndrome and nonverbal learning disorders. Focus Autism Other Dev Disabl 2003; 18(4):257–266.

39. World Health Organization, International Classification of Impairments, Disabilities, and Handicaps: A manual of classification relating to the consequences of disease. Geneva, Switzerland, 1980.
40. Ruble LA, Dalrymple NJ. COMPASS: A parent-teacher collaborative model for students with autism. Focus Autism Other Dev Disabl 2002; 17(2):76–83.
41. Hoagwood K, Burns BJ, Kiser L, et al. Evidence-based practice in child and adolescent mental health services. Psychiatr Serv Sep 2001; 52(9):1179–1189.
42. Glasgow RE, Lichtenstein E, Marcus AC. Why don't we see more translation of health promotion research to practice? Rethinking the efficacy-to-effectiveness transition. Am J Public Health 2003; 93(8):1261–1267.
43. Lonigan CJ, Elbert JC, Johnson SB. Empirically supported psychosocial interventions for children: an overview. J Clin Child Psychol 1998; 27(2):138–145.
44. Schoenwald SK, Hoagwood K. Effectiveness, transportability, and dissemination of interventions: what matters when? Psychiatr Serv 2001; 52(9):1190–1197.
45. Anderson S, Morris J. Cognitive behaviour therapy for people with Asperger syndrome. Beh Cognitive Psychotherapy 2006; 34(3):293–303.
46. Attwood T. The Complete Guide to Asperger's Syndrome. London; Philadelphia, PA: Jessica Kingsley Publishers, 2007.
47. Crager DE, Horvath LS. The application of social skills training in the treatment of a child with Asperger's disorder. ClinCase Studies, 2003; 2(1):34–49.
48. Elder LM, Caterino LC, Chao J, et al. The efficacy of social skills treatment for children with Asperger syndrome. Education and Treatment of Children, 2006; 29(4):635–663.
49. Golan O, Baron-Cohen S. Systemizing empathy: teaching adults with Asperger syndrome or high-functioning autism to recognize complex emotions using interactive multimedia. Dev Psychopathol 2006; 18(2):591–617.
50. Hare DJ. The use of cognitive-behavioral therapy with people with Asperger syndrome: a case study. Autism 1997; 1(2):215–225.
51. Lopata C, Thomeer ML, Volker MA, et al. Effectiveness of a cognitive-behavioral treatment on the social behaviors of children with asperger disorder. Focus Autism Other Dev Disabl 2006; 21(4):237–244.
52. Reaven J, Hepburn S. Cognitive-behavioral treatment of obsessive-compulsive disorder in a child with Asperger syndrome: a case report. Autism 2003; 7(2):145–164.
53. Sansosti FJ, Powell Smith KA. Using social stories to improve the social behavior of children with Asperger syndrome. Journal of Positive Behavior Interventions 2006; 8(1):43–57.
54. Sofronoff K, Attwood T, Hinton S. A randomised controlled trial of a CBT intervention for anxiety in children with Asperger syndrome. J Child Psychol Psychiatry 2005; 46(11):1152–1160.
55. Ozonoff S, Dawson G, McPartland J. A parent's Guide to Asperger Syndrome and High-Functioning Autism: How to Meet the Challenges and Help Your Child Thrive. New York, NY: Guilford Press, 2002.
56. Kransny L, Williams BJ, Provencal S, et al. Social skills interventions for the autism spectrum: Essential ingredients and a model curriculum. Child Adolesc Psychiatr Clin N Am 2003; 12(1):107–122.
57. Rogers SJ. Interventions that facilitate socialization in children with autism. J Autism Dev Disord 2000; 30(5):399–409.

58. Barry TD, Klinger LG, Lee JM, et al. Examining the effectiveness of an outpatient clinic-based social skills group for high-functioning children with autism. J Autism Dev Disord 2003; 33(6):685–701.

59. Barnhill GP, Cook KT, Tebbenkamp K, et al. The effectiveness of social skills intervention targeting nonverbal communication for adolescents with Asperger syndrome and related pervasive developmental delays. Focus Autism Other Dev Disabl 2002; 17(2):112–118.

60. Hwang B, Hughes C. The effects of social interactive training on early social communicative skills of children with autism. J Autism Dev Disord 2000; 30(4): 331–343.

61. Marriage KJ, Gordon V, Brand L. A social skills group for boys with Asperger's syndrome. Aust N Z J Psychiatry 1995; 29(1):58–62.

62. Mesibov GB. Social skills training with verbal autistic adolescents and adults: a program model. J Austism Dev Disord 1984; 14(4):395–404.

63. Ozonoff S, Miller JN. Teaching theory of mind: A new approach to social skills training for individuals with autism. J Austism Dev Disord 1995; 25(4):415–433.

64. Klin A, Volkmar FR, Sparrow SS, eds. Asperger Syndrome. New York: Guilford Press, 2000.

65. Okada S, Goto H, Ueno K. Effect of social skills training including rehearsal of game activities: comparison of children with LD, ADHD, and Asperger syndrome. Jpn Jof Educ Psychol, 2005; 53(4):565–578.

66. Gresham F. Social skills. Conceptual and applied aspects of assessment, training, and social validation. In: Witt JC, Elliott SN, Gresham FM, eds. Handbook of Behavior Therapy in Education. New York, NY: Plenum Press, 1988:523–546.

67. Koning C, Magill Evans J. Social and language skills in adolescent boys with Asperger syndrome. Autism 2001; 5(1):23–36.

68. McGinnis E, Goldstein AP. Skill-Streaming in Early Childhood: Teaching Prosocial Skills to the Preschool and Kindergarten Child. Champaign, IL: Research Press, 1990.

69. Stone W, Ruble L, Coonrod E, et al. TRIAD Social Skills Assessment Manual. Available from: Wendy Stone, Director, Vanderbilt Treatment and Research Institute for Autism Spectrum Disorders (TRIAD), Medical Center South, Nashville, TN.

70. Murray D, Ruble L, Willis H. Congruency between caregiver and teacher report of social skills in children with autism spectrum disorder. (in revision). 2008.

71. McConnell SR. Interventions to facilitate social interaction for young children with autism: review of available research and recommendations for educational intervention and future research. J Autism Dev Disord 2002; 32(5):351–372.

72. Odom SL, Brown WH, Frey T, et al. Evidence-based practices for young children with autism: contributions for single-subject design research. Focus Autism Other Dev Disabl 2003; 18(3):166–175.

73. Frith U. Autism and Asperger Syndrome. Cambridge; New York, NY: Cambridge University Press, 1991.

74. Gray CA, Garand JD. Social stories: improving responses of students with autism with accurate social information. Focus Autistic Behav 1993; 8(1):1–10.

75. Krantz PJ, McClannahan LE. Social interaction skills for children with autism: a script-fading procedure for beginning readers. J Appl Behav Anal 1998; 31(2): 191–202.

76. Buggey T. Video self-modeling applications with students with autism spectrum disorder in a small private school setting. Focus Autism Other Dev Disabl 2005; 20(1): 52–63.

77. Keeling K, Myles BS, Gagnon E, et al. Using the power card strategy to teach sportsmanship skills to a child with autism. Focus Autism Other Dev Disabl 2003; 18(2):105–111.

78. Myles BS, Simpson RL. Understanding the hidden curriculum: an essential social skill for children with youth with Asperger syndrome. Interv Sch Clin 2001; 36: 279–286.

79. Bock M. SODA strategy: enhancing social interaction skills of youngsters with Asperger syndrome. Interv Sch Clin 2001; 36:272–287.

80. Attwood T. Strategies for improving the social integration of children with Asperger syndrome. Autism 2000; 4(1):85–100.

81. McAfee J. Navigating the Social World: A Curriculum for Individuals with High-Functioning Autism and Asperger Syndrome. London: Jessica Kingsley, 2001.

82. Howlin P, Yates P. The potential effectiveness of social skills groups for adults with autism. Autism 1999; 3(3):299–307.

83. Ruble L, Willis H, Crabtree V. Social skills group therapy for autism spectrum disorders. Clinical Case Studies (in press).

84. Adams L, Gouvousis A, VanLue M, et al. Social story intervention: improving communication skills in a child with an autism spectrum disorder. Focus Autism Other Dev Disabl 2004; 19(2):87–94.

85. James L. Review of writing and developing social stories: practical interventions in autism. Child Lang Teach Ther 2004; 20(3):328–329.

86. Baker JE. Social Skills Training for Children and Adolescents with Asperger Syndrome and Social-Communication Problems. Shawnee Mission, KS: Autism Asperger Publishing Company, 2003.

87. Laurent AC, Rubin E. Challenges in emotional regulation in asperger syndrome and high-functioning autism. Top Lang Disord 2004; 24(4):286–297.

88. Bloomquist ML. Skills Training for Children with Behavior Disorders: A Parent and Therapist Guidebook. New York, NY: Guilford Press, 1996.

89. Ghaziuddin M, Weidmer Mikhail E, Ghaziuddin N. Comorbidity of Asperger syndrome: a preliminary report. J Intellect Disabil Res 1998; 42(4):279–283.

90. Gillberg C, Billstedt E. Autism and Asperger syndrome: coexistence with other clinical disorders. Acta Psychiatr Scand 2000; 102(5):321–330.

91. Kim JA, Szatmari P, Bryson SE, et al. The prevalence of anxiety and mood problems among children with autism and Asperger syndrome. Autism 2000; 4(2): 117–132.

92. Clarke DJ, Littlejohns CS, Corbett JA, et al. Pervasive developmental disorders and psychoses in adult life. Br J Psychiatry 1989; 155:692–699.

93. Nilsson EW, Gillberg C, Gillberg IC, et al. Ten-year follow-up of adolescent-onset anorexia nervosa: Personality disorders. J Am Acad Child Adolesc Psychiatry 1999; 38(11):1389–1395.

94. Tantam D, ed. Asperger Syndrome in Adulthood: New York, NY: Cambridge University Press, 1991.

95. Tonge BJ, Brereton AV, Gray KM, et al. Behavioural and emotional disturbance in high-functioning autism and Asperger syndrome. Autism 1999; 3(2):117–130.

96. Attwood T. Framework for behavioral interventions. Child Adolesc Psychiatr Clin N Am 2003; 12(1):65–86.
97. Barnhill GP. Social attributions and depression in adolescents with Asperger syndrome. Focus Autism Other Dev Disabl 2001; 16(1):46–53.
98. Meyer JA, Mundy PC, van Hecke AV, et al. Social attribution processes and comorbid psychiatric symptoms in children with Asperger's syndrome. Autism 2006; 10(4):383–402.
99. Diamond G, Siqueland L. Current status of family intervention science. Child Adolesc Psychiatr Clin N Am 2001; 10(3):641–661.
100. Mabe PA, Turner MK, Josephson AM. Parent management training. Child Adolesc Psychiatr Clin N Am 2001; 10(3):451–464.
101. Sprenger DL, Josephson AM. Integration of Pharmacotherapy and family therapy in the treatment of children and adolescents. J Am Acad Child Adolesc Psychiatry 1998; 37(8):887–889.
102. Lozzi-Toscano B. The "dance" of communication: counseling families and children with Asperger's syndrome. The Family Journal 2004; 12(1):53–57.
103. Stoddart KP. Adolescents with Asperger syndrome: three case studies of individual and family therapy. Autism 1999; 3(3):255–271.
104. Pozzi M. A three-year-old boy with ADHD and Asperger's syndrome treated with parent-child psychotherapy. J of the British Association of Psychotherapists 2003; 41(1):16–31.
105. Josephson AM. Family therapy. In: Lewis M, ed. Child and Adolescent Psychiatry: A Comprehensive Textbook. 3rd ed. Philadelphia, PA: Lippincott Williams & Wilkins, 2002.
106. Josephson AM. Practice parameter for the assessment of the family. American Academy of Child and Adolescent Psychiatry. J Am Acad Child Adolesc Psychiat 2007; 46(7):922–937.
107. McAfee J. Navigating the Social World. Arlington, TX: Future Horizons, Inc., 2002.
108. Baker J. Social Skills Training for Children and Adolescents with Asperger Syndrome and Social-Communication Problems. Shawnee Mission, Kansas: Autism Asperger Publishing Company, 2003.
109. Coyne P. Organization and time management strategies. In: Fullerton A, Cstratton J, Coyne P, et al., eds. Higher Functioning Adolescents and Young Adults with Autism. Austin, TX: Pro-Ed; 1996.
110. Gray CA. Social Stories and Comic Strip Conversations with Students with Asperger Syndrome and High-Functioning Autism. In: Schopler, E., Mesibou, G., Kunce, L., eds. Asperger Syndrome or High Functioning Autism. New York, NY: Plenum Press, 1998.

15

Prognosis of Asperger's Disorder

Saurabh Aggarwal
*Vascular Biology Center, Medical College of Georgia,
Augusta, Georgia, U.S.A.*

Jennie Westbrook
*Department of Psychiatry and Health Behavior, Medical College of Georgia,
Augusta, Georgia, U.S.A.*

Maria E. Johnson
*BrainScience Augusta and Developmental Disability Psychiatric
Consultation-Liaison, Gracewood Hospital, Augusta, Georgia, U.S.A.*

INTRODUCTION

The prognosis of any pathological condition and the factors that influence it are of great value for its proper management. However, many diagnosed with Asperger's disorder and autism spectrum disorder do not consider their condition pathological (1), and may define outcome differently.

Very little is known about the outcome of Asperger's disorder and no specific guidelines have been laid that may help improve the outcome substantially. Further, few studies address what the patients themselves desire for their own outcome. Currently, the study of outcome is based on parameters such as *education, occupation, self-reliance and independence, criminality*, and *psychiatric comorbidity*. These are discussed in detail below.

HIGH-FUNCTIONING AUTISM VS. ASPERGER'S DISORDER

High-functioning autism and Asperger's disorder are highly similar because of overlapping symptoms. Some use IQ as the basis for differential diagnosis, while others use linguistic abilities. Because of the similarity in clinical picture, differential diagnosis is difficult. In studies of outcome they are usually grouped together as more able individuals within the autistic spectrum. Therefore, the data from various studies on individuals with high-functioning autism may be used to assess the outcomes in individuals with Asperger's disorder.

EDUCATION

Data regarding educational qualifications among individuals with Asperger's disorder seem to be quite diverse, and it is difficult to predict the exact possibility of an individual to attend mainstream schools or complete higher education. Let us start by reviewing the data for education from long-term follow-up studies:

Rumsey et al.: From a group of 14 cases [diagnosed with autism on the basis of *Diagnostic and Statistical Manual of Mental Disorders-Third Edition* (DSM-III), with an IQ more than 80], five (35.7%) had attended high school and two attended junior college (2).

Szatmari et al.: Out of 16 cases of autistic children with a mean IQ of 92 (range 68–110), 50% of the children attended special school. The other half attended mainstream school and later attended college or university, with 44% of them obtaining a degree (3).

Howlin et al.: Out of the 19 high-functioning adults, almost half had attended special schools and only three (15%) had attended regular/mainstream schools. Two completed college and obtained diplomas. One person attended university (4).

According to the Maudsley study (5), out of the 68 autistic children with an IQ of 50 or more, 10 attended mainstream schools, 29 (43%) attended special autistic institutions, 9 (13%) attended institutions for children with general learning disabilities, and 16 (24%) attended other special educational institutions. Fifty-three (78%) did not attain any formal educational qualifications. Thirteen children obtained educational qualifications, out of which two obtained diplomas (1 in accounting and 1 in design), two obtained degrees in science or computing, and two completed postgraduate courses (5) (Table 1).

It is quite evident that a considerable number of individuals attended special educational institutions, and only a small fraction of them attended mainstream schools. This may seem paradoxical because special education is recommended only in cases where the child has grossly impaired social skills.

According to Stephan Bauer (6), a developmental pediatrician at the Pediatric Development Center of Unity Health in Rochester, New York, children with Asperger's disorder progress well in the early years of education. He feels that their success in *elementary school* may be due to the fact that they are good

Table 1 Follow-Up Studies Comparing the Level of Education Attained by Individuals with Childhood Diagnosis of Autism or HFA

Follow-up study	N	Diagnosis	IQ	Schooling	Junior college/ college
Rumsey et al. (1985)	14	Autism (DSM-III)	>80	36% main stream schools	14%
Szatmari et al. (1989)	16	Autism	68–110	50% special schools 50% main stream schools	50%
Howlin et al. (2000); Mawhood et al. (2000)	19	HFA	Average performance IQ 93 Average verbal IQ 67	50% special schools 15% main stream schools	10.5% college 5% university
Howlin et al. (2004)	68	Autism (ADI)	≥50	80% special schools 15% main stream schools	10% higher degrees

at memorizing information and are able to develop strong calculative skills. Rote learning is considered an area of strength in children with the disorder. These children may have a problem in developing writing skills/ability. Although they may show some social interest in their peers, there always will be some degree of impairment in social interaction. Children with Asperger's disorder may find it difficult to make friends and keep them. Children tend to be "loners" and may show some traits of obsessive behavior related to their restricted areas of interest.

Dr. Stephan Bauer (6) also feels that the children may face maximum difficulty during the *middle school* period. Problems are mainly related to social skills and not to academic performance. Peer pressure is high, and they try to fit in socially but lack the appropriate skills. Other children may fail to understand their behavior and may tease or bully them. Problems in school may be one of the factors that attribute to high incidence of depression in adolescence in individuals with Asperger's disorder.

As evident from the data listed above, few individuals with the syndrome may attend higher educational institutions. These students usually are highly focused with circumcised interests. Sometimes these narrow intense interests may even be to the extent of an obsession. Such high focus on a narrow spectrum of interest helps these individuals to excel in their areas of interest and outperform their peers. They develop a high level of logic, which makes them very proficient in their field of interest. Case studies have revealed that individuals with Asperger's disorder may be highly gifted people and may go on to become scientists, mathematicians, philosophers, musicians, computer science experts, or even university professors (7).

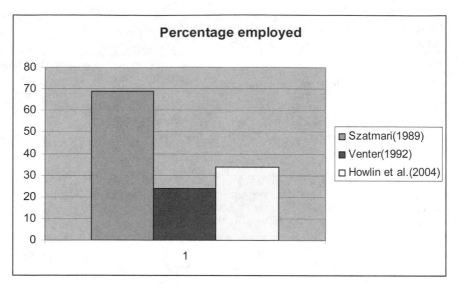

Figure 1 Comparison of the rate of employment among individuals with Asperger's disorder according to different studies.

OCCUPATION/EMPLOYMENT (Fig. 1)

Individuals with Asperger disorder may be employed in a wide variety of fields. The Maudsley study (5) on high-functioning autistic individuals included the following; an individual employed in an oil company, a scientific officer, an electric worker, a cartographer, a postal assistant, factory workers, a grave digger, office/accounts assistant, charcoal burner/gardener, an administrative assistant, a supermarket trolley worker. Other studies also have individuals working in multiple fields.

Studies have researched three types of employment possibilities for individuals with Asperger's disorder:

- Competitive
- Supported
- Secure or sheltered

Competitive employment has no special support system at work and is considered the most independent type of employment. This also includes self-employment or running one's own business.

Supported employment is when the individual is provided with a support system, which allows one to earn a living in a regular work environment. The person may be a part of a team or may work individually on a position specially created for the individual. The job levels are usually higher than the secured or sheltered jobs.

Secured or sheltered jobs have facility-based settings, and individuals usually undergo preemployment training prior to job placement.

Some of the data available provide us with a rough estimate of the rate and the type of employment among individuals with Asperger's disorder.

Szatmari et al. followed up 16 individuals and observed that two people were unemployed, four were in sheltered workshops, three were studying, one worked in family business, and six were in full-time employment. Jobs included sales persons, factory worker, library technician, librarian, and physics tutor (3).

Venter et al. (8) and Lord and Venter (9): Out of the 58 cases they studied, 14 individuals had found jobs. Two had lost jobs later. Jobs were mostly of low level.

Larsen and Mouridsen: Out of the nine individuals in the Asperger group, one individual worked as an insulator although he was a trained gardener, one worked as a driver for several years, then in the fishing industry. At the age of 33 he claimed a disability pension. Four other patients had worked in the labor market as fully paid unskilled workers; currently all were on disability pension. Two patients worked in sheltered card-board box factories. One was put on disability pension when the factory was closed down. The other subject lost his mother and was admitted to a psychiatric institution and did not continue to work further (10).

Howlin et al.: Out of the 68 autistic individuals with an IQ of 50 or more, a total of 23(1/3) were employed. Eight individuals worked independently, one was self-employed, and fourteen individuals worked in supported/sheltered employment. One individual had worked at a factory earlier but was currently unemployed. The cases were followed up by Hutton as a part of a separate study. Hutton observed no increase in the number of people working independently. In fact two individuals who were in independent jobs had shifted to supported employment (1 in accounts, 1 in computing), one individual had resigned and was unemployed, another individual initially working for his father had left the job and was unemployed. The income was poor and a majority of the subjects were in sheltered schemes or occupational programs (Fig. 1) (5).

We may conclude from the multiple data given above that the unemployment rate is relatively high in adults with high-functioning autism/Asperger's disorder. Most of the jobs are acquired through family contacts, mainly parents and not through competitive job markets, and majority of the individuals work in sheltered schemes or occupational programs.

One of the reasons for the high rate of unemployment among these individuals may be lack of workplace accommodations for the special needs of individuals with Asperger's disorder. Decreased educational qualification and low scores on standardized tests may contribute. These individuals may also find it difficult to secure jobs because of poor interview skills. Those who are able to find jobs may be unable to keep them because of social and communication difficulties.

SOCIAL FUNCTIONING

Various researchers have documented improvement in communication and social functioning in individuals with Asperger's disorder or high-functioning autism. In a two-year follow-up study Peter Szatmari et al. noted that children with Asperger's had improved their socialization scores and had fewer autistic symptoms since enrollment (11). Sigman and McGovern felt that individuals with high-functioning autism showed some improvement in cognitive ability and social functioning with age, provided there was early intervention. However, some degree of social impairment does persist throughout their life span. They may be able to maintain relationships with family and friends but may find social interaction difficult (12). Rumsey followed 14 men and none of them were married and all continued to have problems related to social interaction. Only one subject had friends, maintained through his church (2). Szatmari et al. found that 56% of the study group had never experienced a sexual relationship. Only 1 out of 4 of the subjects had dated (13).

According to Larsen and Mouridsen, out of the nine individuals in the Asperger group only two (22%) were married. One of his patients had been married for 19 years and had four children. The other patient had been married for 20 years and had two children. There were two patients who had been married but were divorced later. One had been divorced after 15 years of marriage and the other after seven years of marriage (10).

According to Howlin et al., out of the 68 autistic individuals with an IQ of 50, very few had close sexual relationship. Three were married, out of which one was divorced later. A large majority of the group (56%) had no friends or acquaintances (5).

As evident from data above, individuals with Asperger's disorder may marry but the numbers vary. The low rate of marriage may be attributed to impaired social interaction and dating or a choice to remain single. At times these individuals may decide to get married without dating or the courtship period. Marriage usually does not last long and divorce rates are very high. Some individuals with Asperger's disorder tend to be emotionally aloof, making the social obligations of marriage more difficult or undesirable.

RESIDENTIAL STATUS (Fig. 2)

According to majority of the studies, individuals with Asperger's disorder continue to live with their parents or in supervised living arrangement. In these studies, only some achieved complete self-reliance and lived independently without support. According to Rumsey et al., out of the 14 men that he observed, 6 lived with their parents, 2 lived in supervised apartments, and 1 lived alone (2). In a different study of 16 cases, 10 lived with parents, 5 lived independently, and 1 lived in a group home (13).

Larsen and Mouridsen presented a slightly different picture. Out of the nine cases in the Asperger group, five (56%) had their own homes. Only two

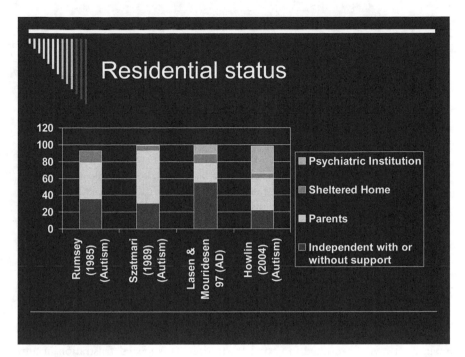

Figure 2 Comparison of the residential status.

lived with their parents and one lived in a psychiatric institution (after his mother expired, with whom he was residing initially) (10).

According to Howlin et al., out of the 68 autistic individuals with an IQ of 50 or above, 3 (4%) lived independently with limited parental support, 4 lived in semisheltered hostel-type accommodation with support, 26 (38%) lived with parents, 14 (20%) lived in specialist autistic provisions, 12 lived in residential settings with little independence, and 8 lived in hospital settings. Data was unavailable for one person (5) (Fig. 2).

FORENSIC PROBLEMS

There is little evidence that criminal offending is increased in Asperger's disorder. Individual case studies (14–18) show a special relationship between the disabilities of Asperger's disorder and certain forms of criminal offending. A large case-control study did not show an increased rate of criminal offending in Asperger's disorder (19), though arson was significantly associated with the diagnosis (19).

Individuals with Asperger's disorder are usually law-abiding citizens, but certain features of the syndrome such as social deficits and obsessive traits could predispose some individuals to criminal offending (5).

Social Disability and Naiveté

People with Asperger's disorder may not understand the social consequences of their actions and may be unaware of the harm their actions may cause the other person (20). Also, individuals with Asperger's disorder may be vulnerable to exploitation by others due to their social naivety (20), and may get involved in criminal offending unknowingly.

It has been accepted by the courts in some cases that the nature of being unable to assess social situations and appreciate another's point of view may be the main cause for criminal behavior (17). In this way individuals with Asperger's disorder who commit certain crimes may be unfit to stand trial and not be criminally responsible though they are not psychotic (17). However, it is important to recognize that in other cases, the unusual idiosyncrasies of a crime may be related to the pervasive developmental disorder (PDD), but the antisocial act was not the result of the PDD (16).

Murrie and colleagues discussed the problems related to interpersonal naivety that may cause these individuals to seek contact through inappropriate ways. For example, in one case, an individual thought that buying a big house would lead to marriage. Murrie also wrote about sexual problems being common; out of six cases, five had sexual problems. He felt that these individuals were unable to get into a relationship and even if they did they were unable to maintain it, which resulted in sexual frustration. This sexual frustration in turn may have caused these individuals to commit sexual crimes (21).

Obsessionality

Obsessionality is another feature of concern, which may perpetuate these individuals to commit crimes such as stalking and compulsive thefts (20). Obsessions with poisons, chemicals, and fire settings may involve these individuals in criminal offenses. Several cases related with arson have been reported in literature (22,23).

Haskins et al. presented theory of mind deficits and preoccupation as two main factors that may predispose these individuals to crime. These theory of mind deficits and preoccupation when combined with social impairment may perpetuate these individuals to commit crime (24). Sometimes a comorbid condition such as attention deficit hyperactivity disorder (ADHD), commonly seen in Asperger's disorder, may be responsible for violent impulsive behavior (20).

Haskins et al. feels that a clearer picture may emerge in the future, as more and more forensic clinicians learn to correctly identify Asperger's disorder (24). There have been several instances when these individuals have been mistakenly diagnosed with various other psychiatric conditions. Hare and colleagues (25) examined 1305 criminal offenders in a special English hospital. Of these 2.4% individuals met the criteria for autism spectrum disorders, but only 10% of the group had been previously diagnosed. Most of the autism spectrum disorders discovered by researchers had been previously misdiagnosed as schizophrenia.

Case Studies

Various cases of violence in individuals with high-functioning autism (HFA)/ Asperger's disorder have been reported. Baron-Cohen (26) described the case of a 21-year-old individual with Asperger's syndrome who had repeatedly attacked a 71-year-old woman whom he called his girlfriend. Mawson et al. (27) reported a man who had violent fantasies and a unique interest in poisons. He was obsessed with the idea of finding a girlfriend and attacked a woman because he did not like her wearing shorts; in another case he attacked a woman with a screwdriver because he did not like woman drivers. He had also attacked babies because he did not like the noise of crying. It is possible that this individual committed these crimes in part because of a lack of understanding of the other person's point of view.

Prevalence of Criminal Offending

We cannot base our conclusions on case studies. To know the exact rate/prevalence of criminal offending in Asperger's disorder, we need a large-scale epidemiological study that involves the total population. At present, we do not have data from such a large-scale study.

Studies in Secure Settings

Scragg and Shah established the prevalence of Asperger's syndrome and autism among the male offenders at Broadmoor Special Hospital in the United Kingdom. Out of a total of 392 offenders, they identified three cases of autism and six cases of Asperger's syndrome, which gave them a prevalence rate of 1.5%–2.3% (28). Scragg and Shah later compared these rates, which were higher than the prevalence rate of Asperger's syndrome in the general population calculated at 0.7% (29). The authors therefore concluded that there was a link between Asperger's syndrome and criminal offending. However, since the study involved a highly selective group in a specialized setting, the results cannot be the basis for any conclusion.

Ghaziuddin et al. reviewed 132 reports of individuals with Asperger's syndrome to determine the link of the disorder with criminality. Out of the 132 cases, only 3 (2.3%) individuals were found to have a clear history of violent behavior. The result obtained was much lower than the figure of 7% who commit violent crimes in the 20 to 24 age-group in the United States (30).

Siponmaa et al. conducted a retrospective study of prevalence of child neuropsychiatric disorders in young offenders. They focused their attention on the patients in the 15 to 22 age-groups who were consecutively referred for presentence forensic psychiatric investigation in Stockholm. A total of 126 individuals were evaluated and a retrospective diagnosis was made, 3% of the total group of offenders matched the DSM-IV criteria for Asperger's syndrome (31).

The studies above seem to contradict each other, Scragg and Shah (28) concluded that there was a link between Asperger's disorder and criminal offending, whereas Ghaziuddin et al. (30) reported the reverse. Scragg and Shah (28) used a highly selective group of individuals for their study, which lowers the credibility of their result.

PSYCHIATRIC PROBLEMS

The increased prevalence of comorbid psychiatric conditions among individuals
with Asperger's disorder likely worsens outcome for those individuals affected.
Please see chapter 4 for information on comorbidity. Figures 3, 4, and 5 summarize
the findings of psychiatric problems in three outcome studies (10,32,33).

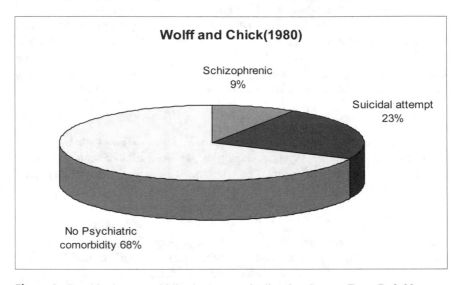

Figure 3 Psychiatric co-morbidity in Asperger's disorder. *Source*: From Ref. 32.

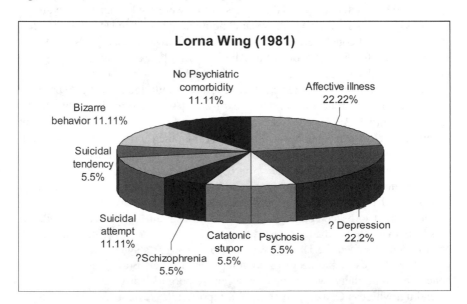

Figure 4 Psychiatric co-morbidity in Asperger's disorder. *Source*: From Ref. 33.

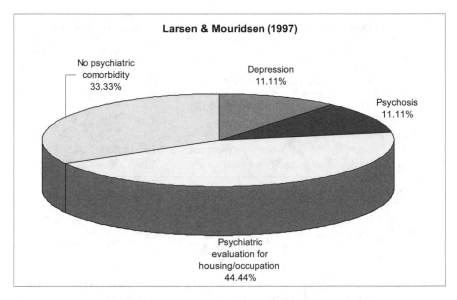

Figure 5 Psychiatric co-morbidity in Asperger's disorder. *Source*: From Ref. 10.

AUTISM VS. ASPERGER'S DISORDER AND THE PREDICTORS OF THEIR OUTCOME

Researchers have tried to ascertain the factors that may influence the outcome or may be used as the predictors of outcome. One such study in this regard is by Peter Szatmari et al. (11). He studied a group of children of four to six years under treatment at the Pervasive Development Disorder Center. Forty-six children with autism and twenty children with Asperger's syndrome were identified on the basis of an IQ test and a diagnostic interview. The children were then administered a set of cognitive, language, and behavioral tests. After a gap of two years the tests were readministered and the results then compared. It was observed that children with Asperger's syndrome showed improvement in social skills and a reduction in autistic symptoms as compared with the children with autism. The researchers, however, were unable to explain the difference in the outcome of the two groups on the basis of IQ or language skills.

Later Szatmari et al. did come to the conclusion that the outcome for the two groups may be different. The predictors, however, of outcome may differ or be the same. He also concluded that early language skills and nonverbal skills were good predictors of outcome later in adulthood (34).

Another important study in determining the predictors of outcome is the Maudsley study (5). They followed 68 individuals (61 males, 7 females) diagnosed with autism confirmed by Autism Diagnostic Interview (ADI) with an IQ of 50 and above, first seen at the age of seven (range 3–15 years); age at follow-up was 28 years (range 21–48). The study showed very good outcome in 12%,

Table 2 Comparison of the Outcome of Follow-Up Studies Based on Study Group IQ[a]

Follow-up study	Group characteristic	IQ	Very good/ good	Fair	Poor/ very poor
Rumsey et al. (1985)	$N = 14$ Autism (DSM-III)	>80	44%	56%	0%
Szatmari et al (1989)	$N = 16$ Autism	68–110	25%	50%	25%
Larsen and Mouridsen (1997)	$N = 9$ Autism	<70	22%	11%	67%
	$N = 9$ Asperger syndrome	>70	33%	45%	22%
Howlin et al. (2004)	$N = 68$ HFA (ADI)	≥50	22%	19%	58%

[a]Predictors of outcome in HFA/Asperger's syndrome.
1. High stability of IQ.
2. Verbal and nonverbal skills.
3. Social competence.

good outcome in 10%, and fair outcome in 19% of the cases. Forty-six percent showed poor outcome and twelve percent, very poor out come.

According to this study individuals with an IQ of 70+ have better outcome, but *IQ was not a consistent factor in determining the outcome*. The study said that some adults with an IQ of 100+ may not function as well as individuals with a much lower IQ of about 70. The predictor of outcome was mainly a high stability of IQ over time. There were high correlations between the child's IQ and social/language abilities. Improvement in communication was seen generally, with time. Forty percent of the subjects who had no language ability when assessed initially at an average age of seven years (3–15 range) were able to develop communication skills over time. IQ and language were not the only predictive factors responsible, rituals/stereotyped behavior and anxiety problems also had a major impact on the outcome in some of the cases (Table 2).

Although results are highly variable for different studies, we may conclude that individuals with Asperger's disorder or the ones with higher IQ have better outcome (35,36) compared with the Autistic group or the ones with low IQ.

INTERVENTIONS

Children with Asperger's disorder have normal or above normal intelligence, and every effort should be made to include them in the mainstream system of education. Teachers need to make an extra effort toward understanding the problems and complexities associated with Asperger's disorder and various principles that may be helpful in managing them.

According to a study conducted by Donna M. Fondacaro (37) where she observed 12 students (10 boys and 2 girls) in the age-group of 8 to 13 years diagnosed with Asperger's disorder, a small teacher to student ratio was the most successful academic intervention, and behavioral modification along with a positive teacher attitude was the most successful behavioral intervention. Higher educational institutions also have taken some positive steps for inclusion of individuals with various forms of pervasive developmental disorders, which also includes Asperger's disorder. Education is a stepping-stone to self-improvement and self-reliance; therefore its importance cannot be undermined.

The important question that arises is how to improve the employment prospects for these individuals? An important study in this regard is a two-year supported employment scheme conducted by Mawhood and Howlin (38), specifically designed for individuals with high-functioning autism and Asperger's disorder. Their aim of the project was to analyze the effectiveness of the supported employment scheme regarding:

- Job placement
- Participant satisfaction
- Cost benefits

The supported group had 30 participants (27 males, 3 females) and the control group consisted of 20 participants (males). After detailed information was obtained for each individual in the supported group, a suitable job was identified. Once employed, these individuals were provided with a full-time support worker for the first two to four weeks, and the assistance was usually tapered off with time; however assistance was available whenever required. The support workers provided their clients with appropriate work-related assistance so that these individuals could perform the tasks related to their jobs successfully. The support workers also supervised and trained these individuals so that they could avoid socially inappropriate behavior at work. They also educated and informed the employers and coworkers how to cope with any potential problems that may occur and how best to avoid such situations.

The results were as follows, over a period of two years, 19 (63%) individuals in the supported group found paid employment out of which three individuals had two jobs each. A total of 22 jobs were found in the supported group. Only five (25%) individuals had found jobs in the control group. The number of hours worked per week did not differ much for both the groups. The mean wage for the supported group (5.71 British pounds) was higher than the mean wage for the control group (4.14 British pounds).

The supported group had a better outcome with regard to the level of jobs acquired. Individuals in the control group had jobs that were mostly of low level, with only one person with an administrative/clerical job, whereas majority of the individuals in the support group had clerical and administrative jobs.

Most of the employees in the study were satisfied and acknowledged the fact that they could not have managed without the support system. It is also interesting to note that the employers were satisfied with the standard of the work. Problems that occurred were not job related or due to professional incompetence but instead mainly due to impaired social functioning.

Although the supported employment program did show promising results for individuals with Asperger's disorder, the program was a very expensive one and job finding was the most costly aspect of the scheme.

Mawhood and Howlin concluded from the overall positive outcome of the study that there was a need for a specialist supported employment scheme. Many individuals who had previously never been employed were able to procure paid employment with the help of the program. The existing system of the disability employment service did not cater to the need of people with high-functioning autism and Asperger's disorder. Many of the people that had been listed with the service had been unable to find jobs for long periods, and many of those who had found jobs eventually were not satisfied with the level of their jobs (38).

The following points from the supported employment scheme by Mawhood and Howlin may help improve the employment prospects for individuals with Asperger's disorder.

- Assistance is usually required by these individuals for finding an appropriate job. At present there is no program being run that specifically caters to the need of the individuals with high-functioning autism and Asperger's disorder. Individuals may contact state employment offices or various social service organizations for this purpose. Family support and expert guidance are definitely of great value in finding the right job.
- The jobs should be meticulously matched after a detailed study of the individual's abilities and limitations. Whenever possible a visit to the job site and meetings with the potential employers should be arranged to analyze the skills required for the job and the obstacles that the individual might face at work.
- Once employed, these individuals should be provided with support workers or job coaches. Initially the assistance should be on a full-time basis, which may be reduced or completely withdrawn with time as per individual requirements.
- Support workers/job coaches are important for the successful employment of these individuals. They teach their clients the skills required for the job. They also educate the employers and colleagues about the potential problems that they might face with their client. This helps avoid misunderstandings and creates a healthy working environment (38).

CONCLUSIONS

These studies of prognosis reveal a wide range of decreased likelihood for employment, independent residential status, higher education, and marriage. Criminality does not appear increased, but when it does occur the social and obsessional disabilities of Asperger's disorder may or may not contribute to the crime. Psychiatric disorders appear to be increased; some of this increase may be secondary to the problems of different social behavior.

People with Asperger's disorder have the capacity to make valuable contributions to society through their unique intelligence (39). In future studies of outcome it will be important to listen to the patients' stated goals (40). Further work will help improve interventions and design accommodations to increase the capacity of the patients and society to interact productively.

REFERENCES

1. Brownlow C, O'Dell L. Constructing an autistic identity: AS voices online. Ment Retard 2006; 44(5):315–321.
2. Rumsey JM, Rapoport JL, Sceery WR. Autistic children as adults: psychiatric, social, and behavioral outcomes. J Am Acad Child Psychiatry 1985; 24(4):465–473.
3. Szatmari P, Bartolucci G, Bremner R, et al. A follow-up study of high-functioning autistic children. J Autism Dev Disord 1989; 19(2):213–225.
4. Howlin P, Mawhood L, Rutter M. Autism and developmental receptive language disorder—a follow-up comparison in early adult life. II: Social, behavioural, and psychiatric outcomes. J Child Psychol Psychiatry 2000; 41(5):561–578.
5. Howlin P, Goode S, Hutton J, et al. Adult outcome for children with autism. J Child Psychol Psychiatry 2004; 45(2):212–229.
6. Bauer S. Online Asperger's Syndrome Information and Support (O.A.S.I.S). 2006. www.udel.edu/bkirby/asperger/as_thru_years.html.
7. Baron-Cohen S. Is asperger syndrome/high-functioning autism necessarily a disability? Dev Psychopathol 2000; 12(3):489–500.
8. Venter A, Lord C, Schopler E. A follow-up study of high-functioning autistic children. J Child Psychol Psychiatry 1992; 33(3):489–507.
9. Lord C, Venter A. Outcome and follow-up studies of high functioning autistic individuals. In: Schopler E, Mesibov GB, eds. High Functioning Individuals with Autism. New York: Plenum Press, 1992:187–200.
10. Larsen FW, Mouridsen SE. The outcome in children with childhood autism and Asperger syndrome originally diagnosed as psychotic. A 30-year follow-up study of subjects hospitalized as children. Eur Child Adolesc Psychiatry 1997; 6(4):181–190.
11. Szatmari P, Bryson SE, Streiner DL, et al. Two-year outcome of preschool children with autism or Asperger's syndrome. Am J Psychiatry 2000; 157(12):1980–1987.
12. Sigman M, McGovern CW. Improvement in cognitive and language skills from preschool to adolescence in autism. J Autism Dev Disord 2005; 35(1):15–23.
13. Szatmari P, Bartolucci G, Bremner R. Asperger's syndrome and autism: comparison of early history and outcome. Dev Med Child Neurol 1989; 31(6):709–720.
14. Kohn Y, Fahum T, Ratzoni G, et al. Aggression and sexual offense in Asperger's syndrome. Isr J Psychiatry Relat Sci 1998; 35(4):293–299.
15. Milton J, Duggan C, Latham A, et al. Case history of co-morbid Asperger's syndrome and paraphilic behaviour. Med Sci Law 2002; 42(3):237–244.
16. Toichi M, Sakihama M. Three criminal cases with Asperger's disorder: how their handicap was reflected in their antisocial behaviors. Seishin Shinkeigaku Zasshi 2002; 104(7):561–584.
17. Katz N, Zemishlany Z. Criminal responsibility in Asperger's syndrome. Isr J Psychiatry Relat Sci 2006; 43(3):166–173.
18. Schwartz-Watts DM. Asperger's disorder and murder. J Am Acad Psychiatry Law 2005; 33(3):390–393.

19. Mouridsen SE, Rich B, Isager T, et al. Pervasive developmental disorders and criminal behaviour: a case control study. Int J Offender Ther Comp Criminol 2008; 52(2):196–205.
20. Berney T. Asperger syndrome from childhood to adulthood. Advan Psychiatr Treat 2004; 10:341–351.
21. Murrie D, Warren JI, Kristiansson M, et al. Asperger's syndrome in forensic settings. IAFMHS; 1:59–70.
22. Everall IP, LeCouteur A. Firesetting in an adolescent boy with Asperger's syndrome. Br J Psychiatry 1990; 157:284–287.
23. Barry-Walsh JB, Mullen P. Forensic aspects of asperger's syndrome. J Forensic Psychiatr Psychol 2004; 15(1):96–107.
24. Haskins BG, Silva JA. Asperger's disorder and criminal behavior: forensic-psychiatric considerations. J Am Acad Psychiatry Law 2006; 34(3):374–384.
25. Hare DJ, Gould J, Mills R, et al. A Preliminary Study of Individuals with Autistic Spectrum Disorder in Three Special Hospitals in England. London: National Autistic Society, 1999.
26. Baron-Cohen S. An assessment of violence in a young man with Asperger's syndrome. J Child Psychol Psychiatry 1988; 29(3):351–360.
27. Mawson D, Grounds A, Tantam D. Violence and Asperger's syndrome: a case study. Br J Psychiatry 1985; 147:566–569.
28. Scragg P, Shah A. Prevalence of Asperger's syndrome in a secure hospital. Br J Psychiatry 1994; 165(5):679–682.
29. Ehlers S, Gillberg C. The epidemiology of Asperger syndrome. A total population study. J Child Psychol Psychiatry 1993; 34(8):1327–1350.
30. Ghaziuddin M, Tsai L, Ghaziuddin N. Brief report: violence in Asperger syndrome, a critique. J Autism Dev Disord 1991; 21(3):349–354.
31. Siponmaa L, Kristiansson M, Jonson C, et al. Juvenile and young adult mentally disordered offenders: the role of child neuropsychiatric disorders. J Am Acad Psychiatry Law 2001; 29(4):420–426.
32. Wolff S, Chick J. Schizoid personality in childhood: a controlled follow-up study. Psychol Med 1980; 10:85–100.
33. Wing L. Asperger's syndrome: a clinical account. Psychol Med 1981; 11(1):115–129.
34. Szatmari P, Bryson SE, Boyle MH, et al. Predictors of outcome among high functioning children with autism and Asperger syndrome. J Child Psychol Psychiatry 2003; 44(4):520–528.
35. Starr E, Szatmari P, Bryson S, et al. Stability and change among high-functioning children with pervasive developmental disorders: a 2-year outcome study. J Autism Dev Disord 2003; 33(1):15–22.
36. Cederlund M, Hagberg B, Billstedt E, et al. Asperger syndrome and autism: a comparative longitudinal follow-up study more than 5 years after original diagnosis. J Autism Dev Disord 2008; 38(1):72–85.
37. Fondacaro D. Asperger Syndrome and Educational Interventions: A Series of Case Studies. Chester, PA: Center for Education Widener University, 2001.
38. Mawhood L, Howlin P. The outcome of a supported employment scheme for high-functioning adults with autism or Asperger syndrome. Autism 1999; 3(3):229–254.
39. Asperger H. Die 'Autisitic Psychopathen' im Kindesalter. Arch Psychiatr Nervenkr 1944; 117:76–136.
40. Aylott J. Understanding and listening to people with autism. Br J Nurs 2001; 10(3): 166–172.

16

Two Case Studies

Donna L. Londino

Department of Psychiatry and Health Behavior,
Medical College of Georgia, Augusta, Georgia, U.S.A.

INTRODUCTION

What a privilege it has been to work with this intriguing syndrome since its inclusion in the Diagnostic Statistical Manual, 4th revision (DSM-IV) in 1994. Through the years, I have seen the interest in and knowledge about this disorder expand in an exponential fashion. Most assuredly, this has contributed to some extent to the increased incidence and prevalence of the disorder in the United States. I received my first referral of an individual with Asperger's disorder in 1996 from a local adult psychiatrist who "had never heard of Asperger's syndrome." Neither had I, but, as a young passionate second-year resident with aspirations of becoming a child and adolescent psychiatrist, I agreed to see this person. Thus began the development of a fervent passion in my clinical and research career that opened up the opportunity for numerous subsequent referrals for evaluation and treatment. Outcomes have been varied and are often dependent upon access to resources, supportive collaboration from the school system, parent advocacy, and commitment to treatment. There has been no greater joy than to witness those individuals with Asperger's disorder that have finally obtained their goals as adults and no greater frustration than confronting obstacles that impede the optimal potential that some could achieve. Two particular cases are outlined below and encompass issues commonly seen for individuals seeking treatment and providers delivering care. Details of the first case have been modified to protect confidentiality. Details of the second case are provided with the informed consent of the individual.

CASE 1

> *"Anxiety, Depression, Frustration, and Anger. The Four Horsemen*
> *of the Mental Apocalypse have plagued me long enough."*

A young adult was referred after a provisional diagnosis made by psychological evaluation and testing requested by the family in an attempt to identify causes of his academic struggles during field rotations in his postgraduate training. Cognitive testing revealed a superior intellect, but with notable strengths in areas of acquired knowledge rather than problem solving or reasoning (Kaufman FSIQ: 128; crystallized IQ: 136; fluid IQ: 112). Always a brilliant student in primary and secondary school, he was ridiculed severely for his lack of compliance with social fashion. His naivete predisposed him to cruel teasing, and his awkwardness and excessive preoccupation with trivia, game shows, and Japanese anime impaired any sustained social relationships with peers his own age. His clumsiness precluded rewarding participation in most team sports. At times, reportedly weary of "having to work so hard," he would become very dysphoric and frustrated. An insightful early revelation was, "I don't seem to know what I need to do to fit in with other people."

Self-stated treatment goals for the patient were as follows:

(Anyone who has provided care for an individual with Asperger's syndrome will appreciate the context.)

- "Work on anxiety, depression, frustration, and anger. The Four Horsemen of the Mental Apocalypse have plagued me long enough."
- "Keep pressures from overwhelming me."
- "Talk less about me, listen, but do not be aloof or nonattentive when not listening."
- To complete graduate school and obtain a job.

Treatment goals as defined by the family were as follows:

- "Fit in better with society, even though he may not be exactly the same as other people."
- "Have peace with himself, especially when 'life isn't fair'. Accept personal limitations."
- "Improve social and communication skills."
- "Apply gray areas instead of seeing things in black and white."
- "Appreciate those accepting him and disregard those rejecting or shunning him."
- "To be skillful enough to complete his degree."

Over the course of the following six years, treatment goals were accomplished. Pharmacotherapy was limited and targeted the identified mood symptoms of depression and anxiety as well as anger outbursts when frustrated. Education on the diagnosis, implications, and management was beneficial for all involved. This included me as the provider, the family, and other systems that ultimately had to be informed for optimal outcome. Individual and group therapy predominantly focused on social skills training. Interventions including directions to hold a clinical update until in the office (instead of the hallway), instructing the patient to limit his use of Clint Eastwood impersonations, and teaching the appropriate use of hugs decreased social oddity and rejection. Social coaching used techniques as simple as responding *yes* or *no* to the appropriateness of observed behavior or accurateness of practiced behavior during structured scenarios.

Education and advocacy facilitated completion of his graduate degree. Three initial job disappointments resulted in the decision to tell the fourth employer. With knowledge of the disorder, this employer modified the work schedule to early evenings to avoid the more rapid pace of daytime business. He also keeps job assignments structured and consistent. The benefit to the employer is an employee who is always on time and excessively conscientious about his work.

CASE 2

"Though I try to be heard seen and accepted I am left alone still."

An adolescent female was referred for evaluation of depression thought secondary to social deficits that had pervasively interfered with the development of friendships. Anger outbursts were problematic at times and mother feared that these occasions might lead to safety risks for her daughter or others. Initial impressions of a female presenting without any makeup or concern for teenage fashion, persistent failure to achieve age appropriate relationships, poor eye contact, social ineptness, and circumscribed interests in wolves and baseball suggested a diagnosis of Asperger's disorder (much rarer in females than in males). Mother and daughter both reviewed the written literature about the diagnosis and noted that "for the first time in their life, they felt that they knew what was wrong." Treatment began with the implementation of pharmacotherapy to target severe dysphoria and irritability. In addition, she was started in individual therapy and referred to my adolescent social skills group. Group therapy was beneficial in normalizing her social deficits by meeting other teenagers with the disorder. In addition, role-play assisted with her ability to better engage in conversations. Anger management targeted more adaptive ways of handling her loneliness and perceived rejection from others (see attached her poem and a drawing of her favorite interest).

Ongoing treatment demonstrated mild to moderate improvement of dysphoria even with relatively poor compliance with medications (sensitivity to side effects, resistance to pharmacotherapy). School support was only fair, and treatment was compromised throughout by financial constraints in the family. She was able to complete coursework to obtain a high school graduate education degree (GED), but has only received partial postgraduate education through Internet college courses. She has yet to be successfully employed in part secondary to her limited motivation in actively seeking a job or completing any employment applications. This is complicated by her lack of self-confidence and perception of failure in other aspects of her life.

As a young adult, her treatment has been compromised by an inability to receive any adjunct financial or health care assistance. The state in which she resides has failed to acknowledge her disorder of Asperger's as criteria for disability and have not deemed necessary requests for assistance for vocational training or evaluation. Her intellectual ability has been utilized as reason to deny assistance despite her consistent demonstration of an inability to sufficiently acquire employment and, in some instances, understand the subtle nuances of providing for her own care and certainly her financial needs independently. She continues to reside with her mother and struggles with severe bouts of depression.

ENDING REMARKS

These cases are representative of clinical aspects of the syndrome and underscore the struggles that these individuals confront as they try to understand the syndrome itself and then work to adapt in educational and vocational systems as well as social relationships. The cases and information presented in this book confirm the need for a continued greater understanding of the etiology, treatment, and prognosis of the disorder. Even more importantly, they represent the absolute importance of a multidisciplinary approach that individualizes treatment on the basis of a person's unique strengths and weaknesses and mandate a charge for advocacy by the families and providers of these wonderful self-defined "neuroatypicals."

17

Social Assimilation in the Classroom

Jeanne Rausch

Columbia County Public School System, Evans, Georgia, U.S.A.

The implementation of the Individuals with Disabilities Education Act (IDEA) and No Child Left Behind (NCLB) Act has revolutionized the way students with disabilities are educated in the United States. Children with disabilities of various types are no longer excluded from mainstream education. Under IDEA, students with special needs must be placed in the least restrictive environment for their education. IDEA brought about the practice of inclusion, a strategy whereby the majority of students with special needs are placed in regular education classrooms in which the teacher coteaches with a special education teacher.

Although students with severe handicaps are still placed in self-contained special education classrooms, most special education students, including those with Asperger's disorder, are now being educated in the regular classroom. Regular education teachers in schools that practice full inclusion must be awar of the new strategies for educating students with special needs.

Having students with Asperger's disorder in the regular classroom creates new opportunities for teaching tolerance and sensitivity toward people who are "different." The regular education students' perception of those with Asperger's disorder is complicated by the lack of clearly discernible physical symptoms seen in some other disorders often found in the classroom, such as Down syndrome. Also, the behavioral symptoms in Asperger's disorder are not immediately apparent. Without solid physical manifestations and often only subtle behavioral symptoms, many of the regular education students may not realize that an autistic student has a disability. The regular education students may simply write that student off as being strange or socially inept. Therefore, it is important to take great efforts in the classroom to encourage sensitivity when a student with Asperger's disorder says or does something inappropriate or unusual.

For example, one student insisted in the pedantic speech that is characteristic of Asperger's disorder (in his case, a voice also quite hypernasal and monotonic) that NASA could not get into space because "the moon was in the way." Explanations that space shuttles could simply steer around the moon could not convince him otherwise. His only consolation was that someone could perhaps drill a hole through the moon, providing astronauts a safe passageway into space. This explanation satisfied him; however, both he and the teacher observed snickers and rolling eyes in the other students. Although they may not notice subtle social cues, children with Asperger's disorder can tell when they are being mocked. He was absent the following day, affording the opportunity to explain to the other students the importance of respecting all people, regardless of their capabilities or behavior.

Many of the teaching strategies that work best for students with Asperger's disorder are fortunately becoming more prevalent in classrooms as they benefit regular education students as well. Engaging the five senses is recognized to improve learning in these students. Teachers now try to engage as many of the students' senses as possible during a lesson. Students do not only hear directions for an assignment—teachers may write them on the board, have students repeat them, and practice the task before performing it. This repetition is beneficial for students with Asperger's disorder who need multiple cues. A growing trend is that of differentiated instruction, which involves teaching the same material in several different ways to appeal to as many learning styles as possible. Teachers who practice differentiated instruction are more likely to have success with students of all disabilities, including Asperger's disorder.

Despite the progressive teaching techniques that are improving the classroom for all students, teaching students with Asperger's disorder can provide its share of logistical problems. Providing a structured learning environment is important for all students, but students with Asperger's disorder need more predictability than regular education students—they thrive with routines. One student had an extreme penchant for consistency. If the desks were rearranged in the room, or the schedule failed to follow the usual daily routine, he panicked and ran to the guidance counselor. Despite efforts to maintain as consistent an environment as possible for the sake of all students, the occasional change to the classroom arrangement or schedule cannot be avoided. However, good preparation could circumvent any anxiety on this particular student's part. With a few days' advance warning that the bulletin board would be changed, or that an assembly that would interrupt the regular routine, he had some time to adjust and handled the changes with relative ease.

Unfortunately, situations such as inconsistency that tend to stress children with Asperger's disorder cannot always be prevented. It is important for educators to designate a "safe place" for their students, a place where they can go if they suffer an outburst or meltdown, where they can calm down before returning to the classroom. The guidance counselor's office is usually a good place for this. Students with Asperger's disorder respond best to a calm, patient voice, so it is essential that a student's safe place have an adult who will treat him or her with respect and understanding. It is also important for the teacher to note what may have triggered the student's anxiety to prevent future problems.

Despite their need for consistency, organization tends to be a problem for students with Asperger's disorder. They may not be able to handle the responsibility of a locker and a notebook for each class. Teachers may have to get one three-ring binder for a student to keep all of his or her work in for every class. It is important for a teacher or parent to go through this binder daily to ensure that papers are placed in the proper section. Making this practice a routine will help the student to maintain a level of organization. Students with Asperger's disorder may also need two sets of textbooks, one to keep in the classroom and one to keep at home. Any effort to streamline the amount of paperwork for which a student has to be responsible will be beneficial.

Just as students with Asperger's disorder are inquisitive, inquisitiveness on the teacher's part is an important skill in working with these students. One student, for no apparent reason, would begin screaming, growling, and stabbing his pencil into his desk. Immediately chiding his inappropriate behavior and sending him into the hallway to calm down did not prevent such occasions from occurring again. After repeated outbursts, the teacher asked him why he was getting so upset. He explained that he had been attempting to twirl his pencil on his fingers unsuccessfully and kept dropping it on the floor. Frustrated with his failure to perform this little trick, he reacted in a way that he did not understand was inappropriate. His disability apparently complicated the process of teaching him the appropriate response to frustration. Interestingly, a simple explanation that if he stopped trying to twirl his pencil he wouldn't drop it had more effect. The explanation was satisfactory for him, and he never had another outburst, at least not for that reason. Again, approaching the issue with a calm, patient voice was essential to success in changing this child's behavior. However, teachers must be aware that the student may not always be able to verbalize his or her emotions or pinpoint the source of stress. For this reason, close observation of the student's behavior is important.

A more severe case of Asperger's disorder can result in nearly nonexistent communication skills and an appearance of complete disconnection from the classroom environment. With this extreme disconnection, prompting may be required to do any and all work. Even the simplest tasks take quite a long time to perform. For example, one student involves himself with class discussion only when it pertains to a movie. Mentioning anything that reminds him of a film he has seen results in an expression of a litany of facts about that movie. It is common for students with Asperger's disorder to display extreme interest in one subject. Because it is such a strong motivator for him, tailoring his assignments to something that will relate to a movie is effective. For example, while other students were writing persuasive essays, he designed an advertisement for his favorite movie.

This final example illustrates that combining the teacher's social skills with the unique gifts of spontaneity, honesty, and specialized knowledge in Asperger's disorder can result in a joyful learning experience. The class activity before Christmas vacation was to write letters to the troops overseas.

A few suggestions as to what to write to the troops were provided to the students. These included hopes for a safe holiday and thanks for their service. Sitting with this particular student, prompting him to write, the teacher asked him to write what he hoped for the soldier. The type of frank naïve honesty seen in Asperger's disorder can be misinterpreted as disrespectful. In this case, the teacher's social awareness, that same awareness that does not come naturally to those with Asperger's disorder, advised her that it was more prudent to keep his letter. His letter read, "Have a Merry Christmas. I hope you don't die."

Into my Soul: A Kaleidoscope of an Aspergian Spirit. Amen.

John Smith Boswell

Medical College of Georgia, Augusta, Georgia, U.S.A.

ASPBERGER'S

"Aspberger's ... Aspberger's syndrome."

"Amen ... Ahh-a-men Ahh-a-men Ahh-a-men Ahh-a-men Ahh-a-men Ahh-a-men. ...

Stop eating your ass burger ... I am not through singing ... Ahh-a-men Ahh-a-men Ahh-a-men Ahh-a-men Ahh-a-men Ahh-a-men Ahh-a-men Ahh-a-men Ahh-a-men Ahh-a-men Ahh-a-men Ahh-a-men Ahh-a-men Ahh-a-men Ahh-a-men Ahh-a-men Ahh-a-men ... *stop*!!!"

The first paragraph is what we silently said to ourselves after our visit to the doctor who proclaimed this syndrome upon us. The latter paragraph is us singing "Ahh-a-men" at a very young unknown age after the family mealtime blessing. Woe to anyone who touched his or her food before the singing was done. No warding could curtail our wrath over that. The last "*stop*" is just what we can only imagine how our family got us to stop singing so they could eat their meal in peace with precious silence. My mother has told me we went through no less than 23 Ahh-a-mens before the family was finally able to start eating. Each Ahh-a-men probably took between three to five seconds of endurance. We are told this is called echolalia, the use of repeating words, an autistic/Aspergian trait.

Nomenclature and its effects on society always fascinate us. You will want to pay very close attention to every single word that I use and its symbolic meaning. The simple choice of using predominately the third person form *we*instead of *I,* until now, might send our doctors who read this running through a maelstrom of thoughts. I now hope that is so, and I do have some idea what those thoughts might be. It is too much fun using your imagination to be more than one person. The sentence fragment, "Grounded in reality" is very foreign to this me. I do not seek any other psychological labels of firmity or infirmity, as you may choose to see it. Asperger's syndrome is enough for this me and probably more than I want aside from my four-letter MBTI (Myers Briggs Type Indicator) profile of INFP (Introverted INtuitive Feeling Perceiving type logic), the idealistic philosopher.

The mind and its decision-making process are universally known as a life mystery. Yet, for humans, there is one fallacy of thought in its ability to deal with the external perception of reality. Our minds take shortcuts through creating dichotomies. The very act of classifying with nomenclature makes us fail to investigate further our reality perception. The investigation itself, however scientific and thorough, should be never-ending, but we make conclusions. A fish is a fish, a dog is a dog; Spot is a dog and Sally is a human. A person might argue with me that the classification system is hierarchical, but the mental shortcut still exists. Stop. You are an Aspergian. *Stop*!

At this point, the mind has already made assumptions as to what you really are, without ever even interacting with you. It is my belief that this is a very dangerous mental fallacy, although not one that is foreseeably surmountable. I think, for a short time, I became more Aspergian-like after this label was stamped into my mind. Our thoughts determine our reality perception, and Asperger's syndrome became more of my reality for a short time after this label was achieved.

METAPHYSICS AND ASTRAL PROJECTIONS

I am an irreligious, but very spiritual, spirit. I enjoy Max Lucado's story, *The Wemmicks,* but a part of my spiritual experience derives from NLP (neuro-linguistic programing) and some of the mirroring philosophies of the German philosopher, Immanuel Kant. One of the tenets of NLP is that we never really know reality; we only know the reality that is represented to our mind through our five senses, touch, taste, hearing, smell, and sight. An example that Bandler and Grinder use is that a bee has a different sensory organization than that of humans. Does this make one sensory perception of this nomenclature that we call reality wrong? No. Both perceptions are different, just as Aspergians are different from normal, extra-bland humans. For this Aspergian, there are 11 sensory modalities, instead of the classic five. The first five, I divide into internal and external sensory perceptions. The external sensory perceptions are those that we gather from our environment. The internal sensory perceptions are those that we create in our mind. Artists, musicians, and Aspergian thinkers like me have a tendency to respond more to the internal sensory modalities. One of my favorite questions to an artist or musician is: "Do you ever see colors that you cannot paint or hear sounds that you cannot replicate because they just do not exist in the external world?" I know for me, my spirit often feels textures, tastes flavors, hears sounds, smells smells, and sees colors in the mind that I believe to be impossible to replicate in the external world. This completes the realm of the five internal modalities of internal touch, taste, hearing, smell, and sight and their contrarian five external sensory perceptions of the same type.

EGO LOGIC

Cosmopolitan thinkers like Wayne Dyer explain this well. Ego logic is the base of humanity, acting in a survival and predatory mode. It is the part of us that seeks the dichotomies of the mind so that it can classify itself as better than and in the realms of having more. At its bases level, ego logic only satisfies the lowest level of Maslow's need hierarchy, the survival needs of food and shelter.

Group Ego Logic

Group ego logic is ego logic on steroids and involves a group of individuals acting on their self-interest. Often, there is one charismatic individual or a small group of individuals who determine the ego agenda. Group ego logic may be a reason I have spurned participation in organized religions and large political and social groups. For an Aspergian, it is usually challenging enough dealing with one other ego at a time.

HARMONIOUS NIRVANA OR JEET KUNE DO SPIRITUALITY

When I meditate, I flip the switch to an off position of all the sensory perceptions that flood my spirit through the shell of this corporeal body, both internal and external perceptions. For this me, the ability to sense inspiration through tuning out the entire sensory perception of reality is the 11th and most important sensory perception. There is no change where no representation of reality exists. I believe this is a mirror of Lau Tzu's thoughts on Taoism.

TODDLER LOGIC—THE DINOSAUR IS ON THE PORCH

My family took a camping trip while I was just learning to speak. I waddled off with my sisters onto a hill. My father shouted, "Bear in the woods." My sisters came running back screaming, "Bear in the woods." I came back shouting, "Dinosaur ... Dinosaur ... on the porch ... on the porch."

RELATIONSHIPS AND ROMANTIC INTEREST

While growing up, people were never my first priority, and I still think this statement is true. In kindergarten, I would eat my lunch and then stare out the window at other kids playing. I had my first and last girlfriend in first grade, a girl named Crystal. Officially, it lasted a full day, as my older sisters' teasing put a stop to my desire to mention that to the family. Unofficially, Crystal was my first grade quartz jewel . . . Check yes or no? *Yes.* There is something I love about the innocence of youth that keeps things simple, and there are absolutely no sexual prowess pressures involved as there are as in adulthood. When I was shamed by others for urinating in the trashcan at the back of the classroom because my bladder and knowledge of the toilet betrayed me, at the end of the day, Crystal was still my friend. Today, at age 29, I question whether adults of the opposite sex can really be this thing people call "just friends." I know that I have no women like Crystal in my life now, and no man or woman calls me for an emotional friendship check. There is an irony to this since INFPs are natural counselors. It seems to me that people end up being something called "friends with benefits" or married, both of which are beyond my current emotional comprehension.

In seventh grade, I won the state conservation essay contest, and this was the year I met Little Badger. Little Badger is not her real name, but I now find a fondness for naming people with terms of endearment, if I really care about them or just see them as really special. I take little credit for this as another Aspergian, John Robinson, has convinced me of the benefits of this method. As I see it, the name Little Badger suits her indomitable spirit and her positive, can-do life energy. Little Badger approached me in the gymnasium and asked me with these little badgerette eyes, "Who do you really like?" To which I responded, "I do not know." I got a really giddy feeling at that point, and from that moment on I knew I liked Little Badger, but I had no idea how to tell her that. I also had a fear of what to do next if she told me that she liked me. Later that summer, Little Badger ended up being the first girl I danced with, which to this day is a beautiful memory. Seasons change, and I would not see Little Badger for another year as she was a year older than I, and that meant she would be at the high school while I was at the middle school for another year. I would often dream of Little Badger, but I lacked the confidence and social ability to interact with her. Either way, I seemed so confident and secure in the knowledge that she knew I liked her, everything else did not matter. I was sure that osmosis and telepathy would take care of the rest. I wrote Little Badger letters of endearment through the course of high school and stuffed them in a shoebox, which later in life I destroyed, and I would sing the lyrics of a song by Starship over and over just because it had her name in it. By the time I got to high school, Little Badger had a new boyfriend, Brian, and I still had no clue as to how to interact with her or any of her friends. All through high school, I never used the telephone to call any girl for absolutely any reason. I was sure that if I called Little Badger and talked to her, she would see this as something special and that I really liked her. So I did it; I called Little

Badger and talked to her. It filled me with bliss just to hear her voice. I was all ready to tell her that I liked her until I heard her sister laughing. I thought it was Little Badger's friend as her sister and her friend have the same name, which I did not know at that time. Either way, my ability to say what was in my soul was lost in that moment. I now see that we had a nice chat, but we did not create any emotional connections. Brian made extra efforts over the next week to make sure that I made no other calls to Little Badger. How he found out, I will never know. I certainly did not call him. I had made a decision. If Little Badger did not show any interest in me after this point, then I must move on, no matter how much it hurt. Time would heal any heart wounds and make me forever forget that Little Badger held any sway over my spirit. My social inadequacies with people in general and especially Little Badger led to depression, my first psychological doctor, and a new round of prescription medications, mainly ritalin and wellbutrin.

I just attended my own funeral. Although there was someone else in that coffin, the husband of a friend that Little Badger and I mutually shared, I was sure it was I. After more than 10 years out of high school, I finally saw Little Badger again at this funeral, and I finally had the ability to tell her the words that were in my soul, "Little Badger, I really had the hots for you." Little Badger exclaimed an incredulous, "What? I never knew." All I could say was "Yes, that has been ages ago," and her reply was "No, it is not." I finally knew that Little Badger cared about me. She even reached out and touched my elbow, and touching is something very, very, very, very special to this Aspergian, but probably not as big an issue to most normal, bland people. Ralph Waldo Emerson would have told me, "One very is enough." I thought time would wash away my feelings for Little Badger, but I know this is not true. I know I still care for Little Badger. I know that to this day Little Badger knows how to ensnare my attraction senses, but I can only wish her a happy life without me as she has this bond called marriage with another man. It saddens me that this prevents us from having any real probability of some sort of social contact. If not lover, I certainly would be happy to call Little Badger my sister and treat her like I do the sisters I grew up with and I am confident that she would like that as well.

Unlike Little Badger, I made every effort for over three years to make Choo-choo my girlfriend, and I made her very aware of it, and in my mind she was, and that was probably enough. I met Choo-choo after high school. I made her a beaded bookmark and thought about her as often as I did about Little Badger. It is my belief that I treated Choo-choo as the image of my fantasy girl. This is not an image that she could live up to, nor could she or I have truly wanted her to. Nevertheless, it put Choo-choo in the position of her being on a pedestal, not as an equal in a mutually rewarding relationship. I now see that we never achieved any degree of friendship and our personal interest was very different. I can at least relax in the knowledge that I spared Little Badger the torment of my relentless undying affections, unlike Choo-choo. Simply put, I am in a position to have a conversation with Little Badger if by some remote chance of fate we were to see each other again.

I am wiser regarding relationships after my experiences with Little Badger and Choo-choo. Little Badger and Choo-choo are life's paradoxes and parables for me. I think often now of the twin paradoxical short stories, *Three Feet from Gold* in Napoleon Hill's book *Think and Grow Rich* and Price Pritchett's story of the fly in *You Squared*. Are we the fly that a simple change in strategy of flying out the open window instead of trying to pierce the glass pane could change our destiny, or in the process of changing strategy, do we often stop three feet from gold? I am slowly beginning to have the paradigm shift that the world is an ocean of abundance in all life areas and that often we do stop three feet from gold just so we can be the fly who takes a new strategy to land in a different vein of life abundance. As long as I follow my definite major life purpose and recognize when I am really the fly trying so vainly to pierce the windowpane, I will meet with Thoreau's definition of success, "If one advances confidently in the direction of his dream, and endeavors to live the imagined life, a person will meet it with uncommon success in common hours."

Mike's words echoed in my ear again, "Find them, Fuck them, Forget them!" That was his philosophical viewpoint of women when I knew him. I knew I could never treat women in this manner. I valued the sacred feminine too much to embrace this viewpoint, and I had no misogyny toward women. An adult at age 29, I had just finished reading Neil Strauss's book, *The Game,* and the entire thought of treating women as a score was an abomination to me. However, I saw inside the book that these men had the social skills with women and men that I and so many other Aspergians desperately lack. I had to find a way to rationally separate the wheat from the chaff after reading this while still maintaining my inner personal identity. I would not become a social robot. As I was growing up, there were no classes on some of the most important life skills in high school, mainly financial management and social development. No matter how much I despised Neil's book, this book along with other readings has launched me onto a path of social experimentation and development. I now pay more conscious attention to what people call body language. I can smile at people in passing and take pleasure at them smiling back at me. I can watch lateral eye movement (LEM) and know more about how to interpret it. I can do magic tricks and some ventriloquism. I have renewed past interest in art, Latin dance, and origami. I have delved deeper into the psychological interests of neurolinguistics and hypnosis. I also know that when my mother tells me, "You are Perking," I am probably doing something in that moment that would be socially unacceptable in most situations. Psychiatric doctors can place pictures of people with different facial expressions and I can tell a smile from a frown, but it is a big challenge to tell you what a smile or a frown means. Even if you told me a story about why someone was smiling or frowning, the interpretation of the body gesture would still be a mystery, and I do not think there is any psychological test for this. Social skills are an art form, and I have only now picked up my social paintbrush to see what I can paint. I was a rosebud where others were roses in bloom. Now they are wilting and I am blooming. There is a season for everything, and now is my season. Just like learning to ride a bicycle, I will fall and bleed numerous times but I, like Thomas Edison, will discover 250,000 different ways of how not to ride a bicycle or invent a light bulb or, in my case, create meaningful social relationships. In the end, I will figure out the social algorithm just like I discovered the way to perform perfectly on the Wisconsin Card Test. For a time, I believe that I will indulge in what some people will perceive as social overcompensation and will have to be aware of this. It is great to travel through the desert until you finally reach the oasis; however, it is not wise to drink from the oasis until you choke. The world will just have to be mindful of eccentric Aspergian logic when we really start to apply our intellect to the social enigma.

PERSONAL JOURNAL ENTRY

In my childhood, religion created two dichotomous views of sexuality, holiness, and evil. My mother always valued the holiness of sex, the striving for all things pure and chaste in a relationship. I know it now to be a pedestal that no mortal human can achieve. I strived for this gift of holiness anyway. I knew that if I ever faltered into the realms of adultery and licentiousness of a love relationship, I could never wash that stain back to holiness. I was broken because the holiness of sex would never allow me to acknowledge the humanity of sex. My path in fervent religious holiness never allowed me to expose myself to opportunities for true intimacy. I deprived my own self of love, which in itself is holiness.

Now, it seems to me that painting sex into holiness and evil does neither element justice. I could never feel the holiness of sex in any other form than an abstract approval of God's creation, and I also never truly appreciated the dark, destructive capacities of sex except as a source of personal guilt. If I can restore both the holiness and the real darkness—for paradox is usually a sign of the presence of spirit—then I might be able to more fully enter the mystery that is sex, and find in it a genuine route to intimacy, both within myself and with others.

THE BUS RIDE

The most significant childhood event in my life aside from running Daniel's dirt bike straight into an oak tree at 35 mph, helmet not included, and shooting myself in the left index finger with a .177 caliber air rifle pellet had to be the bus ride. The only significant difference is that the first two events were of my own volition, the events on the bus ride were not. In eighth grade, I enjoyed playing tennis and joined the school tennis team. To my joy, I would get to ride the bus with the high school–age boys to a tennis match. To be blunt, for more than three hours, I was hazed and physically molested by the young men I rode this bus with. I never even got off the bus to play tennis. Danny, the bus driver, tennis coach, and high school chemistry teacher blatantly neglected the actions of the young men molesting me, and he never checked to see that I even played tennis. I ended up in the hospital that night. I can say that like Tim Robbins's character Andy Dufrense in *Shawshank Redemption,* I put up a fight, and some of those young men had a few bruises themselves. I chose not to pursue legal action against these individuals, but my trust in them is forever violated. The school district did end up paying for me to see a psychiatric counselor after this event. Danny went on to become the high school principal and district administrator. To this day, I have not played tennis since that time. Life has its little twists.

MUSINGS CONCERNING PSYCHIATRIC SPECIALISTS

I will now tell you how to get rid of your psychiatric specialist forever!!!

This method might have you seeing so many different psychiatric specialists that you will no longer have any stable psychiatric help. For the psychiatrically challenged who really do not like their psychiatric specialists or licensed certified social workers (LISWs), all you have to do is heighten the sexual tension between you and your psychiatric counselor and proclaim your sexual interest in them. There usually seems to be a policy in the psychiatric community against personal relations between psychiatric professionals and their clients. "It taints the therapy session," stated one psychiatric professional who unintentionally found out that I found her attractive. For more information on how to rid yourself forever of psychiatric help even if you need it, we sell the entire above paragraph as a personal e-mail for $1.99 a copy. Don't you just love our consumer smut-oriented world? A smile is here.

These were the very first words to the psychiatric doctor who so graciously allowed me to join the Society of Aspergians, "You are my new Hermes, that phallic rise out of the earth that ejaculates wayward travelers towards the right path," making a gesture of quotation marks on my right side, the doctor's left side. "No, I meant right path," repeating the quotation mark gesture on my left side, the doctor's right side. It made me feel like I was Tom Wingo sitting with Dr. Lowenstein in the Pat Conroy book, *The Prince of Tides*. The only thing is I had no contemptuous feelings toward the doctor who first said, "Asperger's Syndrome," and I was not in the habit of having sex with mules or donkeys either.

I have spelled world backward more times than I want to count. I want to ask, "What do psychiatric professionals think a dlrow is anyway?" I have a thought on this. Maybe a dlrow is that unexplained realm of harmonic sanity that these professionals themselves are trying to achieve, like Maslow's self-actualized individual. Either way, ask someone interested in psychology, and I bet they can tell you they know the word "dlrow," although they probably do not know what it means. I tried entire sentences with the words turned around, and these professionals did not get it. "I drove my truck around the world" became "I evord ym kcurt dnuora eht dlrow." I started talking their social language and all I got was blank stares. I was sure they would recognize at least the word dlrow. Can we please get dlrow added to the dictionary like evoo (extravirgin olive oil) was added?

Thank you! Ahh-a-men! Ahh-a-men!. . . .

CAREER

Today, at 29 years of age, creating a meaningful career for me is a life challenge. I take solace in the knowledge that, like Emerson and Thoreau, I am at least dancing to the music of my own spirit. I believe that I have made the mistake of trying to work out of my own ego in fields that really do not match my personality, blinded by greed and the "What's in it for me" mentality. I believe Carl Jung described this as warrior mode, and that was the stage of life that I was in for a time. I now know some simple life truths. As Harvory Mackey said, "Find something you love to do and you'll never have to work a day in your life". I have many beautiful skills that can be used to serve humanity and I will manifest my career purpose. I am a writer, philosopher, and poet of my own time. I am wise enough to see the rules of work constantly changing, as we see China demanding a higher standard of living, the shift toward a more global economy, and economies of scale continuously changing the need for certain jobs. I also see opportunities for people as the career experience of the baby boomer generation attritions out. The effort of many elderly in menial jobs because their retirement planning somehow failed or never occurred saddens me. Equally saddening is to see people in a state of entitlement, never engaging in self-improvement, where many choose to live off of government subsidies instead of contributing to humanity. Our governments have a vested interest in keeping a certain segment of the population marginalized. The attitude is, "Let's keep them sheep grazing on just a small pasture so that their basest needs are satiated. We can have the big pasture all to ourselves." Are our economies of scale becoming too efficient as to allow people to endure a life of brooding? On a personal note, I know that I certainly cried the day I applied for government disability based on Asperger's syndrome. I can and will be more than just an entitled individual in a small pasture. Through all the work I have had, I was self-actualized the most when working as a runner on the Chicago Board of Trade. The psychological aspects of observing frenzied open pit futures trading and crowd logic really appeals to me. I absolutely know that I could excel as a futures trader as I wrote a business plan for this at one time, and I have completed much of the psychological work that Dr. Van Tharp produced. I also believe that I can become a spiritual guide, a quadoshka and tantra healer with proper training. My skill with computers, programming, and GNU/Linux-based operating systems could lead me for a time into the technology field and will be highly useful in any career area. Perhaps, even my writing skills will educate people about Asperger's syndrome. Now, I believe that my ultimate calling is in one of these fields since most of them require my strong intrapersonal intelligence versus my weaker interpersonal intelligence. This is all I have to express about this subject for now.

THE ASPERGIAN

We are someone special; we will build monuments of memory into people's hearts and minds, and for us that will always be enough. Our footsteps will not be in sand where winds and tides sweep away the lore of a lived life, but in stone. We will be able to quote Douglas McArthur's last lines from his poem, "Build me a Son" ... "I have not lived in vain."

Me. I am someone special; I will build monuments of memory into people's hearts and minds, and for me that will always be enough. My footsteps will not be in sand where winds and tides sweep away the lore of a lived life, but in stone. I will be able to quote Douglas McArthur's last lines from his poem, "Build Me A Son" ... "I have not lived in vain."

Ahh-a-men ... Ahh-a-men ... Ahh-a-men. ...

Index